HOOF PROBLEMS

Rob van Nassau

HOOF PROBLEMS

Hoof Construction
Trimming and Shoeing
Solutions for Common Issues and Ailments

With more than 1,000 illustrations

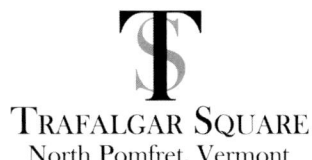

TRAFALGAR SQUARE
North Pomfret, Vermont

First published in the United States of America in 2007 by
Trafalgar Square Books, North Pomfret, Vermont 05053

Printed in China

Originally published in 2004 in the Dutch language as *Hoef Problemen* by
Forte Uitgevers bv
Postbus 1394
3500 BJ Utrecht, NL

© 2004 Forte Uitgevers bv, Utrecht
© 2007 English translation by Kenilworth Press

All rights reserved. No part of this publication may be reproduced, stored in a retrieval system, or transmitted in any form or by any means, electronic, mechanical, photocopying, recording or otherwise, without the written permission of the publisher.

ISBN 978-1-57076-382-3

Library of Congress Control Number: 2007928140

Disclaimer of Liability
This book is not to be used in place of veterinary or farrier care or expertise. The author and publisher shall have neither liability nor responsibility to any person or entity with respect to any loss or damage caused or alleged to be caused directly or indirectly by the information contained in this book. While the book is as accurate as the authors can make it, there may be errors, omissions and inaccuracies.

English translation by Nina King

Photograph Credits
All photographs and illustrations are those of Rob and Antoon van Nassau except the illustrations on pages: 15, 37, 38, 39, 40, 41, 42, 43, 44. The illustrations on these pages have been borrowed from the book Equine Atlas of Clinical Equine Anatomy and Common Disorders of the Horse by R. J. Riegel, DVM and S. E. Hakola, BS, RN, CMI, published by Equistar Publications Ltd, Ohio.
  The X-ray pictures were provided by the veterinarians at the veterinary hospital at Visdonk in Roosendaal except for the photos on pages: 80 (right, above), 107 (right, below) 215 and 220 (right, centre). These were produced by E. Digit.
  The illustrations on pages 45 and 172 have been borrowed from the book Tickners Hippische Encyclopedie by J. Tickner, published by Forum Boekerij, Den Haag.
  Cover photos: Rob van Nassau, Oud Gastel.
  With thanks to: HAS Den Bosch, Leonoor Los, Drs Ben Boschker and Drs Paul de Vries.

CONTENTS

FOREWORD
by Simon Curtis FWCF, HonAssocRCVS   7

PREFACE   8

PART 1
The Hoof

1 THE HORSE

Joints and Bones	11
Muscles, Tendons and Ligaments	15

2 THE HOOF

Construction of the Hoof	19
Hoof Mechanism	27
Hoof Shapes	29
Foot Axis and Limb Conformation	34

3 HOOF CARE AND HORSESHOES

Hoof Care	45
Horseshoes	47
Trimming and Shoeing	53
The Hoofcare® Breakover Shoe	63

PART 2
Disorders of the limbs and hooves in relation to hoof care and horseshoes

1 THE LIMB

Arthrosis	71
Wire Wounds	74
Stringhalt and Spasms	76

2 THE LOWER LIMB

Splint	78
Bone Spavin	79

3 THE LOWER FOOT

Outside	85
Over-reaching	85
Deformed Hooves	87
Greasy Heel	89
Over at the Pastern	91
Pes Equinus and Club Foot	93
Inside	97
Cyst	97
Keratoma	99
Low and High Ring-bone	106
Ostitis	110

4 THE HOOF

Coronary Band	113
Irritation of the Coronary Band	113
Damage to the Coronary Band	115
Sandcrack	118

4 THE HOOF CONTINUED

Horny Wall — 123
Poor Quality Horn, and Chipped Hooves — 123
Complete Horny Wall Cracks — 126
Grass Crack — 128
Rings of Horn — 132
Seedy Toe — 133
False Quarter — 135
Separating Walls — 137
Superficial Horny Wall Cracks — 142
Full Thickness Horny Wall Cracks — 144

Toe — 150
Long Toes and Low Heels — 150
Inflammation of the Toe — 157

Heels — 162
Rolled-Under Heels — 162
Under-Run Heels — 164
Inflammation of the Heels — 166

Frog — 171
Thrush — 171
Canker of the Frog — 173
Inflammation of the Frog — 179

Sole — 181
Dropped Sole — 181
Puncture Wound — 182
Bruised Sole — 186
Cracked Sole — 188

Hoof Capsule — 190
Infected Crack — 190
White Line Disease — 191

Pedal Bone — 197
Chip Fracture of the Pedal Bone — 197
Pedal Bone and Navicular Fracture and Fissure — 200
Laminitis — 202
Sinker — 211
Encapsulated Bone Fragment — 213
Side-bone — 215

Navicular — 217
Navicular Disease — 217

INDEX — 223

FOREWORD

Rob van Nassau's book, *Hoof Problems,* is a much needed text that can be studied and enjoyed by farriers, veterinary surgeons and horse owners. Books have been written on the subject of horseshoeing for more than 500 years. Fiachi published his treatise in 1556. However, they have rarely been written by a practising farrier and seldom with such detail. Farriery, although fundamentally the same craft for a thousand years, has been undergoing a renaissance since the 1970s. This book reflects the fact that we are no longer shoeing, in the main, working or military horses but are mostly concerned with leisure, sports and athletic horses. These horses bring a different set of problems to the horse owner and farrier.

The illustrations are detailed without obscuring the basic anatomy. There are many examples comparing various conformational faults which affect the equine leg and foot. Rob covers a very wide range of horse types and breeds. He has a chapter devoted to conformation in which he shows the link between the less than perfect leg and its effect upon the hoof capsule. This book also demonstrates how the farrier needs to take into account the breed when assessing conformation and gait, as this often differs, and therefore farriers must adapt their techniques accordingly.

One piece of advice that I give to farriers is always to carry a camera and to make sure that they photograph the horse's foot before they work on it. It's too late when you have completed the job and you have just a picture of the finished foot. Rob has obviously carried a camera for a long time. *Hoof Problems* is full of good case histories with 'before' and 'after' photography.

Simon Curtis FWCF, HonAssocRCVS

PREFACE

A horse with bad hooves is of little value; not for nothing do we often say, 'No foot, no horse'. This book is a treasure trove of information about every aspect of horses' hooves.

Part 1 provides general information about the hoof, hoof care, conformation of the limbs, and horse shoeing.

In Part 2, more than fifty common hoof problems are discussed, with chapters giving information about the characteristics and cause of each disorder, the making of a diagnosis, the treatment, the shoeing and the prognosis. Various new methods of treatment for serious disorders are described as well as a thorough look at some of the farriery techniques we have developed ourselves.

With our thirty years of professional experience one of our goals is to train and to provide further education for farriers both young and old, at home and abroad.

Many hoof problems can be prevented by good hoof care. This does not so much mean tarring and oiling or feeding all kinds of food supplements; rather it means ensuring plenty of exercise, keeping the horse under natural conditions and, above all, employing a skilled farrier.

We hope that the acquisition of more knowledge about horses' hooves will lead to better care and to speedier treatment, and thus to an improvement in the well-being of the horse.

> More information on hooves and hoof care can be found on Rob and Antoon van Nassau's website: www.hoofcare.nl

Part 1

The Hoof

1 THE HORSE

Joints and Bones

A joint is a moveable connection between two or more bones. Joints are found everywhere in the horse's body. Their function is to enable the horse to move.

STRUCTURE
Joints are held together by strong ligaments (e, shown left) attached to the bones.

So that friction between the bones is minimised, joint lubricant

Example of a joint.
a. Bone end
b. A layer of cartilage on the bone ends
c. The joint cavity containing synovial fluid
d. The joint capsule
e. The ligaments

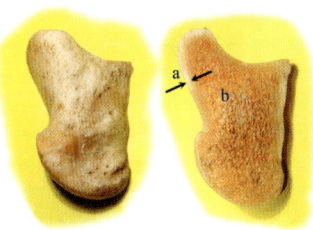

A bone is made up of a very hard covering (a) and a core that is built up from weaker bone tissue with an open structure (b).

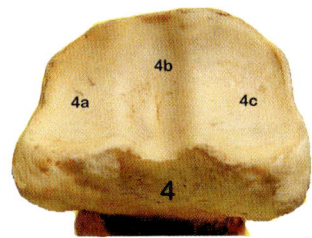

The head of the cannon bone fits exactly (4a, 4b, 4c) into the joint surfaces of the long pastern bone. All joint surfaces are covered with very smooth cartilage. The synovial fluid in the joint capsule (the synovial bursa, or mucus pouch) ensures that this cartilage is lubricated, enabling supple movement of the joint.

(synovial fluid) is secreted into the joint cavity (c, above left) which is contained within an elastic joint capsule (d, above left). The bones fit neatly together with the thin layer of lubricant between them.

Cartilage (b, above left) attached to the bones absorbs concussion caused by the horse's movement.

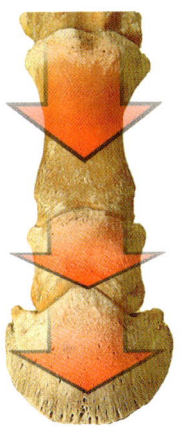

There are only ginglymus joints in the lower foot. Ginglymus joints can only move backwards and forwards.

TYPES OF JOINT
There are several kinds of joints such as ball-and-socket joints, ginglymus joints and pivot joints.

In the lower limb, a horse has only ginglymus joints. These joints consist of two unequal parts which fit together closely with an elevation in the middle, thus allowing the bones to move only backwards or forwards. Rotation is limited, which explains why the cause of so many problems in the lower foot arises from faulty movement and the weight bearing on the joints. In this way, the pastern joint can fill with excess fluid (synovia) and attachment problems of the ligaments, or inflammation of the joints, can arise.

INFLAMMATION OF THE JOINTS

Inflammation of the joints can be caused, for example, by overtaxing of the joints. The joint fills up with fluid, which causes so-called joint fissures to develop. In acute cases, the horse becomes lame. Inflammation of the joints can also arise from infection via the blood. Where there is chronic inflammation of the joints, the joint cartilage can be destroyed. Such inflammations can even lead to arthrosis. In this disease, uncontrolled bone growth appears in and around the joints. As the arthrosis develops, the lameness of the horse increases. Recovery is usually no longer possible.

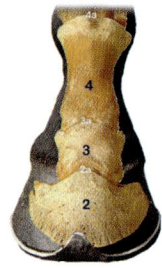

2. Pedal bone; 2a. Hoof joint
3. Short pastern bone; 3a. Coronary joint
4. Long pastern bone; 4a. Pastern joint

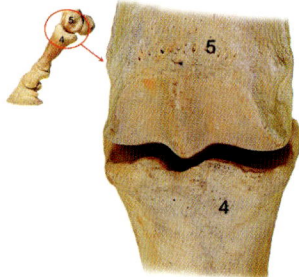

The pastern joint consists of the cannon bone (5) with the long pastern bone underneath (4). The bones fit into each other in such a way that they can move only backwards and forwards, and not sideways.

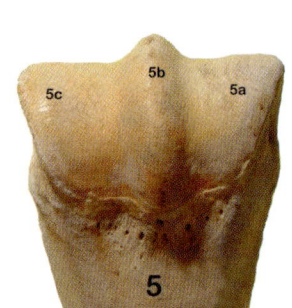

The joint head of the cannon bone (5) consists of two smooth surfaces (5a and 5c) and a raised part or elevation (5b). The largest gliding surface is always on the inside (medial) of the limb.

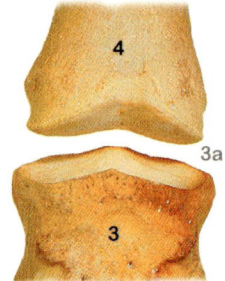

The elevation of the pastern joint (3a; between (3) short pastern bone and (4) long pastern bone) is significantly flatter than the long pastern joint and it has two gliding surfaces.

FOALS

Many foals are born with defective limb conformation. This mostly rectifies itself within weeks and the foal stands squarely on its four legs. There are, however, foals whose limb conformation remains defective because of an inherited disorder such as club foot.

Defective limb conformation such as knock knees or bow legs can also arise if growth at the epiphysis is uneven. If, for example, the epiphysis of the cannon bone grows more quickly on the inner side of the bone, it causes a defective situation in the pastern joint.

Usually a minor defect can be helped by paring the foal's hooves very regularly. In extreme cases the hooves can be fitted with extensions or horseshoes. In this way, the conformation can be forced to change a little. In some cases, however, an operation is necessary.

Good hoof care is of great importance for all foals.

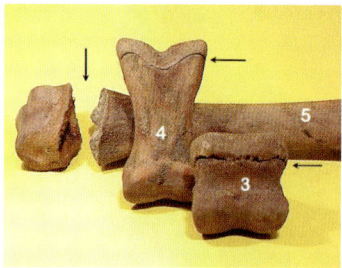

All young bones have growth plates (see arrows) at the epiphyses. When the bone has grown to its maximum length the plates ossify. The growth plates in the bones of the lower leg ossify at different ages, from approximately six months to two and a half years; growth plates of other bones ossify at up to three and a half years. If a horse is taxed at a too young age, there are harmful consequences for the growth plates.
3. Short pastern bone; 4. Long pastern bone; 5. Cannon bone.

TECHNICAL JARGON

The limb parts are called:

- **Limb.** The whole leg, including (fore limb) the shoulder blade
- **Upper limb.** The part between the shoulder joint and the elbow joint
- **Lower limb.** The part from the elbow to just above the knee
- **Lower foot.** The part down to and including the pastern joint
- **The hoof of the foot.** Parts in the hoof capsule and the capsule itself
- **Hoof capsule or capsule.** Only the horny parts of the hoof
- **Lateral.** The outer side of the horse's limb
- **Medial.** The inner side of the horse's limb
- **Dorsal.** The front side of the horse's limb
- **Palmar.** The rear side of the horse's front limb
- **Plantar.** The rear side of the horse's hind limb
- **Proximal.** Nearer to the horse's body
- **Distal.** Away from the horse's body

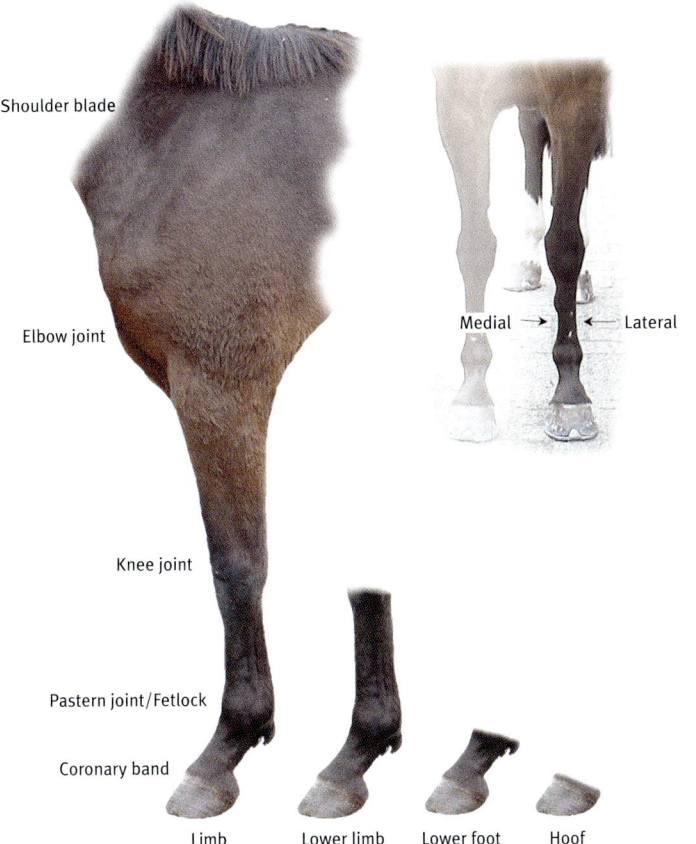

The nomenclature of the various joints in the horse limb is:

- **Knee joint.** The joint between the radius and the cannon bone
- **Pastern joint (fetlock).** The joint between the cannon bone and the pastern
- **Coronary joint.** The joint between the long pastern bone and the short pastern bone
- **Hoof joint.** The joint between short pastern bone and pedal bone

The Horse

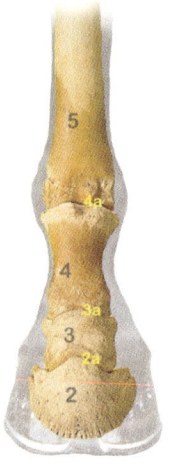

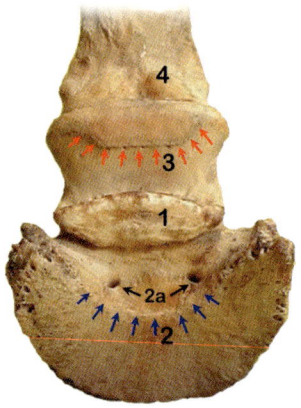

The lower limb of the horse, seen from the front:
2. Pedal bone; 2a Hoof joint
3. Short pastern bone; 3a Coronary joint
4. Long pastern bone; 4a Pastern joint
5. Cannon bone

Lower foot of the horse, seen from behind and lifted up:
1. Navicular bone
2. Pedal bone; 2a. Hoof arterial channels
3. Short pastern bone
4. Long pastern bone

Blue arrows: where the deep digital flexor tendon attaches.
Red arrows: where the superficial digital flexor tendon attaches.

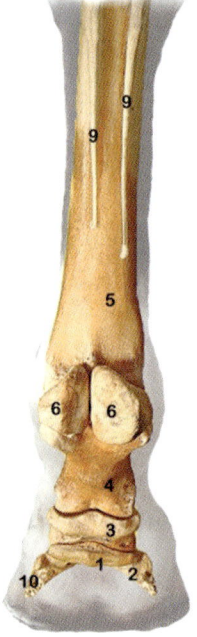

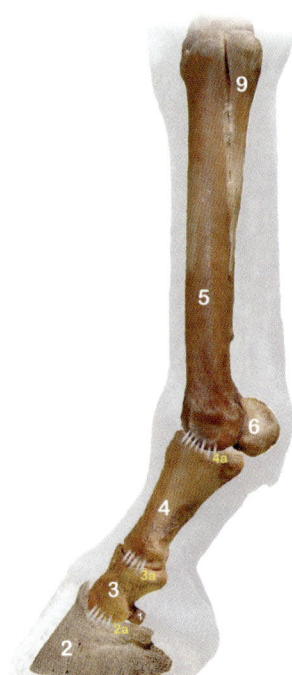

The same lower limb of the horse, seen from behind:
1. Navicular bone
2. Pedal bone
3. Short pastern bone
4. Long pastern bone
5. Cannon bone
6. Sesamoid bone (two pieces)
9. Small metacarpal bone (two rudimentary pieces)
10. Pedal bone lateral cartilage

The lower limb of the horse, seen from the side:
1. Navicular bone
2. Pedal bone; 2a. Hoof joint
3. Short pastern bone; 3a.Coronary joint
4. Long pastern bone: 4a. Pastern joint
5. Cannon bone
6. Sesamoid bones (two pieces)
9. Small metacarpal bone (two rudimentary pieces)

Muscles, Tendons and Ligaments

A muscle is a bundle of tissues that makes it possible for the horse to move. A horse can intentionally contract its muscles.

THE CONSTRUCTION AND WORKING OF MUSCLES

The muscles are securely attached to the bones by tendons. Each muscle is built up of a number of muscle bundles, bound together by connective tissue. A muscle bundle consists of a large number of muscle fibres; muscle fibre is composed of thread-like cells with many nuclei which can only be seen by using a microscope with a minimum enlargement of 400.

Each muscle fibre has a spur (axon) of a motor nerve cell. This spur leads to the end plates that lie on the muscle fibre. The decision to move a muscle is made in the brain or spinal column. For movement, first an impulse (surge of current) is sent via the spur of a nerve cell to the end plates of the muscle fibre, causing a chemical to be released by the muscle fibre that makes the muscle contract. When the muscle contracts, it becomes thicker and shorter, drawing the two points where the muscle is attached to the bone (by tendons) towards each other.

Directly after contraction – which is caused by just one single impulse – the muscle relaxes. But when impulses follow in rapid succession, the muscle fibre has insufficient time to relax completely, and so remains contracted for the duration of the impulse burst.

In order for the bone to return to its original position, another muscle must be contracted. This situation is called antagonism.

There are three different kinds of muscular tissue: horizontally striped muscular tissue (also known as the voluntary muscles, because the horse can activate them at will, for example when contracting the back muscles); smooth muscular tissue (also known as the involuntary muscles, because the horse cannot consciously activate them, for

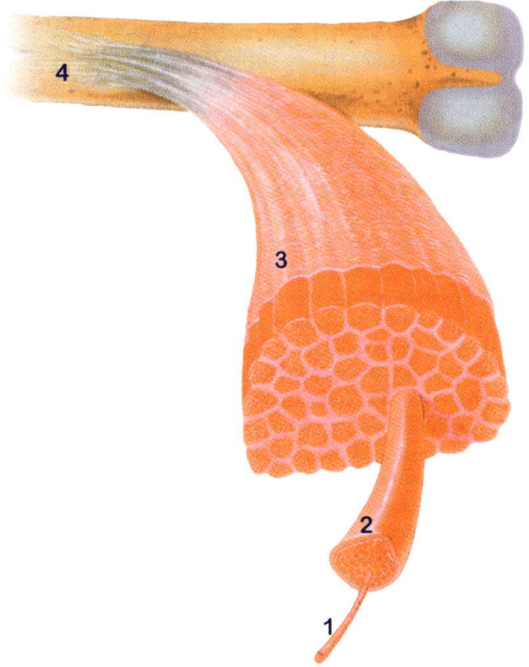

Muscles are firmly attached to bones by tendons and are encased by a layer of connective tissue (4). A muscle is built up from a number of muscle bundles (3). Between the muscle bundles is connective tissue. A muscle bundle is built up from a great number of muscle fibres (2). Muscle fibres are thread-like cells with many nuclei (1).

example the tiny muscles in the vascular system and in the intestines peristalsis); and heart muscular tissue (horizontally striped muscle that is involuntary, thus in a separate category). On horizontally striped muscular tissue, rings can be clearly seen; smooth muscular tissue has no rings. Muscle fibre is made of horizontally striped muscular tissue.

When the horse moves forward there is continuous antagonistic muscle activity, allowing balanced and harmonious movement of the limbs.

TENDONS

Tendons attach the muscle to the bone. They are situated at each end of the muscle. In the lower foot of the horse, the tendons are an extension of the muscles that produce the backwards and forwards movements. A tendon is made up of bundles of sinuous fibre. The sinuous fibre is bound together by connective material. In various places, the tendon is enclosed by a tendon sheath filled with lubricating fluids (synovial fluid). There are very few blood vessels in the tendon, which limits the supply of nutrients and the removal of waste matter. This explains why a tendon injury heals extremely slowly. A tendon does not contract like a muscle, and does not stretch: its function is to transfer the force of traction.

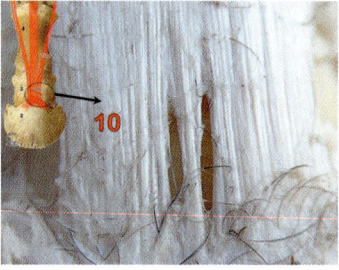

A macro registration of the extensor tendon or the toe extensor with its strong tendons (10) which are attached to the coronary protuberance of the pedal bone.

TENDONS IN HORSE LIMBS

In the forelimb, the transition from muscle to tendon starts at the height of the knee (the wrist joint), and in the hind limb at the height of the hock. The lower limb is completely 'wrapped' with tendons and ligaments that criss-cross over each other. These ensure absorption during the enormous release of force in locomotion and jumping.

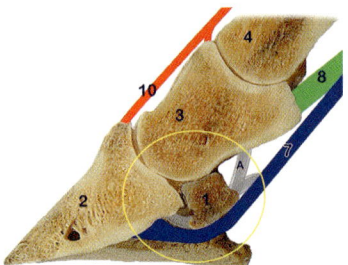

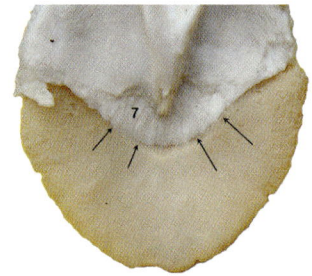

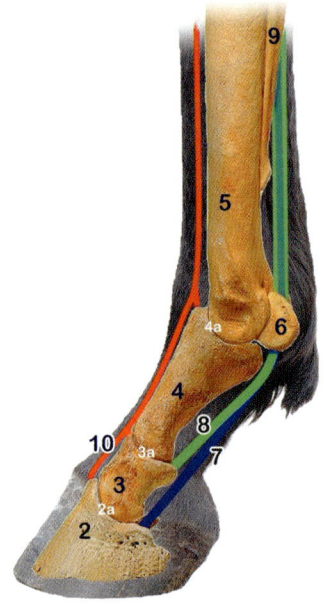

Shown in blue (and 7 on the adjacent diagram), the deep flexor tendon glides over the navicular bone (1) and is attached to the underside of the pedal bone (2). In this area (circled) the tendon glides over the navicular bone like a pulley.

The deep flexor tendon attaches at the semilunar crest under the pedal bone.

2. Pedal bone; 2a. Hoof joint
3. Short pastern bone; 3a. Coronary joint
4. Long pastern bone; 4a. Pastern joint (fetlock)
5. Cannon bone
6. Sesamoid bones (2)
7. Deep flexor tendon, or pedal bone tendon
8. Superficial flexor tendon, or short pastern bone tendon
9. Small metacarpal bones
10. Extensor tendon

The most important tendons in the lower limb of the horse are:
- **Extensor**. The extensor tendon, otherwise known as the pedal bone extensor. This is found at the front of the limb.
- **Deep flexor tendon**. The deep flexor tendon, otherwise known as the pedal bone flexor tendon. This tendon, together with the superficial flexor tendon, ensures the backwards and forwards movement of the lower foot.
- **Superficial flexor tendon**. The superficial flexor tendon; otherwise known as the short pastern bone tendon, because it is attached to the upper rear of the short pastern bone. At the height of the pastern joint, the superficial and the deep flexor tendons glide between the sesamoid bones.
- **The two collateral ligaments**. These ligaments combine with the extensor tendon, enclose both sesamoid bones and run behind the knee to make the transition to muscle. The enclosure of the sesamoid bones is otherwise known as the apron ligament or annular ligament. This extremely important ligament serves as a sort of hammock that ensures that the pastern is supported.

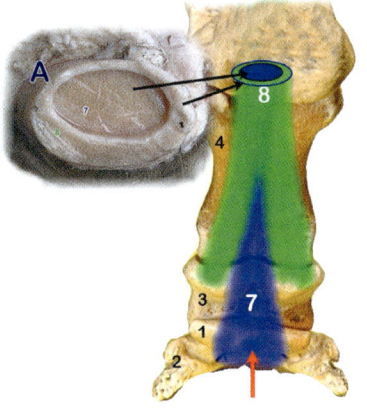
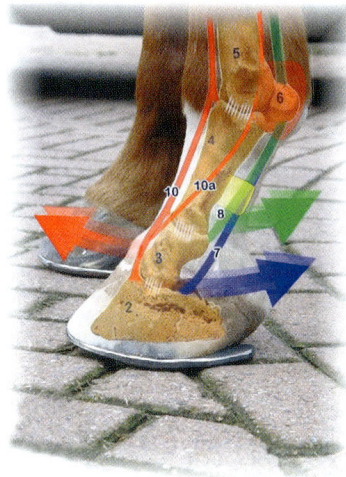
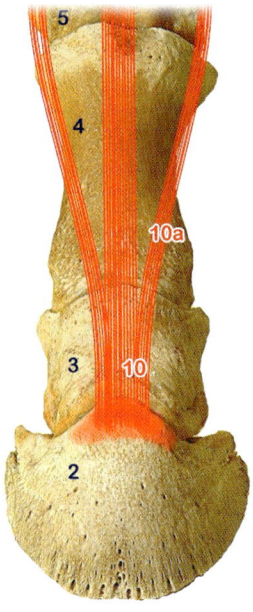

The deep flexor tendon and the superficial flexor tendon stretch from the knee together as a 'tube with content' (A); the deep flexor tendon (7) slides into the superficial flexor tendon (8).
The superficial flexor tendon divides, attaching itself to the rear topside (parapet) of the short pastern bone (3) and allowing the deep flexor tendon to pass through and attach under the pedal bone (red arrow).

The extensor tendon (10) enables the lower foot to be rotated forward (red arrow). It attaches to the lateral cartilages of the pedal bone (2).
The deep flexor tendon (blue, 7) and the superficial flexor tendon (green, 8) enable the lower foot to be rotated backwards (blue and green arrows).
The deep flexor tendon (7) is attached to the under surface (the semilunar crest) of the pedal bone (2).
The superficial flexor tendon (8) is attached to the rear topside of the short pastern bone (3).

The extensor tendon (10), attached to the parapet of the pedal bone (2), enables the hoof to be rotated forwards.
This tendon has two side branches (10a) that run from the annular ligament of the fetlock (5) via the long pastern bone (4) to the side of the coronary band (2). The annular ligament of the fetlock is thus supported.

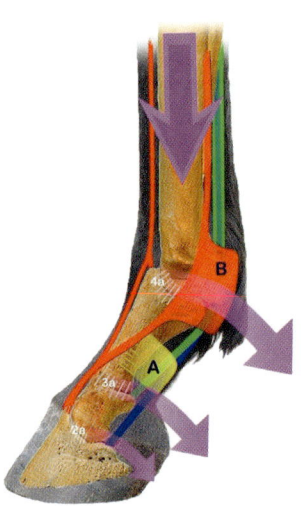
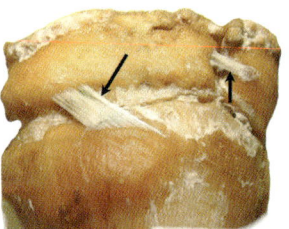
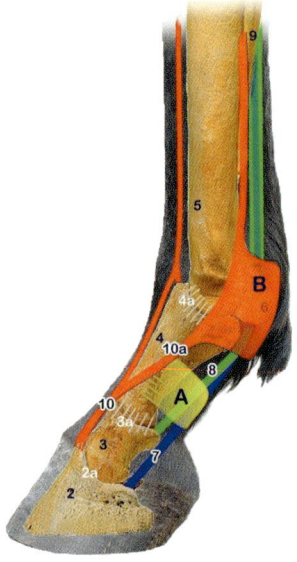

At the back of the fetlock joint there is an annular ligament, a very strong cuff-shaped strengthening band (B).
There is also an annular ligament in the pastern cavity (A).
The function of ligaments is to hold all the parts together, strengthen the joints and keep bones in the correct position, and to bear the forces (purple arrows) that are released when weight is borne by the lower foot.
The bones are also held together by small ligaments or strengthening ligaments (2a, 3a, 4a). These are very stiff but pliable.

An illustration (front of fore knee joint) of the stiff but pliable strengthening ligaments (black arrows) that keep the bones in place.

2. Pedal bone; 2a. Hoof joint
3. Short pastern bone; 3a. Coronary joint
4. Long pastern bone; 4a. Pastern joint (fetlock)
5. Cannon bone.
6. Sesamoid bone (hidden behind B)
7. Deep flexor tendon (pedal bone tendon)
8. Superficial flexor tendon (short pastern bone tendon)
9. Small metacarpal bones.
10. Extensor tendon; 10a. side branches

A. Annular ligament of the pastern cavity
B. Annular ligament of the fetlock (apron ligament)

JOINT LIGAMENTS

The joint ligaments are supporting bands of extremely strong connective tissue. These bands are bendable but very tough. Their function is to strengthen the joints, holding the bones together in the correct position. Joint ligaments are found in all sorts of joints, for example at the back of the pastern and hoof joint. At the back of the fetlock joint, and in the pastern cavity, there is an extremely strong cuff-shaped annular ligament supporting band.

2 THE HOOF

Construction of the Hoof

'No foot, no horse' is a well-known saying. It illustrates well how important the hooves of a horse are and how necessary it is to keep them in good condition. This section examines each part.

THE HOOF CAPSULE

One of the most important parts of a horse's hoof is the hoof capsule. The proposition that horses do not stand, but instead hang by their pedal bone in the hoof capsule, is indeed true. Thus it is not surprising that the hoof capsule must always be in top condition for a horse to function well.

To get a good idea of a horse's hoof, we can compare the lower foot with our finger tip. Our nail is, for the horse, the horny wall, our phalanx the pedal bone.

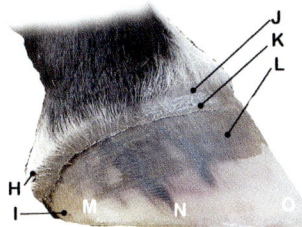

Seen from the side:
J. Coronary suture
K. Periople
L. Horny wall
M. Heel part
N. Side wall (or quarter)
O. Toe

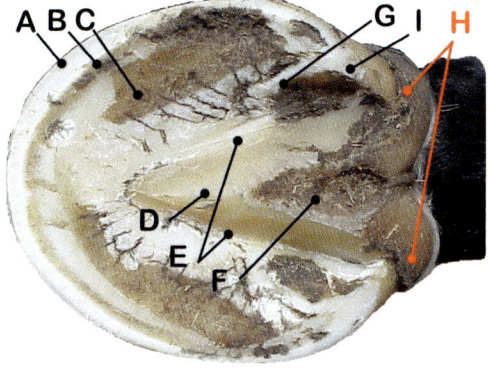

Seen from the back:
H. Bulbs
I. Heel
P. Central groove
Q. Pastern cavity

Seen from underneath:
A. Weightbearing edge
B. White line (or nail line)
C. Sole
D. Frog
E. Lateral grooves
F. Central groove
G. Bars
H. Horny bulbs
I. Heel

The Hoof 19

The horn of the hoof capsule has five characteristics:
1. The horn wall is a closed entity that does not absorb oil, hoof lubricant or substances other than water.
2. The percentage of water and fat has a great influence on the elasticity of the horn. A high percentage of water and fat makes the hoof elastic and shock-absorbent. If the hoof dries out severely and shrinks through evaporation, the horn becomes hard and atrophies or crumbles away. This can be the cause of poor quality hooves and sheared heels.
3. Ammonia – for example from urine – affects the horn. Ammonia is soluble in water, has a deleterious effect on the horn, and can even dissolve it. This can result in thrush or a separating wall.
4. Horn is extremely resistant to the effects of corrosive substances such as acids.
5. Horn is a bad conductor of heat, and therefore the inner parts do not freeze in snowy or frosty conditions. As a bad conductor of heat, the hoof is protected against the hot fitting of horseshoes.

The hoof capsule is composed of carbon (about 50%), oxygen, nitrogen, hydrogen and sulphur. The horn wall contains 10% water; the solar surface 30%; the frog 42%. The average percentage of fat in the wall is 0.75%: in the solar surface 0.25%; in the frog 0.50%.

To prevent the drying-out of the hoof capsule during dry periods, the horse can have its hooves placed in wet sand. The sand should be made wet a few times a week, and each time kept wet for several hours by using, for example, a garden hose.

Alternatively, the straw in the stable can be dampened with a watering can. Water absorption by the hooves is a very slow process.

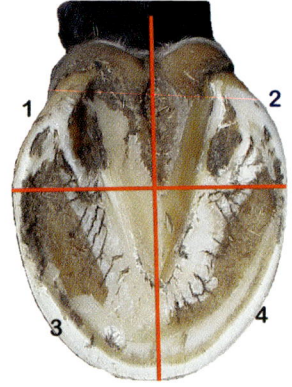

The underneath is divided into four parts, making it clear which part is being referred to. The outer side of the hoof is always wider and longer than the inner side.
1. Inside heel quarter
2. Outside heel quarter
3. Inside toe quarter
4. Outside toe quarter
1–2 Back half
3–4 Front half

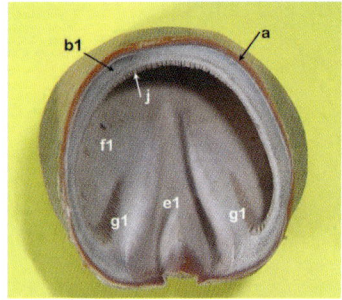

The hoof capsule is composed of:
a. The edge
b1. The horny wall
e1. The frog cushion
g1. The bars
f1. The sole
j. The insensitive laminae into which the sensitive laminae fit

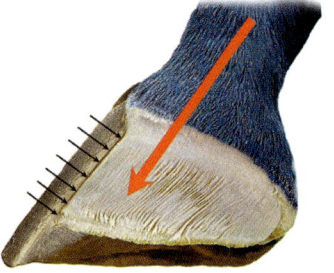

The weight that is borne by the hoof (red arrow) is held by the tightly-knit attachment of the laminae in the hoof capsule (black arrows). Thus a special kind of hanging attachment is created.

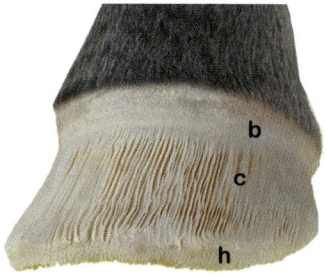

The epidermis changes to the coronary corium (b); it is necessary for the development of the sensitive laminae (c). The sensitive laminae change structurally at the end, becoming a kind of soft horn (h).

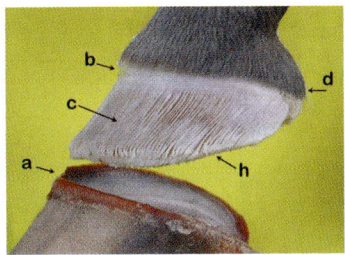
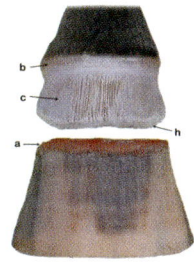
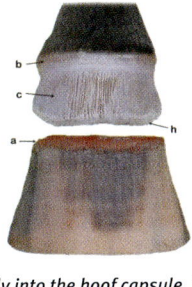

The pedal bone, with the sensitive laminae (c), fits exactly into the hoof capsule. The sensitive laminae are intricately bound with the insensitive laminae that are present on the inside of the hoof capsule.
a. Coronary suture
b. Coronary corium
c. Sensitive laminae
d. Bulb corium
h. Formation of white line

The insensitive laminae (j) lie neatly side by side on the inside of the horny wall (b1).
a. Periople.

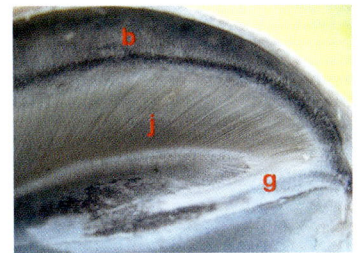

On the sides of the hoof capsule, the insensitive laminae are shorter (j) where they recede into the turning (g) next to the frog – here they are called the bars. Horny wall (b).

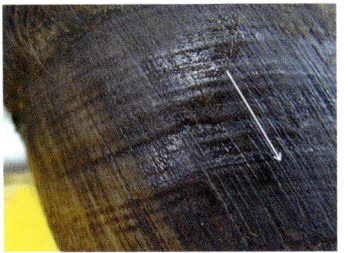

A hoof capsule; the horny tubules can be clearly seen.

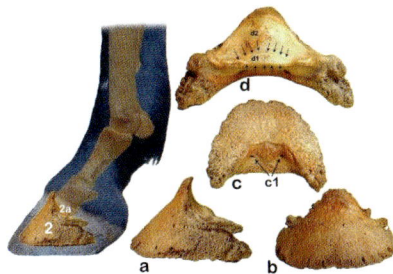

The pedal bone consists of:
a. *The side wall surface. The wall surface is highest at the front, with the coronary prominence above; it is slanted and lowest at the heel.*
b. *The front surface.*
c. *The underside. This has a semilunar crest where the deep flexor tendon is housed. There are two channels (c1) for the main arteries.*
d. *The pedal bone has two joint surfaces: the joint surface of the navicular bone (d1) and the joint surface of the short pastern bone (d2); together they form the hoof joint.*

THE PEDAL BONE

The pedal bone is enclosed by the hoof capsule. As the pedal bone with the sensitive laminae (fleshy plates) is fixed to the insensitive laminae (horny plates) of the hoof capsule, it hangs in the hoof capsule.

The pedal bone is made up of three surfaces:

1. **The wall surface.** This has the same form as the outside of the hoof capsule. The wall surface is highest at the front and, above this, is the coronary prominence.
2. **The side surfaces of the pedal bone that narrows toward the back.** The hoof cartilage is attached to the narrowest part (the lateral cartilages of the pedal bone).
3. **The solar surface with the accompanying joint surfaces.** The solar surface is concave. Inside the concavity is a crescent-shaped surface where the deep flexor tendon is situated. There are also two openings in this area. The end sections of the digital artery come through these to the inside, forming a loop in the pedal bone. The digital artery is split into many small branches that go through the pedal bone to the outside via the many small holes in the wall surface. The joint surface is made up of two surfaces: the larger surface over which the short pastern bone glides, and the smaller surface where the navicular bone is situated.

THE NAVICULAR BONE

In the horse's hoof, the navicular bone is a small bobbin-shaped bone, which lies against the back of the joint between the pedal bone and the short pastern bone.

The navicular bone has three surfaces:
1. The joint surface with the pedal bone.
2. The joint surface with the short pastern bone.
3. The tendon surface over which the deep flexor tendon glides. The tendon surface is covered with cartilage which makes the surface extremely slippery.

A bursa filled with the joint-lubricating synovial fluid lies between the navicular bone and the deep flexor tendon. The deep flexor tendon runs over the navicular bone like a cord over a pulley.

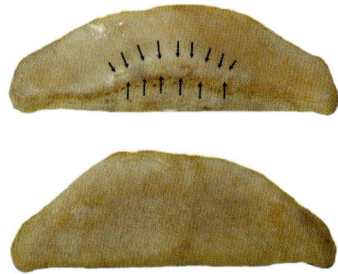

The navicular bone is a bobbin-shaped bone over which the deep digital flexor tendon glides. The navicular bone has three surfaces: the joint surface with the pedal bone; the joint surface with the short pastern bone; the gliding surface of the deep flexor tendon.

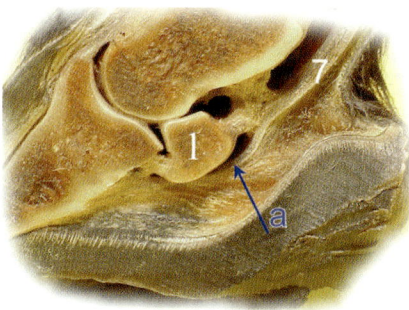

Between the navicular bone (1) and the deep flexor tendon (7) there is a synovial bursa (a). The deep flexor tendon runs over the navicular bone like a cord over a pulley.

THE BLOOD VESSELS

In and around the pedal bone there is an extremely dense network of fine blood vessels. Blood is pumped into the hoof by two arteries. The blood provides the hoof with all kinds of substances, such as nutrients and building materials. As soon as the blood has deposited the materials, it is discharged via the veins.

THE NERVES

The hoof has numerous nerves which split into many branches from the fetlock. Within the hoof they are further divided into many extremities which end in the laminae. These are microscopically small organs that take care of touch and the feeling of pain. The hoof is, thus, a very sensitive tactile organ.

There is a dense network of blood vessels with numerous nerves encasing the pedal bone – thus the hoof is a sensitive tactile organ.

DEVELOPMENT OF THE HOOF CAPSULE

The transition from the hide to the hoof is called the coronal suture. The soft hide changes into the hard hoof with the elastic periople in between. Just above the coronal suture is the periople corium that produces the periople. The periople consists of thin elastic horn. It is 1 to 2 cm wide and spreads itself over the horny wall below as a very thin varnish-like

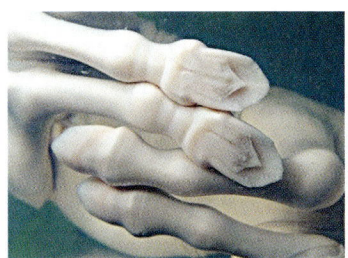

The foal's hooves are already correctly formed in the womb.

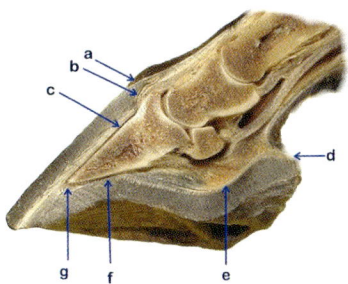

The combined hoof corium is:
a. periople corium
b. coronary corium
c. wall corium
d. heel corium
e. frog corium
f. sole corium
g. development of the white line

covering of hard horn. This thin layer of exceedingly hard horn ensures the protection of the horny wall and covers it for about 5 to 10 cm from above to below. At the coronal suture, the long coronary hairs form the end of the hide. The hide continues into the hoof as the hoof corium.

THE HOOF CORIUM

When the epidermis changes into the coronal suture, the name changes from hide to hoof corium or pododerma. The hoof corium covers the whole hoof. The name already indicates exactly where the hoof corium is – just as do the coronary, wall, frog, sole and bar corium. Every hoof corium produces horn.

The hoof corium forms the hoof capsule. The hoof capsule is composed of several parts that form the whole. The hoof corium has, unlike the epidermis, no fat or sweat glands: only in the sensitive frog can a number of sweat glands be found. As the hoof corium contains many blood vessels and nerves it is very sensitive. The hoof corium is thus known as 'the quick' or 'the flesh'.

THE PERIOPLE CORIUM

The periople corium develops a thin layer of horn that has the function to partly cover and protect the horny wall.

THE CORONARY CORIUM

The coronary corium (germinating layer) is found at the coronal suture and develops the horn in the form of horny tubules that lie side by side and on top of each other and which grow downwards along the pedal bone. The coronary corium also secretes horn between these tubules. This secretion is a semi-horny substance and has the function of keeping the tubules adhering together.

As well as the development of horny tubules, the coronary corium also develops the insensitive laminae at the transition to the laminal surface against the pedal bone. These insensitive laminae cover the whole interior of the hoof capsule. They go from above to below, parallel with each other; they are only a couple of millimetres wide, and contain no blood.

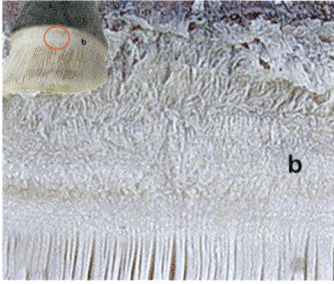

The coronary corium (b) is where the hoof capsule – in the form of horny tubules and insensitive laminae – is developed. These tubules are cemented together by a semi-horny substance.

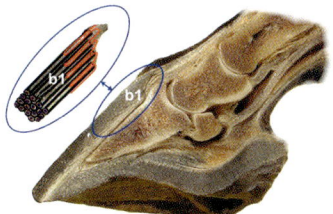

The coronary corium develops tiny tubules (b1) that lie neatly together; combined, they form the horny wall.

The coronary corium has about twenty-five insensitive laminae per centimetre in the toe part, about fifteen insensitive laminae per centimetre at the heel, about ten insensitive laminae per centimetre in the bars, and about six hundred insensitive laminae in a middle-sized hoof. These laminae are known as the primary sensitive laminae.

On every primary lamina there are side laminae that grip each other ensuring a better connection. These side laminae are known as the secondary laminae.

The horny wall with the horny tubules and the insensitive laminae all grow downwards together.

THE WALL CORIUM

The wall corium develops between the insensitive laminae and the sensitive laminae. There is practically no subcutaneous connective tissue present under the wall corium. Thus this corium lies on the bone membrane of the pedal bone.

Sensitive laminae have the same form as the insensitive laminae but they are vascular. They lie alternately between the insensitive laminae – like folded hands, where the fingers of one hand intertwine with the fingers of the other hand. This connection is extremely strong, and especially so when under pressure.

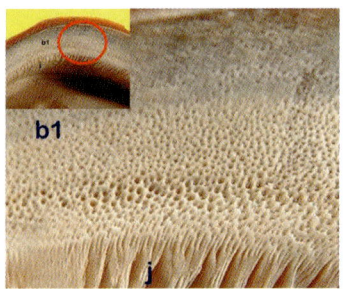

The horny tubules (b1) that are developed by the coronary corium have a long core; they are visible on the horny wall as holes.

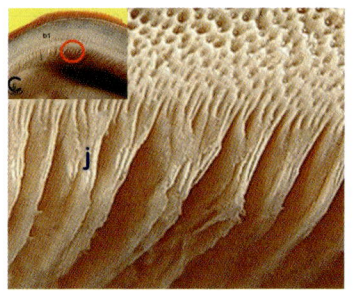

The insensitive laminae are on the inside of the horny wall (j); these are bloodless. The sensitive laminae are between the insensitive laminae.

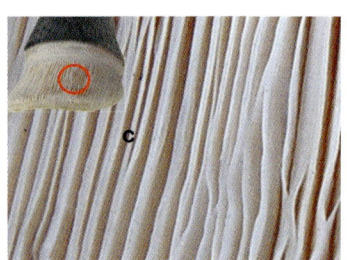

The sensitive laminae (c) on the pedal bone are interspersed between the insensitive laminae and thus form an extremely tough connection, especially when pressure is applied.

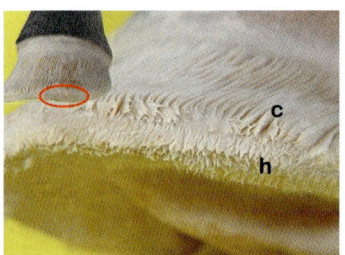

At the pedal bone edge, the sensitive laminae (c) form a very fibrous mass (h) that develops another kind of soft horn.

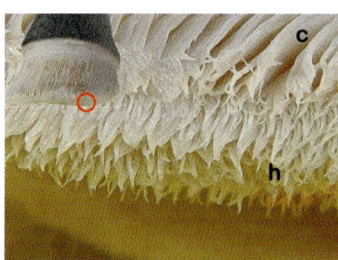

This fibrous mass forms a soft horn that fills up the growing horny tubules and thus forms the white line.

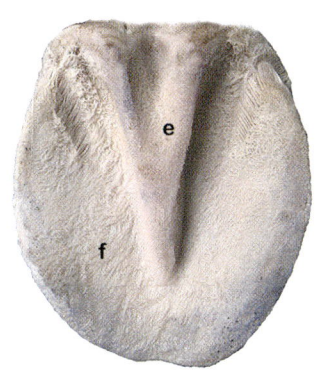

Under the pedal bone, the solar surface is developed by the sole corium (f). Just as with the wall corium, there is little subcutaneous connective tissue present. This sole corium fits to the bone membrane of the pedal bone. The frog corium (e) has more subcutaneous connective tissue.

The sensitive laminae that lie on the pedal bone do not grow downwards, although the insensitive laminae do. At the edge of the pedal bone, the sensitive laminae change into a strong mass of tissue that develops another sort of soft horn. This soft horn fills out the space between the insensitive laminae that are growing downwards and thus the white line – also known as the nail line – is formed. The white line is easily visible between the horn wall and the sole.

THE SOLE CORIUM

Under the pedal bone, the solar surface is developed by the sole corium. Just as in the wall corium, there is very little sub cutis connective tissue present; the sole corium also lies on the bone membrane of the pedal bone. The sole corium has a soft fibrous structure. The structure of the horn that is developed by the sole corium is robust and extremely pliable; this is necessary for the hoof mechanism of the hoof.

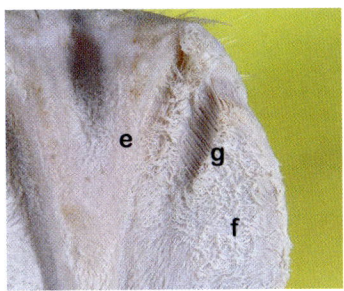

The sole corium (f) has a soft fibrous texture. The structure of the horn that the sole corium develops is rough and extremely elastic. This is necessary for the hoof mechanism of the hoof. The frog corium (e) consists of a firmer but fine fibrous tissue, and it develops the digital cushion. The illustration also shows the bars (g).

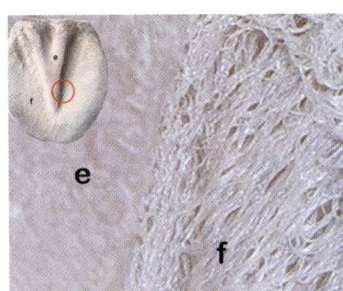

The fibrous structures of the frog corium (e) and the sole corium (f) are very different and as a result have different horn structures.

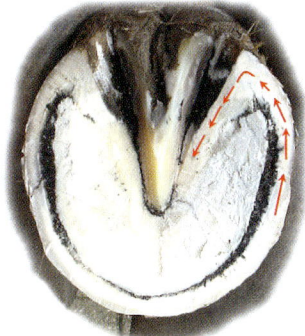

The horny wall turns inwards at the heel, parallel to the lateral groove, and is an important strong part of the hoof capsule.

THE BULB CORIUM

The bulb corium is situated at the back of the hoof; it is divided in the middle by the groove between the heel bulbs. It consists of a strong, stiff connective tissue cushion which runs across the central cleft.

THE FROG CORIUM

The frog corium has somewhat more subcutaneous connective tissue. It consists of a fine, fibrous tissue with a rather fixed structure. The frog corium develops the frog cushion. This is seen by the triangular or V-shaped form of the central cleft together with the two lateral clefts. The frog has a robust structure with many fat and cartilage islets. The frog cushion is extremely elastic. The frog plays an important role in the hoof mechanism, allowing the back half to expand under the pressure of foot-all and serving as a protection and as a buffer for the internal parts.

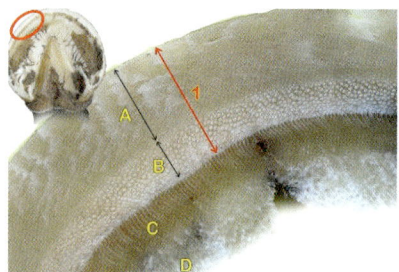

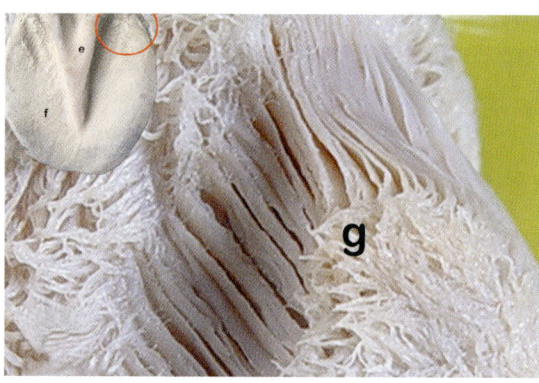

Underneath the hoof are:
1. The horny wall
A. Horny tubules of the first kind (small and narrow)
B. Horny tubules of the second kind (big and wide)
C. The white line, insensitive laminae with the semi-horny substance between that is developed on the underside of the sensitive laminae
D. Sole

The turn-in of the heels, the bars (g), consists partly of sensitive laminae; they give extra firmness to the hoof capsule.

THE BAR CORIUM

The wall corium turns at the rear of the hoof at an angle and returns towards the front, forming the bar corium. The bar corium ensures extra firmness at the rear underside of the hoof. Thus the hoof capsule and the bars form a whole.

HOOF CAPSULE PIGMENTATION

The hoof capsule can be pigmented or without pigment. The colour of the epidermis regulates the colour of the hoof capsule. Horses with white marks on the limbs (for example a sock or white coronet) in general have hooves without pigment. If the lower limb is dark, the colour of the hoof capsule in the direction of the horny tubules is also often dark. If there are dark flecks on a white coronet, then these flecks usually continue downwards in the form of dark stripes on the white hoof capsule. People generally think that pigmented hooves are stronger than those without pigment: chemical analysis has proved that actually there is no difference in the composition of the horn and thus also not in the strength of the

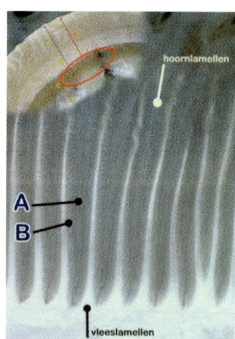

The insensitive and sensitive laminae are intertwined in the white line. On every primary lamina (A) there are side laminae (B) that grip the secondary laminae providing a strong connection.

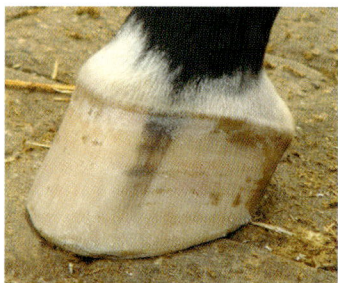

A white hoof capsule is just as strong as a black one.

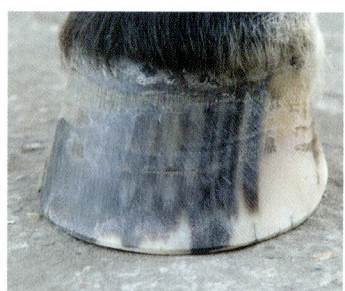

It has been suggested that a pigmented (black) hoof capsule is stronger than a non-pigmented (white) hoof capsule. This is untrue – pigment has nothing to do with the quality or hardness of the horn.

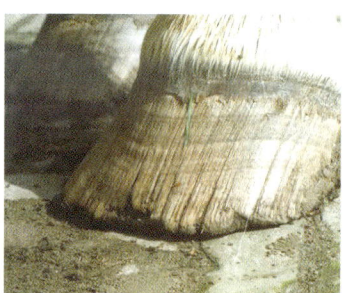

Under the influence of ultraviolet light, cracks can appear on the horny wall of older horses. This is caused by the disappearance of the semi-horny substance that holds the horny tubules together: it has no deleterious effect.

horn. Black merely gives us the impression of robustness and strength; perhaps white is associated with weakness, just as we associate red with warmth and fire and blue with chill and cold.

Amongst older horses, there are often small cracks caused by ultraviolet radiation on the surface of the horny wall. Ultraviolet radiation causes a mild disintegration of the horny material between the tubules that keeps them together. These little cracks in the horny wall are harmless.

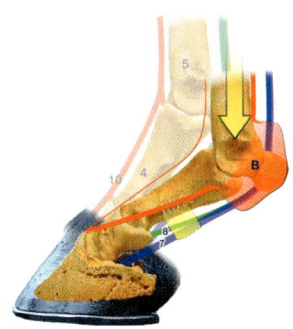

The horse's movement, and the take-off of the hoof, cause enormous energy to be released which is partly absorbed by the annular ligament of the fetlock (B). Thus the pressure necessary for hoof mechanism is brought to bear on the hoof capsule.
4. Long pastern; 5. Cannon; 7. Superficial flexor tendon; 8. Deep flexor tendon; 10. Extensor tendon

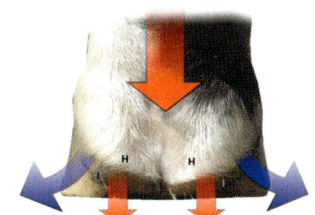

When a horse puts its hoof to the ground, the body weight will flatten both heel bulbs (H) and the digital cushion. This causes the heels (I) to be spread outwards.

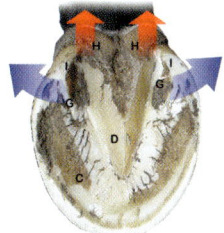

When there is weight on the hoof, both heels are pushed outwards (blue arrows), and when there is a release of pressure they return to normal position.
C. Sole; D. Frog; G. Bars; H. Bulbs; I. Heels

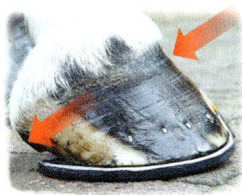

When bearing weight, the front of the hoof capsule is pulled back and it becomes flatter.

Hoof Mechanism

What is understood by hoof mechanism is the change in form that takes place in the hoof when it is set down or lifted up. The moment before the hoof is lifted from the ground – the last moment before take-off – is when the pressure on the hoof is at its greatest. At that moment, the following changes in form take place:
1. The solar surface becomes flatter.
2. The bars lie flatter.
3. The frog is pressed downwards.
4. The pedal bone with its horny wall growth attached is pressed down – that is to say, the pedal bone rotates.
5. The angle of the wall with the ground becomes more acute because of the above-mentioned changes, and the hoof becomes wider.

BLOOD CIRCULATION IN THE HOOF

The supply and discharge of the blood in the hoof is regulated by the change in shape that the hoof undergoes when being set down or lifted

The Hoof

up. The alternate weightbearing and release of the hoof works like a suction pump for the veins in the hoof.

The arterial blood, the blood supply bringing nutrients to the hoof, streams into the hoof by its own weight and the heart's thrust – and then, because of the change in form, the blood from the arteries in the hoof is sucked out. When under weightbearing pressure from the hoof, the blood– which now no longer contains nutrients, but carries waste matter from the hoof – is squeezed out through the network of veins in the hoof into the two side veins which carry the blood away. As soon as the hoof is relieved it resumes its original shape again and the blood would naturally return into the veins; however, this reversal of the blood is prevented by valves in the veins. These valves are also known as shunts. The mechanism can be compared to a door that only opens one way: you can open the door and go through it, but you can neither push back the door nor go through the other way. The result is that the blood is always being pushed in the correct direction.

It is important that the hoof has good blood circulation. The advantages are:

1. The more regular the flow of blood, the more blood containing nutrients (oxygen and nourishment) supplies the hoof and the more the parts of the corium can be nourished.
2. Horn growth and the quality of the horn are improved.
3. The horn grows faster and more fluid is supplied.
4. The horn becomes elastic.
5. A hoof mechanism that works well absorbs shock well.
6. Good blood circulation promotes the horse's elasticity of gait.
7. Good blood circulation prevents fatigue.
8. Good blood circulation reduces the chance of hoof and bone defects.

Ideally, horses should not be in stables; they are in their element when they are on the move all day. This is when the hoof mechanism is at its best, as is the growth and the quality of the hoof.

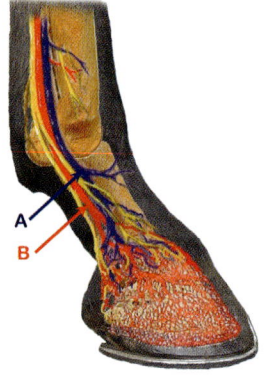

The alternate weightbearing and pressure release of the hoof works like a suction pump for the veins that are in the hoof. The arterial blood (A) is pushed in by its own momentum, and because of the change of form the blood is sucked out of the hoof. When there is pressure on the hoof, blood from the veins is forced into the two side veins that then discharge the blood (B).

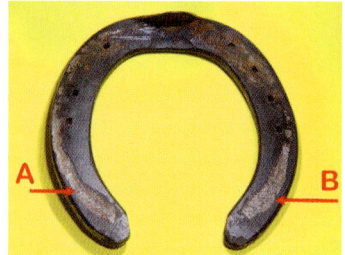

Wear can clearly be seen on this horseshoe on the places where the heels have stood and spread.
A. Inside branch; B. Outside branch

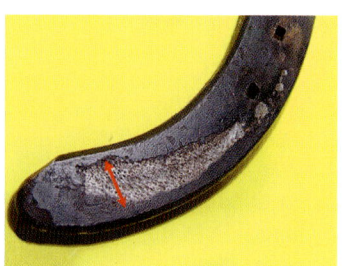

A big enough shoe is one of the most important things for a properly functioning hoof mechanism; after eight weeks, the heels should still be supported by the horseshoe.

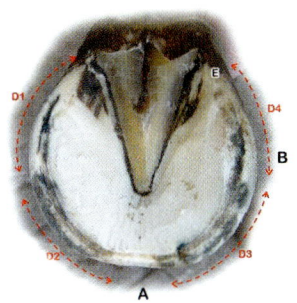
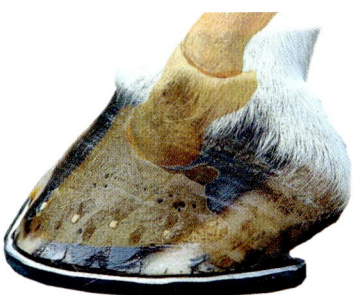
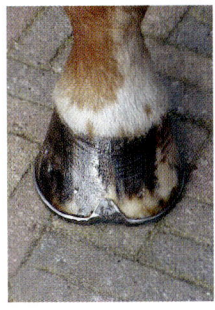

The fore hoof is round and is divided into the toe section (A), the outer section (B), and the the inner section, and is divided into four quarters: the inner heel quarter (D1); the inner toe quarter (D2); the outer toe quarter (D3) and the outer heel quarter (D4).

The angle of the horny wall on a fore hoof is, at the toe, about 45 to 50 degrees; it is steeper toward the back.

A normal fore hoof. The coronary band indicates the hoof shape.

Hoof Shapes

THE NORMAL HOOF

There is no general norm for a horse's hoof shape, proportion and structure as these are dependent on the different types of horse or pony breeds.

The fore hoof:
1. The fore hoof has a rounded shape.
2. The horny wall is at its longest at the toe and at its shortest at the back of the heel. The ratio is about 1:2, which means that at the toe the horny wall is about twice as long as it is at the heel.
3. The hoof capsule is divided into five parts:
    a. The front part, called the toe
    b. The lateral (outer) side of the hoof capsule
    c. The medial (inner) side of the hoof capsule
    d. The horny wall is divided, for simplicity, into four, also known as quarters
    e. The heel wall, also known as the heels
4. The angle of the horny wall at the toe is about 45 to 50 degrees, and becomes steeper toward the back; the inner wall is a little steeper than the outer wall.
5. The horny wall is thickest at the toe and becomes thinner toward the back (in a ratio of about 2:1).
6. Small, evenly-spaced ridges (rings) appear on the horny wall down from the coronet due to changes in feed rations, seasonal changes, or through the giving of medicine.
7. At the back of the heel, the horny wall makes a sharp angle inwards toward the middle of the solar surface (the bar angle) where the bars change over to solar surface.
8. The solar surface is clearly concave.
9. The frog is big and widely developed.
10. The middle and lateral clefts are not too close to each other and are not too deep.

The Hoof

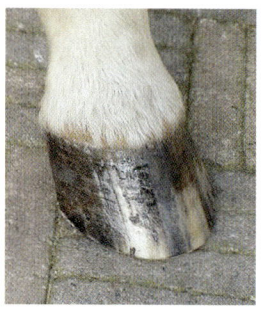

A normal hind hoof. The coronary band indicates the hoof shape. The hind hoof has a triangular shape.

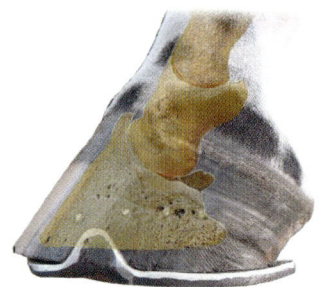

The hind hoof – with an angle of 50 to 55 degrees – is mostly a bit steeper than the fore hoof.

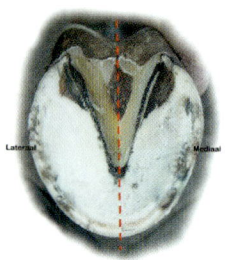

By dividing the hind hoof into two, it is clear to see that the outer side (lateral) is broader than the inner side (medial).

The same norms count for the hind hoof, with the addition of:
1. The hind hoof is mostly 50 to 55 degrees, steeper than the fore hoof.
2. The heels are longer (higher).
3. The hind hoof is triangular in shape.
4. The hind hoof is smaller than the front hoof.

Both the fore hoof and the hind hoof have an outer (lateral) half that is wider than the inner (medial) half.

DEFECTIVE HOOF SHAPES

Defective hoof shapes can arise from a defective limb conformation. Horses can also have defective hoof shapes from birth or through sickness. However, most hoof shapes are related to the limb or the foot axis of the horse.

THE WIDE HOOF

The characteristics of a wide hoof are:
- A big, but above all, wide circumference of the hoof
- Less upright walls than the normal hoof shape
- Short and low heels that in some cases can be under-run (heels that lie under the hoof)
- A flat solar surface with very little concavity
- Broad and low heel bulbs

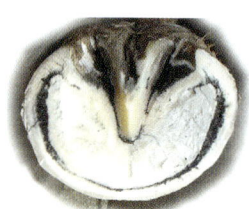

A wide hoof has a large and, above all, broad circumference; the walls are also less sheer than a normal hoof shape.

THE NARROW HOOF

Characteristics of the narrow hoof are:
- The oval form
- High and upright heels
- Elongated side walls giving a narrower frog
- A concave sole – that is to say, more concavity than a normal hoof.
- Narrow heels that can become sheared heels (see Sheared Heels)

With these shapes, the hoof mechanism can function less well and be restricting. Some of these shapes are more common in certain breeds such as Andalusians and Arabs.

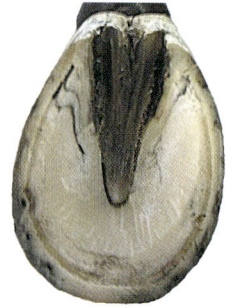

A narrow hoof has an oval form with upright heels; the side walls are long and the frog is narrow.

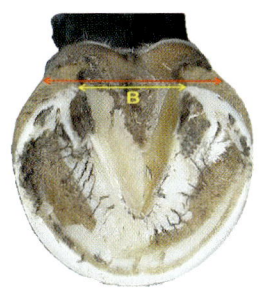

Under-run heels. The horn at the heels is turned in a little (B). The heels are turned in by the pressure the horse puts on the wall.

UNDER-RUN HEELS

Characteristics for this form are:
- The heel wall is turned somewhat underneath
- The pressure put on the heels by the horse causes the walls to be pushed inwards
- Thus the walls roll under the vertical line of the heel

THE FLAT FOOT

Characteristics of the flat foot are:
- A flat solar surface
- The heels lie low and flat under the hoof
- A rather more horizontal horny wall
- An extremely flat frog

A flat foot has a bigger chance of painful bruising, for example by walking on stones; lameness can result.

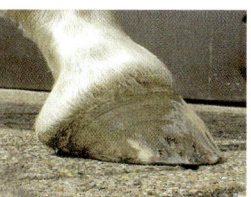

A flat foot has a flat solar surface and heels that lie low and flat under the hoof.

SHEARED HEELS

Characteristics of the hoof with sheared heels are:
- The back half of the hoof is extremely narrow
- The heels are very high
- The side walls are steep and are close to being vertical. The wall can turn under due to this narrowing of the heel part

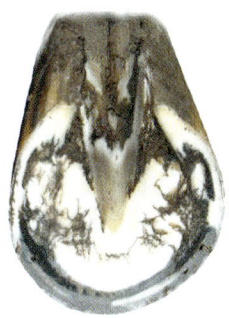

The hoof with sheared heels has an oval shape and both heels lie within the vertical line. Sheared heels result in a strongly reduced hoof mechanism.

Sheared heels lead to a strongly reduced action of the hoof mechanism, and thus to a lesser blood circulation. Less blood circulation leads in turn to less horn development. Less horn development leads to a narrow and small hoof, and a small hoof limits the hoof mechanism. Thus the horse falls into a vicious circle and there is more chance of thrush.

A widening shoe can be a solution: in this shoe, both branches of the shoe are forged so that they are angled outwards, so that the hoof can no longer narrow down. Unfortunately this shoe has the disadvantage that it can push the heels outwards when weight is borne.

A shoe for sheared heels; the weight-bearing surface of both branches of the shoe are forged to slant outwards so that the heels cannot slide inwards.

THE MALFORMED HOOF

A malformed hoof is not actually a defective hoof form, because it results from the conformation of the limb. It is mostly seen when a horse has a toe-out conformation or a toe-in conformation. The farrier should respect the conformation.

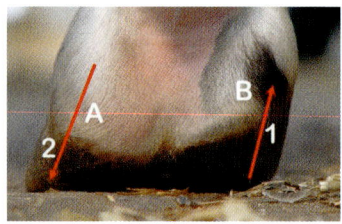

In a malformed hoof, the inner horny wall (1) is parallel to the outer wall (2). The extreme pressure of the hoof on the ground will cause the outside heel bulb (A) to be positioned lower than the inside bulb (B).

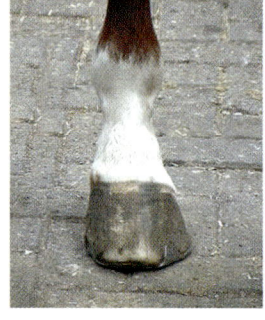

A malformed hoof. This is actually a deviation of the hoof shape, as the malformed hoof is a result of the conformation of the limb and lower limb. The coronary band is not horizontal but slants to the outside.

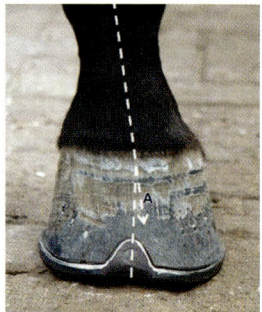

Malformed hooves should not have their position changed, as the hoof joint is, generally, broken to the outside. The weightbearing from the limb will put pressure on the outside half of the hoof (A). A horse with a malformed hoof shape will place it on the ground with equal all-round pressure.

THE CURVED HOOF

If a horse has a base-narrow conformation as well as a toe-out or toe-in conformation, the pressure on the outer horny wall will be great. Thus the hoof is pushed inwards and it will grow downward in a curve.

THE DIAGONAL HOOF

The characteristics of a diagonal hoof are two relatively straight lines (see blue lines) and two curved lines (see red lines) opposite each other. A diagonal hoof is mostly the result of a toe-out or toe-in conformation. In a toe-in conformation the hoof has a tendency to roll over the outer edge (outside front quarter); the opposite occurs with a toe-out conformation.

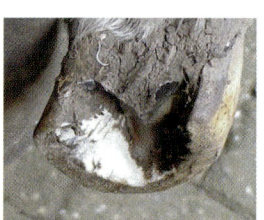

The curved hoof. Where there is both a base-narrow and toe-in (bow-legged) conformation, a curved hoof can result. The outer and inner walls grow curved inwards.

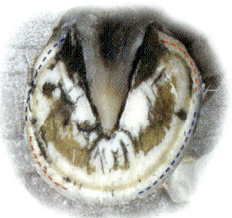

The diagonal hoof. This hoof shape has two relatively straight lines (blue line) and two curved lines (red line) diametrically opposed. The diagonal hoof is usually the result of the toe-out or base-narrow conformation.

THE UPRIGHT HOOF

The characteristics of an upright hoof are:
- The angle at the toe wall is greater than 55 degrees
- The horny wall is, at the toe, more than 55 degrees and has the same steep angles of wall

The toe of an upright hoof continues to get steeper and can result in club foot.

CLUB FOOT

The characteristics of a club-footed hoof are:
- The horny wall at the toe can reach an angle of as much as 90 degrees

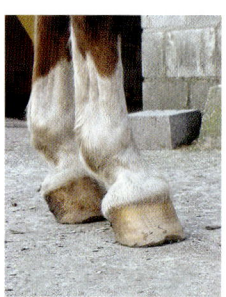

The upright hoof. Here the angle of the toe wall is greater than 55 degrees. Generally, the foot axis is also sheer, as are the heels.

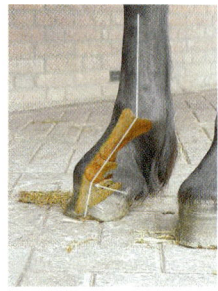

The club-footed hoof has an upright toe wall which can even be vertical.

- The axis of the foot is broken forwards in the hoof joint

Horses with one or more club-footed hooves need extra attention. A club foot can lead to pes equinus.

DROPPED SOLE

We speak of a dropped sole if the sole is convex and bulges out from the weightbearing edge. This is mostly seen in horses that have had laminitis and the horny walls can no longer be restored to good condition.

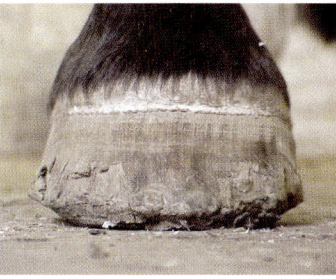

In the dropped sole hoof, the sole has descended and is lower than the weightbearing edge. This causes lameness.

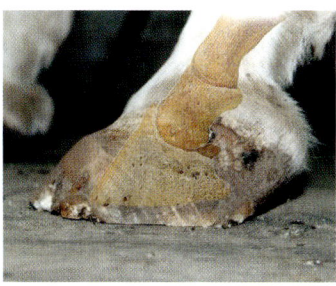

If a horse has had laminitis, there can be a deviant growth of the horny wall. If the farrier leaves the toe wall too thick, a deformed hoof can result.

THE DISTORTED HOOF

If a horse has had laminitis, a deviant growth can develop on the horny wall. If the farrier has left the horny wall of the toe too thick, a distorted hoof can result. This hoof shape causes the horse unnecessary problems and should be removed (see also laminitis section).

THE FOAL HOOF

Newly-born foals have long threads of extremely soft horn coming from the solar surface and the frog. These threads quickly dry out and in a very short time the hoof assumes a normal shape.

The shape of the hooves of a foal is determined by heredity.

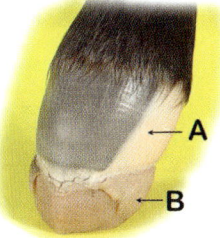

This foal hoof is one minute old. The hoof capsule (A) is very soft, and underneath is a spongy tissue (B) to protect the hoof and the womb. This tissue quickly dries and falls off.

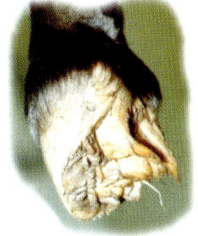

After several hours, the foal hoof assumes a proper shape: the horny wall hardens and the soft under part dries out and breaks off so that a normal sole is created.

A FREAK OF NATURE

A foal was once brought to us with one of the small metacarpal bones developed as a full foal hoof at a point where there was a protuberance of the bone not visible from the outside. The little extra hoof was removed just above the pastern joint so that the foal would not be bothered by it later.

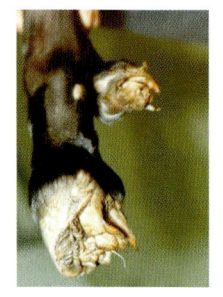

A freak of nature: the extra little foot has a hoof and a short and long pastern bone.

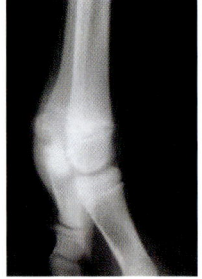

The X-ray clearly shows the 'double' bones.

Foot Axis and Limb Conformation

When judging foot axis and limb conformation we start from the point of the ideal example. However, horses do not often conform to the ideal. The reality is quite different and a deviant limb conformation does not necessarily mean a wrong conformation.

EVALUATING LIMB CONFORMATION

In order to assess the limb conformation of a horse or pony it must be standing squarely on a flat surface – with both fore and hind limbs exactly next to each other. It is important that the horse stands squarely because in this way its body weight is evenly distributed over all four legs. During the evaluation the horse should not rest any of its legs.

The horse must be viewed from the front, the back and the side in order to properly evaluate the foot axis and the limb conformation. In evaluating, an imaginary vertical line is dropped dividing the limb in two.

A defective foot axis is often caused by a defective limb conformation. It is through defective foot and limb conformation that the tendons and ligaments in the limb have an extra load locally and the joints wear unevenly. The horse can have problems with this as it gets older.

FOOT AXIS

The hoof of a horse must always be shod according to the foot axis. The foot axis is an imaginary line that begins in the middle of the pastern joint, then goes through the axis length of the three bones of the underfoot and parallel with the toe wall. Thus the long pastern, the short pastern and the pedal bone – which are on this imaginary line – are an extension of each other. A foot axis is looked at from the side and from the front.

In a normal foot and limb conformation, the hoof is loaded in proportion with equal pressure on the ground. As soon as the angle of the foot axis changes, thus also does the pressure of the foot on the ground. If the hoof joint is broken backwards, the heels are more loaded as compared to a normal foot axis where the load is equal all round. The consequence of uneven loading is disproportionate wear. This can influence the paces of the horse and the quality of the hooves.

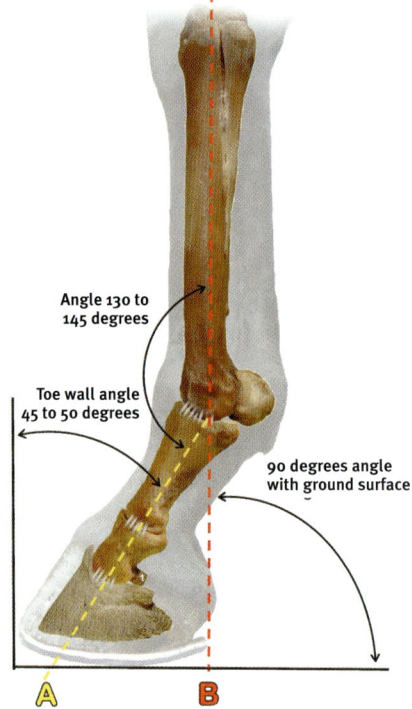

A foot axis (A) is an imaginary line that starts at the centre of the pastern joint. It can be drawn through the axis length of the three bones of the lower foot and is parallel with the toe wall. The long pastern, short pastern and pedal bone are thus an extension of each other.

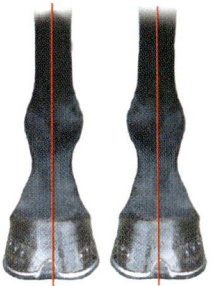

A foot axis seen from the front.

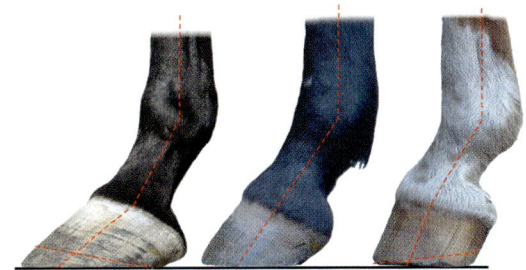

1. Foot axis broken toward the back in the hoof joint
2. Normal foot axis
3. Foot axis broken toward the front in the hoof joint

If a horse is not correctly pared or shod according to the normal foot axis, problems can arise.

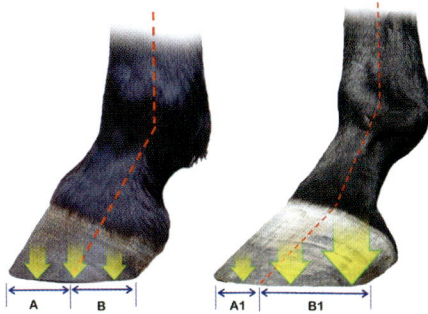

A normal hoof is evenly weighted and there is an equal pressure on the ground surface (A and B). When the foot axis is changed, the weight of the hoof on the ground will change (A1 and B1). Therefore we see that a hoof with a foot axis broken toward the back in the hoof joint shows more weight on the heels than would be borne by a normal foot axis where the weight is evenly distributed. Uneven weightbearing results in uneven wear that can affect the paces and the quality of the hoof. (The bigger arrows indicate added weightbearing).

Seen from the side, there are three different kinds of foot axis:

1. **A weak foot axis.** The angle between the horny wall and the ground is less than 45 degrees. This is also called 'weak pasterned'. Thus the pastern joint is also loaded and sinks low – sometimes nearly to the ground. This leads to extra stress and the wearing out of the flexor tendons. Horses with a weak foot axis can also be long-pasterned, that is to say the length of the pastern is longer than normal and the loading of the pastern joint becomes even greater.
2. **A normal foot axis.** The normal foot axis is at the same angle to the ground as the horny wall; at the fore hooves it is 45 to 50 degrees and at the hind hooves 50 to 55 degrees.
3. **An upright foot axis.** Here, the angle of the horny wall to the ground is greater than 45 degrees. This is also called 'steep pasterned'. An upright conformation is less able to absorb shock, which gives extra wear to the joints as a result. A horse with an upright foot axis can be short pasterned – the length of the pastern is shorter than normal. Horses with a steep shoulder often have an upright foot axis.

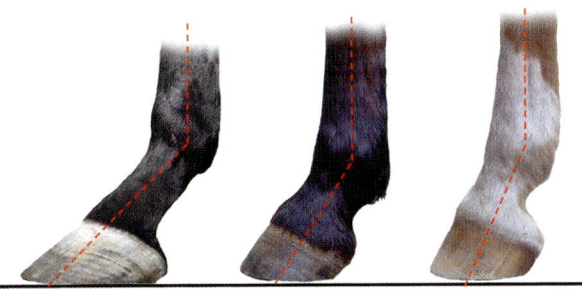

Seen from the side, there are three kinds of foot axis.
1. weak foot axis; 2. normal foot axis; 3. upright foot axis

The Hoof

If a horse has not been well trimmed or shod according to the normal foot axis, problems can arise. Two faults:

1. **A foot axis broken to the rear in the hoof joint.** Here, the farrier has left the toes of the horse too long. The weight on the heels is thus very great, which can result in under-run or low heels. This can result in big problems with the flexor tendons.
2. **A foot axis broken to the front in the hoof joint.** This can arise if the farrier has not trimmed the heels enough. It can also appear 'naturally' in horses that over-reach. Through this, the movement can deteriorate.

TOE-IN AND TOE-OUT CONFORMATION

Two defective conformations that originate in the foot axis are the toe-in conformation and the toe-out conformation.

In the toe-out conformation, the limbs are vertical and parallel to each other to the fetlock. From the pastern, the hooves turn out. The outer side of the hoof capsule is wide and long, as it bears less weight than the inner side. The inner side is steep and short, as it bears more weight than

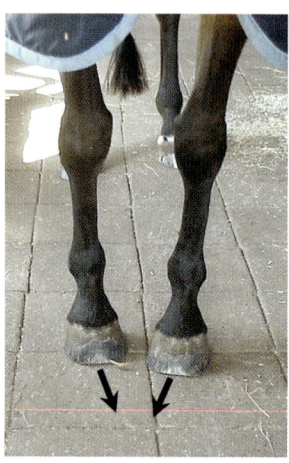

The toe-in conformation. The limbs are vertical and are parallel with each other as far as the fetlock. From the fetlock, the hooves turn inwards. The outer side of the hoof capsule is upright and short as it bears more weight than the inner side. The inner side is wide and long as it bears less weight.

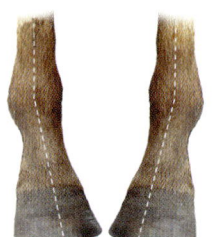 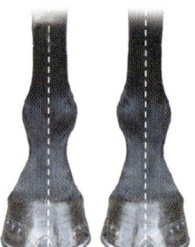 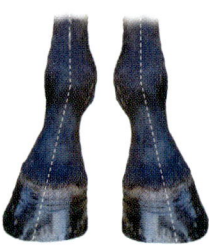

Toe-in conformation   Normal conformation   Toe-out conformation

Foot axis seen from the front: toe-in (outer edge upright and short, inner edge wide and long giving a cutting gait) and toe-out conformation (outer edge wide and long, inner edge upright and short giving a dishing gait) with, in both cases, a straight axis. These conformations begin at the pastern joint (fetlock) and must not be corrected.

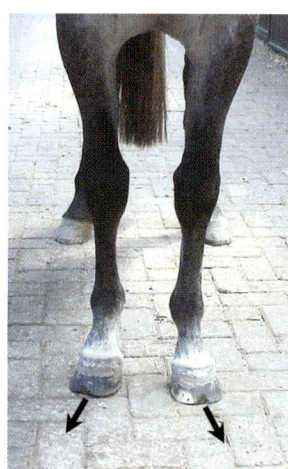

The toe-out conformation. The limbs are vertical and parallel with each other as far as the fetlock. From the fetlock, the hooves turn outwards. The outer side of the hoof capsule is wide and long as it bears less weight than the inner side. The inner side is upright and short as it bears more weight than the outer side. The foot axis is straight but from the fetlock the line runs outwards.

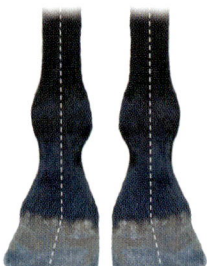 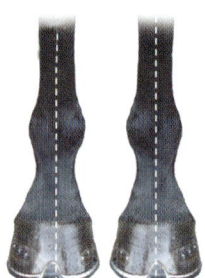 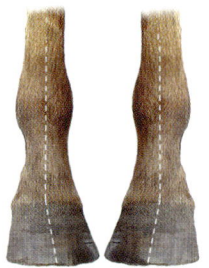

Foot axis broken to the   Normal conformation   Foot axis broken to the
outside in the hoof joint   inside in the hoof joint

Foot axis broken to the outside in the hoof joint, normal conformation, foot axis broken to the inside in the hoof joint.

Deviations in foot axis seen from the front. These are broken inwards or outwards from the hoof joint and have slanted hooves and have faulty weighting of the joints as a result.

Part 1 – The Hoof

the outer side. The foot axis is straight, but from the fetlock follows a line outwards. This position produces a cutting gait whereby, in movement, the lower limb swings inside and can strike the other limb. The hoof has a tendency to roll over at the inside front quarter.

Defective foot axes, as seen from the front, which are broken inwards or outwards from the hoof joint down cause malformed hooves and faulty weightbearing of the joints.

LIMB CONFORMATION

The fore limbs of a horse can be assessed from two viewpoints:

1. **Viewed from the front.** In an ideal postition, vertical lines run from the chest downwards through the middle of the fore limb and hoof. The distance between the hooves must be a minimum of one hoof width.
2. **Viewed from the side.** In an ideal position, the vertical line starts at the upper two thirds of the shoulder blade, goes straight down through the under arm and the cannon bone and ends behind the hoof.

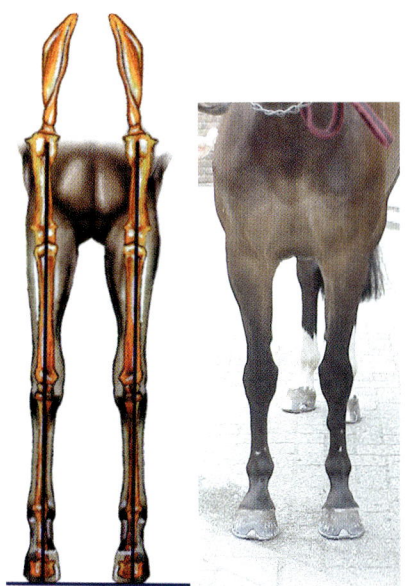

In an ideal limb conformation, seen from the front, vertical lines run from the chest downwards through the middle of the fore limb and hoof. The distance between both hooves should be a minimum of one hoof width.

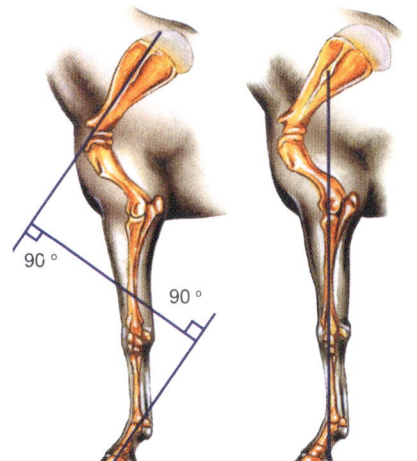
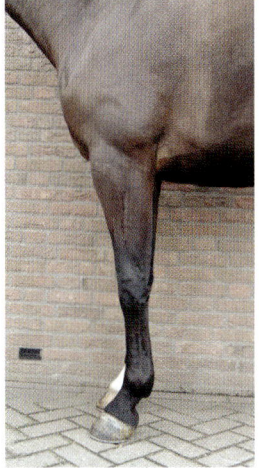

An ideal limb conformation, seen from the side. The vertical line starts at the upper two-thirds of the shoulder blade and runs straight down through the under arm and cannon bone, and ends behind the hoof. The line of the shoulder blade and the foot axis should be parallel.

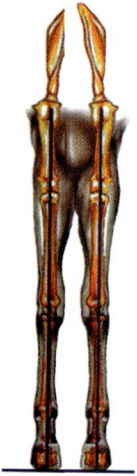 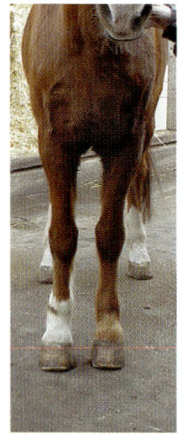 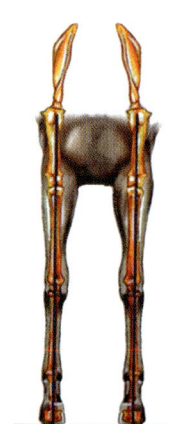 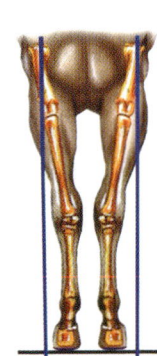 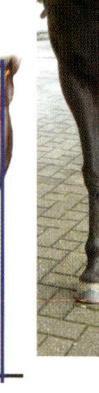

A narrow conformation. In this conformation, the vertical lines run true and parallel, but the limbs are extremely close together. These horses often have a narrow chest.

A wide conformation. In this conformation, the limbs are parallel, but they are too far apart. These horses often have a broad chest; the elbows are often turned somewhat out.

A base-narrow conformation. In this conformation, from the shoulder joint the bones of both limbs slant toward each other within the vertical line (converging). The space between the hooves is small; the foot axis is straight.

Defects of the fore limb, as viewed from the front:
1. **A narrow conformation.** In this conformation, the vertical lines are correct and run parallel to each other, but the limbs are placed too close together. The horse often has a small chest.
2. **A wide conformation.** Here, equally, the limbs are parallel but are too far apart. The horse has a broad chest. Mostly, both elbows are slightly turned out.
3. **A base-narrow conformation.** In this conformation, from the shoulder joint the limbs slant inside the vertical line, toward each other (converging). The space between the hooves is small. The foot axis is straight.
4. **A base-wide conformation.** Here, from the shoulder joint the limbs slant outside the vertical line away from each other (diverging). The distance between the hooves is big, and the foot axis is straight.
5. **Bow-legged conformation.** In this conformation, the imaginary line that goes through the knees is broken to

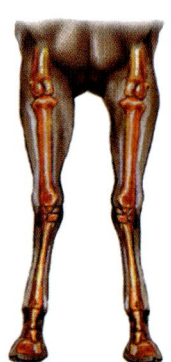 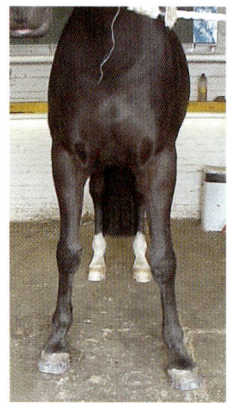 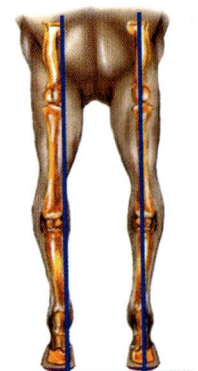 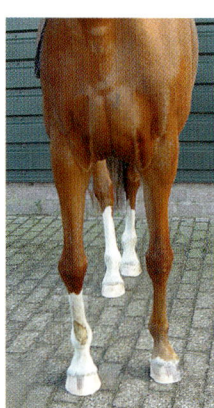

A base-wide conformation. In this conformation, from the shoulder joint the bones of both limbs slant away from each other, outside the vertical line. The distance between the hooves is large; the foot axis is straight.

A bow-legged conformation. The knees are broken outwards and fall outside the vertical line. The distance between the knees is greater than the width of the chest and of the distance between the hooves.

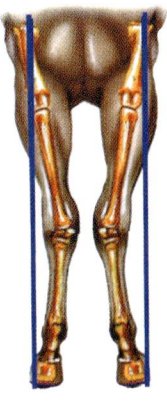
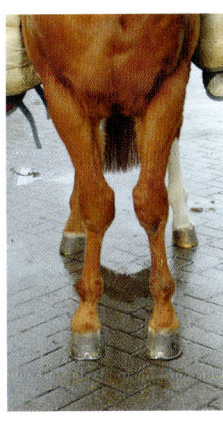

A knock-kneed conformation. The knees are broken inwards and fall within the vertical. Unlike the bow-legged conformation, the distance between the knees is smaller than the width of the chest and of the distance between the hooves.

the outside, where the knees fall outside the vertical line. The distance between the knees is greater than that between the hooves and the chest width. The inside of the knee joint bears the most weight. The inner side of the hoof is longer, as it bears less weight than the outer side; the outer side is shorter, as it bears more weight than the inner side.

6. **Knock-kneed conformation.** Here, the imaginary line that goes through the knees is broken to the inside where the knees fall inside the vertical line. The distance between the knees is smaller than that of the chest width and that between the hooves. Here, the outside of the knee joint bears the most weight. A knock-kneed conformation often causes problems. The inner side of the hoof is lower and steeper because it bears more weight than the outer side. The outer side of the hoof is higher because it bears less weight than the inner side.

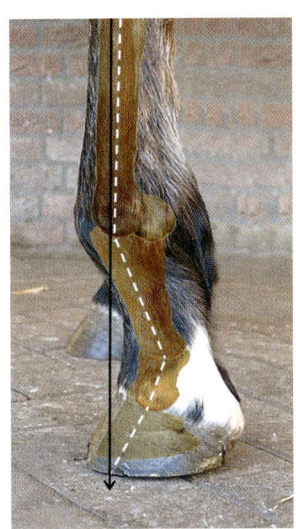
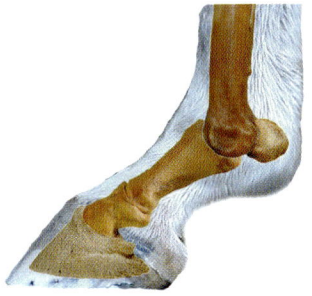
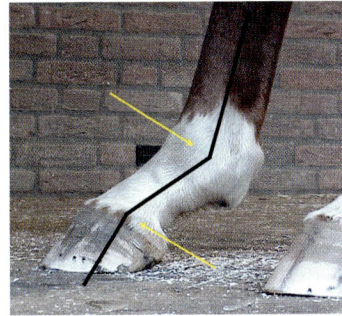

A 'bear paw' conformation. This conformation displays a combination of a foot axis broken forward and a hoof joint with a weak pastern. This conformation should never be rectified.

'Over at the pastern' conformation and way of going. In an upright pastern conformation, when the long pastern and the foot axis are practically an extension of each other, the chance is great that, in movement, the pastern joint will fold forward. This is called 'over at the pastern, way of going'. If the fetlock folds forward when standing still, it is called 'over at the pastern'.

Defects in the fore limb, as seen from the **side**:
1. **'Bear paw' conformation or badly broken-back pastern axis.** This is a combination of a foot axis broken forwards in the hoof joint and a weak pastern. This defect is detrimental for the movement of the horse. The hoof will, however, wear down normally and should thus not be changed.
2. **Over at the pastern: stance and way of going.** When there is an upright pastern conformation, where the long pastern and the foot axis are nearly the extension of each other, there is a big chance that the pastern buckles forward when the horse moves. This is called 'going over at the pastern'. When this happens when the horse is standing still it is then called 'over at the pastern' conformation. In this conformation the foot axis can be broken backwards. This can be a birth defect; the prognosis is not favourable.

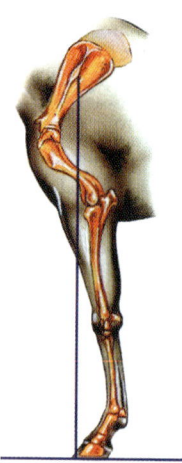 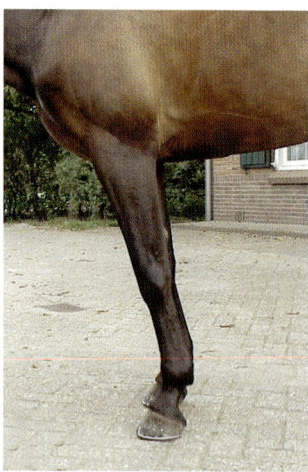 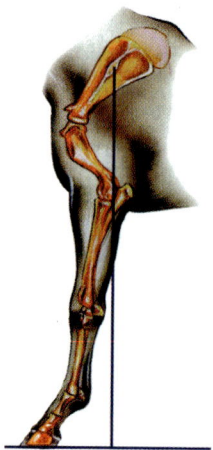 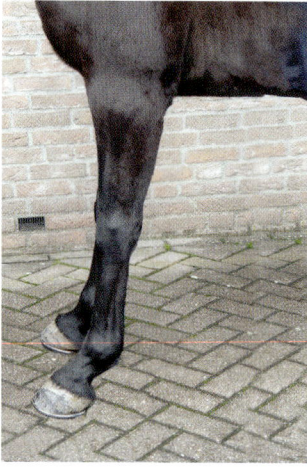

An undershot conformation. The fore limbs stand behind the vertical. The vertical line falls in front of the hoof, which has a short toe and a long heel.

The stretched stance. The fore limbs are in front of the vertical. The vertical line falls behind the hoof, which usually has a long toe and a short heel. This conformation is frequently seen in horses with laminitis.

3. **Undershot stance.** The fore limbs stand behind the vertical, and the vertical line falls in front of the hoof. The fore limbs have to carry a greater weight, for example because of pain in the back part of the hoof. In this conformation, the hoof has a short toe and long heel.
4. **The stretched conformation.** Here the fore limbs are in front of the vertical. The vertical line falls well behind the hoof. This conformation is common in laminitic horses. Generally, the hooves then have long toes with short heels.
5. **Over at the knee.** This is also known as 'knee-sprung' conformation. The knees are bowed forwards. This position can be congenital or be caused, for example, by a horse that had to work too hard when young.
6. **Weak knees.** This is also known as 'calf knees'; in this conformation the knees are bent backwards. This position can be congenital or appear at a later age. The knee joints take extra strain in this conformation. The consequences of weak knees are more serious than the consequences of a knee-sprung conformation.

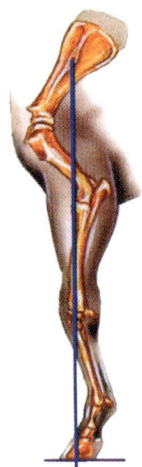 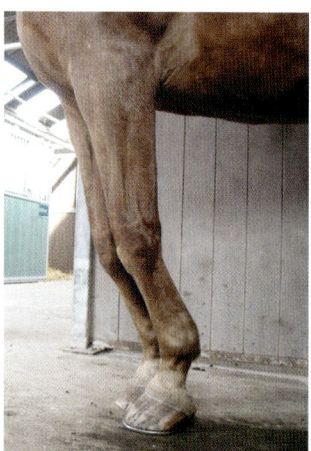 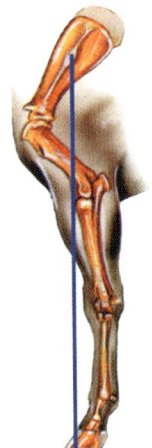 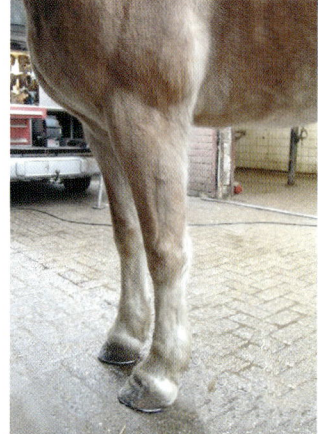

Over at the knee. Here the fore knees are bowed forward. This conformation can be congenital or due to too much hard work at a young age.

Weak knees or calf knees. The fore knee is now bent backwards. This conformation is congenital or appears in old age.

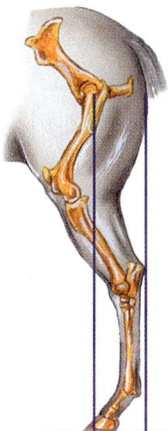 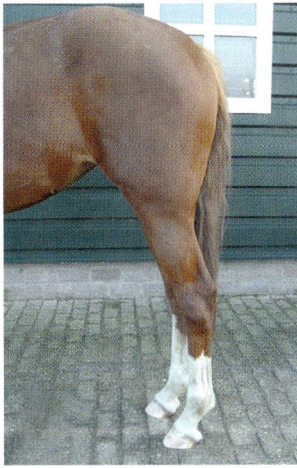 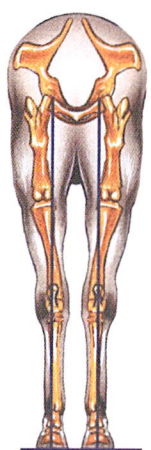 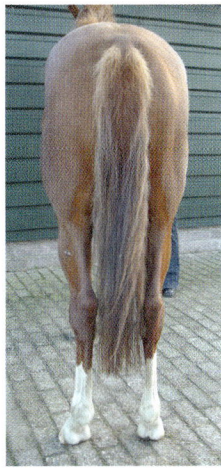

Limb conformation of the hind limb seen from the side. Here the vertical line begins at the ischium and goes straight down just behind the cannon bone and behind the hoof.

Limb conformation of the hind limbs seen from behind. It is clear to see in the illustration how the vertical line begins at the ischium and goes down next to and parallel to the cannon bone.

The hind limbs of a horse can be assessed from two sides:
1. **Viewed from the side.** The vertical line starts at the ischium and runs straight down. The line runs just behind the cannon bone and touches the ground behind the hoof.
2. **Viewed from the back.** The vertical line starts from the ischium and runs straight down. In so doing the line should run close to and parallel with the cannon bone.

Defects of the hind limb as viewed from the **side**:
1. **The upright conformation.** This is also called 'straight in the hock'. Here the angle of the tarsal joint is more than 145 degrees – which can cause hock problems. It is possible that the vertical line falls behind or in front of the hock. The horse has slow movement, as it is unable to bring its hind limbs well forward. Above all, the tarsal joint does not flex enough. The hoof has a short toe and a long heel.
2. **The straight conformation.** In this very unusual conformation the angle at the hock is absent, the vertical line runs directly down from the ischium and the angle at the hock and the heel are also absent.

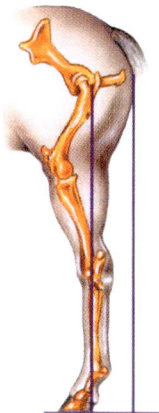 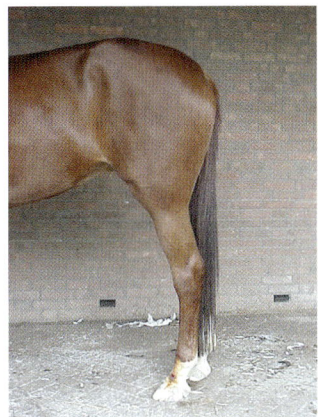 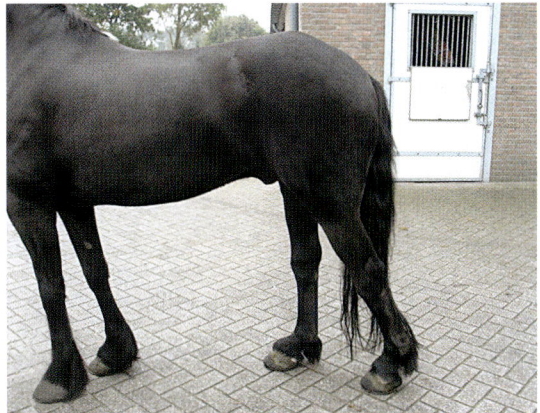

The upright limb conformation or 'straight in the hock'. The angle of the hock joint is greater than 145 degrees. Sometimes the vertical line runs behind or next to the hock. The hoof has a short toe with a long heel.

The straight conformation. The angle at the hock is non-existent – just as are the angles of the hock and the tarsal joint. The vertical line of the hind limb goes straight down from the ischium. This conformation is seldom seen.

The Hoof

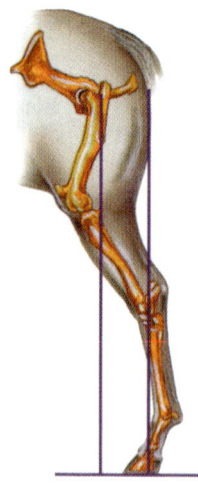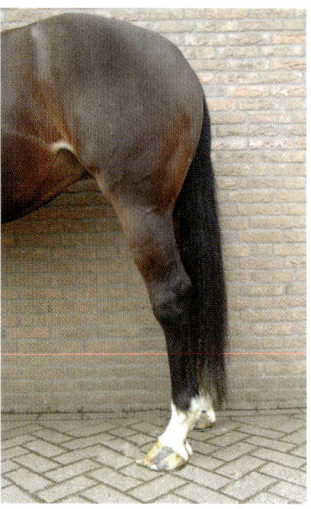 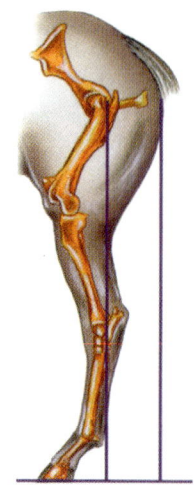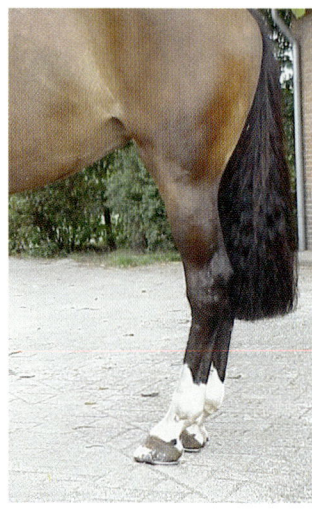

A stretched conformation. The horse places its limbs behind the vertical. The vertical line falls in front of the tarsal joint and the cannon bone, resulting in a bigger angle at the hip joint. The hoof has a short toe and a long heel.

An undershot conformation. Here the horse places the limb too far forward and in front of the vertical line. This conformation is often congenital. The hoof has a long toe and a short heel.

3. **The stretched conformation.** In this conformation the limbs are placed behind the vertical. The vertical line thus falls in front of the hock and the cannon bone, so that the angle of the hip joint is large. The hoof has a short toe and long heels.
4. **The undershot conformation.** In this conformation the limbs are placed in front of the vertical; the whole leg stands too far forward. This conformation is often seen with horses that have pain in the fore limbs, for example horses with laminitis. The undershot conformation is mostly a defect of birth. The movement does not have scope, and forging is often seen. The hoof has a long toe and low heels.
5. **The sickle hock conformation.** Here the angle of the hock is less than 145 degrees. This conformation is also called 'sickle legs'. Problems with the hock can arise due to excessive wear such as a thickening in the middle of the back part of the hock or bone spavin (arthrosis on the inner side of the hock). In a sickle hock conformation the hoof is normal in shape.

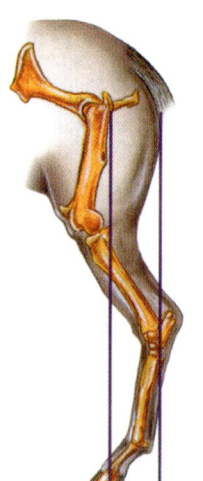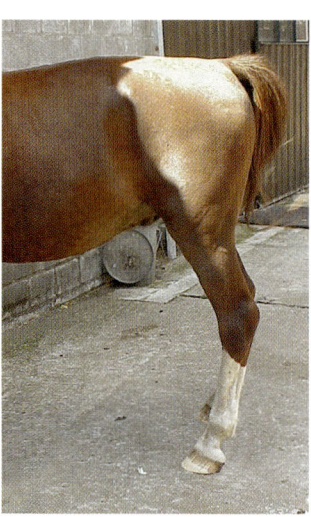

A sickle hocks conformation or curved limb. The angle of the tarsal joint is less than 145 degrees. The hoof is a normal shape.

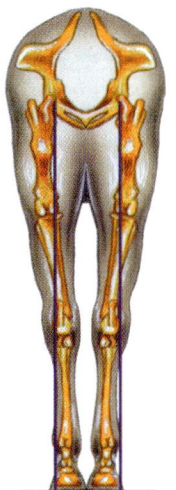 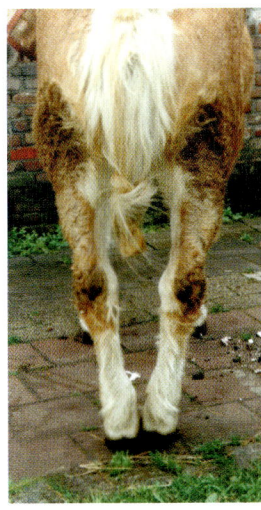 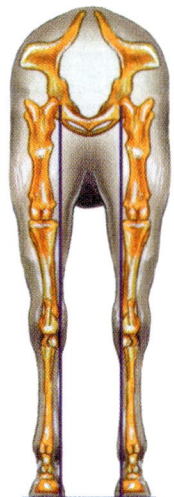 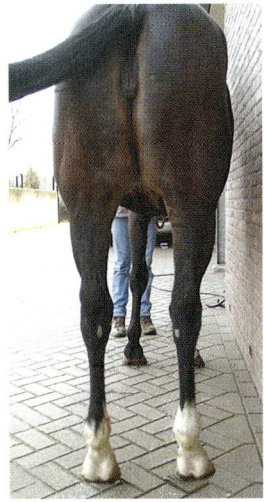

A base-narrow conformation. The limbs stand close together and within the vertical line. In movement, the hooves are placed in front of each other and the limbs strike each other. The hoof is slanted but must not be rectified.

A base-wide conformation. The limbs are far apart and outside the vertical line. The horse waggles when moving. The hoof has a normal shape.

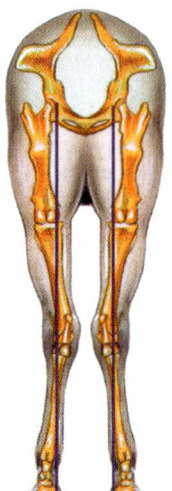 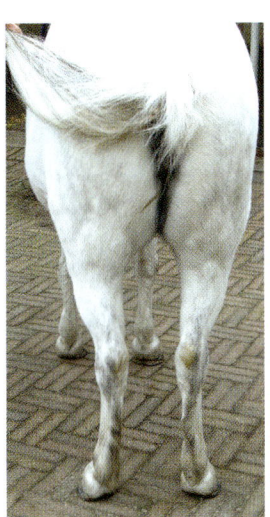

A cow hocks conformation. The hocks are close together and are broken to the inside of the vertical line. The cannon bone slants outwards from the hock joint so that the hooves are turned outwards.

Defects of the hind limb, viewed from the **back**.

1. **Base-narrow conformation.** Here the legs are close together and inside the vertical line. When moving, the horse's back hooves strike each other and the hooves are set down in front of each other. The outer side of the hoof is crooked but may not be changed otherwise the joints will be under strain.
2. **Base-wide conformation.** Here the legs are wide apart and outside the vertical line. The horse has a waddling movement. The hooves have a normal shape.
3. **The cow hocks conformation.** Here the hocks are extremely close together, and they are broken in toward the vertical line. Cow hocks are the cause of great strain on the hock joint. The cannon bone turns out from the hock joint – this is the so-called toe-out conformation. When the leg moves forward, the hoof is placed straight ahead and then the lower leg turns outwards. Cow hocks are rather common. The hoof has a low inner side and a high outer edge. This conformation should not be corrected under any circumstance.

The Hoof

4. **The bow-legged conformation.** This conformation is also sometimes called 'wide in the hocks'. In forward movement, the hocks turn inwards and the hooves are put straight on the ground, then the legs turn inwards once more. The hoof is also turned inwards under weightbearing. It is wrong to try to correct this; a shoe with fixed studs to reduce the twisting is thoroughly advised against. In this conformation a horse can strike its own limbs.

CONSEQUENCES OF LIMB CONFORMATION AND HOOF SHAPES

There is clearly a connection between limb conformation, hoof shape, and the gaits of a horse. A correct limb conformation is twinned to a correct gait and correct hoof shape: thus no problems arise. Deviant limb conformation leads to wrong weightbearing of the hooves, which in turn causes deviant hoof shape that again leads to deviant gaits.

It is impossible to determine whether a deviant hoof shape and/or limb conformation causes lameness. Actually, there are numerous horses with deviations that have never been lame. What can be determined is where the most wear is and where the most strain is. In shoeing, this must be taken into account. Unfortunately, there are many farriers who try to 'correct' a normal shape or conformation – resulting in a lame horse.

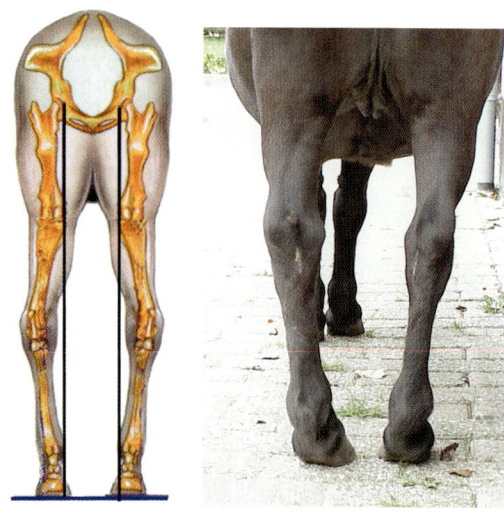

A bow-legged conformation, or wide in the hocks. When moving forward, the horse puts its hooves straight on the ground and turns the hocks in. Then the limbs twist inwards. The horse can sometimes strike its own limbs. When weight is borne, the hooves turn in.

FOOT AXIS AND LENGTH OF STRIDE

The foot axis determines the gait of the horse.
1. The hind limb makes the movement of a flattened arc with a normal foot axis of 45 degrees.
2. When the hoof has a long toe – angle less than 45 degrees – the hoof needs more time to roll over at the toe. This means that the horse must lift its hoof up more; then the hoof is set down on the heel part first. The stride is longer but slower, which limits the movement of the horse.
3. An upright hoof – angle greater than 55 degrees – is quicker because it rolls over faster at the toe and is lifted higher before being set down; thus the stride is shorter and more rapid.

A farrier can change the stride length by shoeing in a specific way. For example, it is possible to prevent forging, where the hind hoof strikes the heels of the fore hoof shoe.

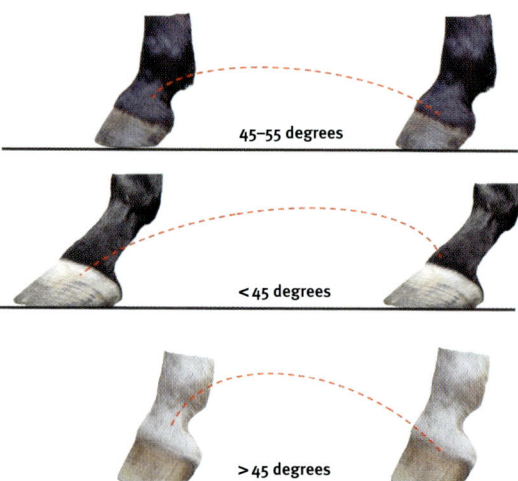

A normal hoof, a hoof with a long toe, and an upright hoof.

3 HOOF CARE AND HORSESHOES

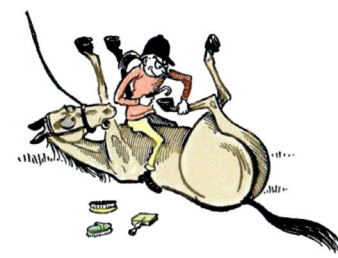

Caring for the hooves.

Hoof care

Care is crucial to achieving and maintaining a strong and well developed hoof capsule.

WATER

In order to keep a horse's hooves elastic and resilient, they must regularly come into contact with water. Water is actually one of the most important elements of a horse's hoof – the horn capsule of the hoof is made up of 40% water. Good elasticity of the horn will prevent it from cracking or from becoming friable.

There are various ways of making the hooves wet:
- Let the horse walk regularly through water, for example by going through puddles in the woods or in the outdoor school
- Make the straw in the stable a little damp
- After a ride, clean the horse's hooves with water and a soft brush
- If the horse is in a field, keep the area around the drinking trough wet so that the horse will get its hooves wet several times a day while drinking

EXERCISE

Many hoof capsule disorders result from inadequate and incompetent care. Many sport horses have hooves that grow insufficiently due to being kept wrongly. This problem is mainly the result of too little movement: the hoof mechanism can only function if the horse exercises – that is to say, moves – and not if it stands still.

The hoof mechanism works like a valve for the supply of nutrients and the removal of waste products. When the hoof mechanism is working well, the hoof receives plenty of nutrients, whereby the horn – and thus the hoof – can grow well.

Horses that live in the open air have fewer hoof problems than horses that are stabled and rarely go outside. It is for this reason that, when it comes to hoof care, stabled horses deserve more attention.

BEDDING

It is important that stabled horses are mucked out regularly, and that an adequate top layer of clean straw is added, so that hooves stay clean and dry. Straw is the best stable bedding. Straw is coarse, does not cling to hooves, and has a capillary action whereby urine is absorbed and the straw stays dry.

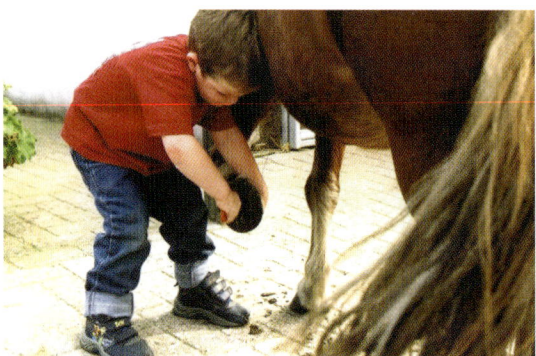

Starting them young!

Beddings such as sawdust, wood shavings and shredded paper draw moisture from the hooves. Sawdust clings to hooves because it has a solid structure; urine is not absorbed but remains on top – thus the horse is constantly standing in its own urine and, because it contains ammonia, this affects the hooves.

One can test the effects of various bedding very simply. Make the hands wet; then in one hand make a ball of straw and in the other a ball of sawdust. One quickly notices that the hand with sawdust feels warmer and dryer than that with the straw. This is because sawdust draws moisture out of the hand – which is not good for the hooves.

OILING

Many people regularly apply oil to their horse's hooves. The intention is well meant and it looks smart, but actually oil is not good for hooves. The oil cannot penetrate the hoof because of the varnish-like layer on the horny wall. Many people still think that the hoof should first be wetted before a layer of oil is put on, assuming that a layer of water would remain under the oil and would supply the hoof with moisture.

Alas, this is not true. Oil cannot be spread on water, as both elements repel each other. If a wet hoof is oiled, the water is wiped away and the oil stays on the hoof. An oiled hoof cannot absorb water, as the oil closes the hoof surface and it takes a few days before the oil disappears. In other words, oiling hooves is pointless. It is useful, however, to apply oil every now and then to the coronary band to keep it supple.

These days, there are countless remedies available for the prevention or curing of hoof splits, hoof cracks or poor quality of horn; remedies that promise to improve quality; that will harden or soften; remedies with laurel oil, mane oil, lanolin, biotin and all sorts. However, of all the hoof care remedies that claim to stimulate growth, cure poor quality of hoof or strengthen the horny wall, not one has yet been proven to work.

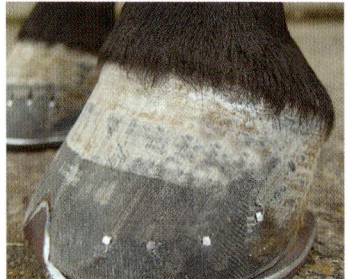

Horn tissue is produced by the perioplic ring. The varnish-like layer ensures the protection of the horny wall – also from oil!

TARRING

There are also varying opinions on the tarring of hooves. The hoof's frog must not be too hard, as it is part of the movement of the under foot – the hoof mechanism – that needs to be soft and elastic. If too much tarring takes place, the horn and the frog dry out, and the horn becomes too hard. This encourages thrush. When there is thrush, the farrier must cut away the frog until all affected parts have been removed. The hoof is subsequently treated with iodine.

If a hoof with thrush has tar applied, there is a chance that the problem may be made worse. By tarring, the inflammation caused by the thrush gets closed in. As the bacteria need no oxygen they can continue to develop. Where a horse has been treated for thrush, after riding the frog should be cleaned with water and occasionally treated with iodine or hydrogen peroxide. Lastly, a layer of antiseptic ointment can be thinly applied.

CONCLUSION

Good care, lots of movement and good shoeing will result in healthy hooves for all horses.

Horseshoes

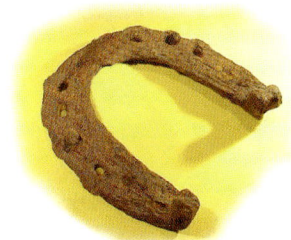

Horseshoes were already being used by the Celts. It is remarkable that about 2000 years ago, and maybe even earlier, they came upon the idea of putting iron shoes on their horses – especially when you know that our horseshoes are more or less the same.

The use of horseshoes goes back a very long way. The Celts were expert workers of iron and were the first to discover that it was possible to apply horseshoes by fixing the shoes with nails into the insensitive part of the hoof. Horseshoes have changed little over time. There have been attempts at improving the horseshoe by changing the thickness and width and by using other materials such as synthetics. Hoof shoes have also been developed.

Although horseshoes have remained fairly unchanged, the working methods of farriers have changed dramatically. In former times, the client had to bring the horse to the farrier; today the farrier comes to the horse. Many farriers work in cooperation with a horse clinic where they regularly treat horses with hoof problems.

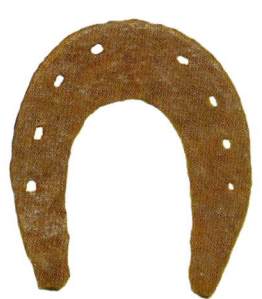

The Romans developed and changed horseshoes further. This is a broad shoe, especially at the front. After hundreds of years, this model is still being used, although in a somewhat more modern version.

Horseshoes have several purposes:
1. They protect the hoof from too much wear.
2. They protect the condition of the hoof, or prevent deterioration of the condition.
3. They can be used for correcting the limb conformation of young horses.
4. They can improve the horse's gait.
5. They can solve lameness or associated problems.
6. In equestrian sports such as jumping and eventing they provide the horse with more of a grip by use of studs.
7. They help support the horse in its work in the various disciplines.

MATERIALS AND TOOLS

The farrier's van is fitted out with an anvil, an oven, tools and materials. When doing his work the farrier uses various special tools:

1. **Turning hammer.** With this a horseshoe can be forged. Different hammers have different weights.
2. **Hoof knife, hoof hammer and drawing knives.** These are used for the paring and trimming of the weightbearing edge, the sole and the frog. The knives are used for cutting away the frog and for checking the hoof.
3. **Farrier's pincers.** There are four kinds of pincers:
   - Nippers. When a horse has extremely long walls it is inconvenient to trim them with a knife thus the farrier uses nippers to cut back the walls.
   - Pull-offs. With these, the farrier removes the horseshoe from the hoof without damaging the hoof.
   - Clench pull-offs. When a nail is deeply embedded or stuck in the fullering of the horseshoe, the farrier uses this to grip and remove the nail. They are used when nailing the horseshoe, to support the nail head when clenching up (bending the protruding point of the horseshoe nail in the horny wall).
4. **Nailing hammer, clenching tongs and clench groover.** The farrier uses a special nailing hammer for driving the nails into the hoof wall. The long head of the hammer is balanced in a way that concentrates the force centrally on the nail – thus the farrier need not hit hard upon the hoof. With the clench groover he removes a tiny bit of horn where the nail protrudes. The nail protruding from the wall is then cut off short and is pulled down into this little hollow with the clenching tongs so that the extremity – the 'clench' – is embedded in the horny wall.

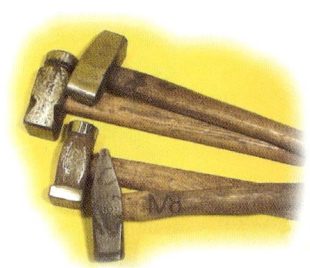

Nailing hammers of various weights and types.

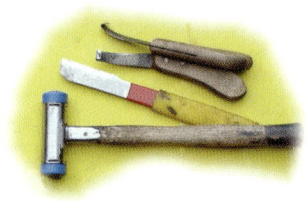

Tools for trimming hooves. From below: hoof hammer, hoof knife and drawing knives.

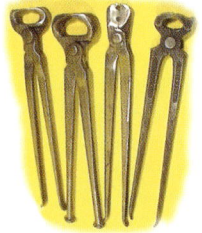

Various hoof pincers. From left to right: hoof nippers for clipping horn; pull-off pincers for removing shoes; clench pull-offs for pulling nails out by the head; clenching tongs for completing the nailing of the shoes.

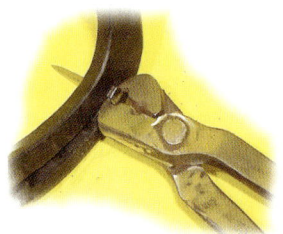

With the clench pull-offs the nails are pulled by the head from the horseshoe.

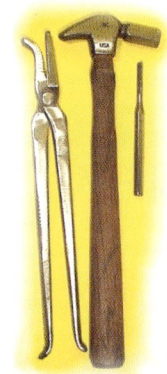

From left to right: clenching tongs to pull the 'clench' (the clipped-off nail protruding from the wall) from the horny wall; a nailing hammer; a clench groover to make the indentation under the clench.

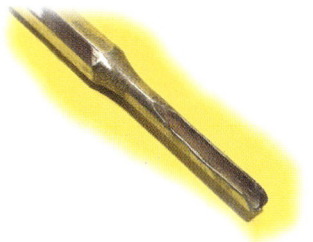

With a clench groover the farrier removes a tiny bit of horn from under the nail protruding from the wall. The 'clench' can then be set in the hoof wall.

5. **Hoof rasp.** A horse's hooves are filed down with special hoof rasps that are extremely sharp. Farriers usually use two files: one is for the hoof and the other for the finishing of the shod hoof.
6. **Fuller and stamp.** The fuller makes the groove in the horseshoe. The stamp makes a square hole in the groove, in the correct place, for the nail head to fit. To shoe a horse's hoof well, every farrier should have had lessons in forging skills.

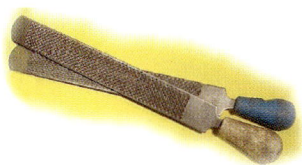

The horse's hooves are filed down with a special hoof rasp.

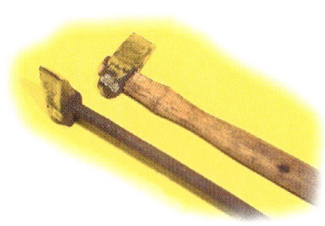

With a fuller, a crease can be made into the horseshoe so that the driven-in nails can easily be removed with clench pull-offs.

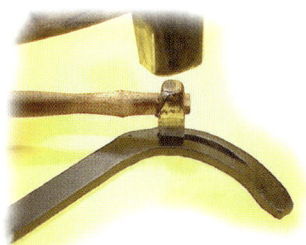

The fuller is hammered into the hot shoe with a special chisel.

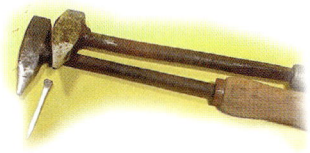

Square holes are made in the correct places in the fuller with a punch, where the nail heads will fit. Each size of nail requires a different punch.

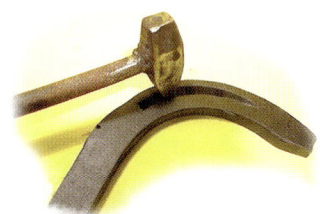

The punch is hammered almost right through the horseshoe, in the crease; the nail heads will then fit exactly.

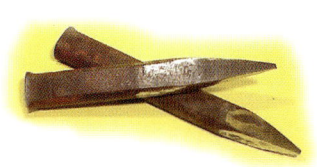

The nail holes in the horseshoe are opened up with a pritchel.

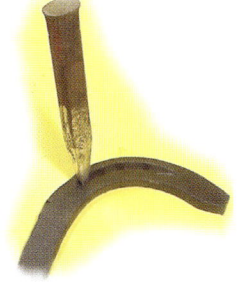

When punching the nail hole, a square hole is made in the foot surface of the horseshoe.

Hoof Care and Horseshoes

THE HORSESHOE

The horseshoe consists of a toe part and two branches, which consist of an inner branch and an outer branch. The horseshoe must be forged into the shape of the hoof capsule. The outer branch is always a bit wider than the inner branch.

Characteristics of a horseshoe are:
1. Each horseshoe has an upper side (foot surface) and an under side (ground surface).
2. A horseshoe has an outer side and an inner side.
3. The horseshoe must be completely flat.
4. The foot surface must be broad enough to support the horny wall of the hoof, the white line and a small part of the sole.
5. In the ground surface there is a crease, the so-called fuller. The nail holes are situated here. In factory-made horseshoes this crease is often pre-fabricated. The inner side of the fuller should be extremely steep or upright and the outer side sloped. The fuller is absent at the toe part to give more strength to the toe part of the horseshoe. Moreover, it is not necessary to have a continuous fuller as there are no nail holes in the toe part. The depth of the fuller should be about two-thirds the thickness of the horseshoe.
6. The two front nail holes – the toe nail holes – are situated either side of the toe and are about one and a half to two times the width of the horseshoe apart from each other. Behind these, on both sides, are two or three nail holes. In the fore shoe, the last nail hole is situated no further than halfway along the branch, so that the hoof mechanism is hindered as little as possible. In the hind shoe, the last nail hole is situated further back.
7. In the heel parts, the shoe is generously fitted, so that the weightbearing edge of the hoof capsule can be completely supported when it spreads under the pressure of the hoof mechanism. The horseshoe branches are fitted wider and longer than the hoof,

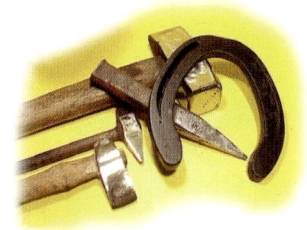

Tools to make the shoe.

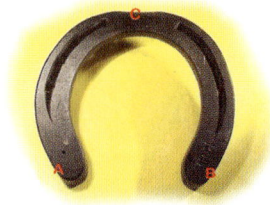

The shoe consist of a toe part (C) and two branches made up of an outer branch (A) and an inner branch (B). The shoe should be forged to the shape of the hoof. The outer branch (A) is always a bit wider than the inner branch (B).

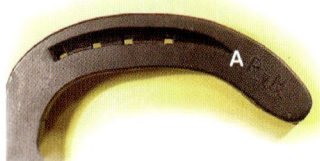

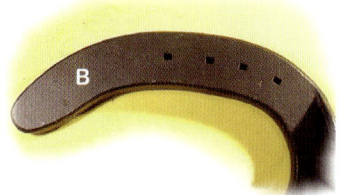

The under surface (A), the surface that touches the ground (also called the ground surface) has the fullering which holds the nail heads.

The upper surface (B), the surface that the hoof stands on (also called the foot surface) is completely flat. The square holes where the nails emerge can be clearly seen.

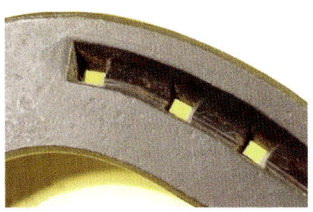

The fullering and the nail holes must be positioned so that they come exactly against the white line.

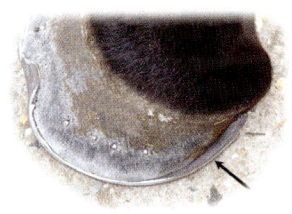

In the heel area, the shoe extends wide of the hoof so that the horny wall, when expanding with the hoof mechanism, is still carried by the shoe.

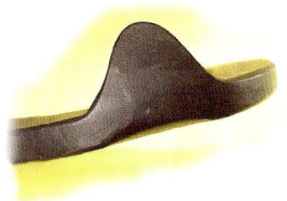

A shoe with a clip.

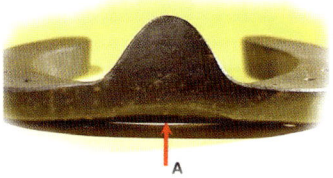

In order that the hoof can easily move forward, a rocker toe is forged into the toe of the shoe. A rocker toe is an upward curve in the toe section (red arrow, A).

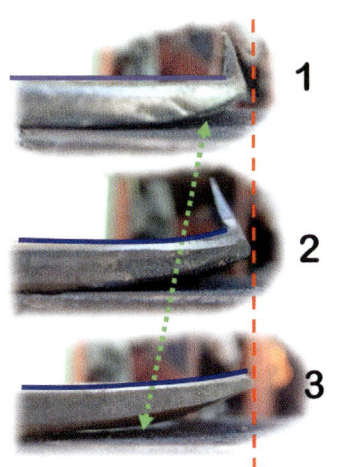

The aim of the rocker toe is to allow the hoof to move forward more easily. The green line shows the point where the hoof rolls forward.
1. *No rocker toe. The horse has worn down the toe area.*
2. *A normal rocker toe.*
3. *A Hoofcare® Breakover shoe, where the roll over point comes further back underneath the hoof.*

because the weightbearing edge of the hoof, under pressure, is spread backwards and sideways by the hoof mechanism; fitting of a shoe longer and wider is called extension.

8. A shoe can have one or more clips. These are sometimes already present in pre-fabricated shoes.
9. The farrier usually makes a clip on the horseshoe himself, which is called 'drawing a clip'. The toe clip is one and a half to two times the thickness of the shoe in its height and is designed to prevent the shoe from shifting.
10. On the hind shoes, two side clips are often drawn, either side of the toe. These are also known as 'brushing shoes'. It is much better however that only one toe clip is drawn on normal hind shoes.
11. Fore shoes are often given a rocker toe. This is an upwards sloping of the shoe in the toe part, in both the ground surface and the foot surface. This curve allows the hoof to breakover more easily at the toe; thus it is often applied to fore shoes. A rocker toe is not often applied to hind shoes. The function of the rocker – to allow easier 'breakover at the toe' – is, due to the way a horse moves, mainly necessary in the fore hoofs.

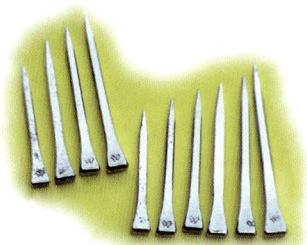

Nails come in various sizes and in various thicknesses and lengths.

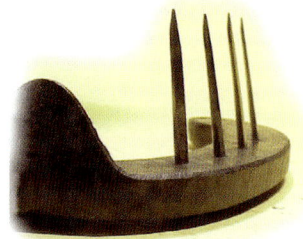

The nails must be placed in exactly the right position, and slightly at an inward angle.

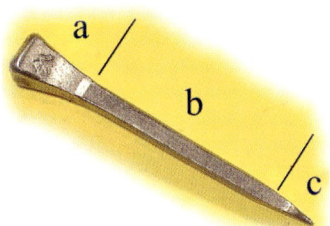

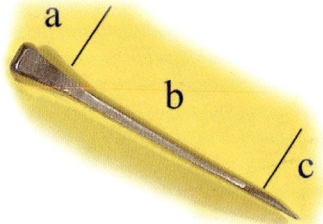

Two nails:
a. The head (a). A plug-shaped part that is wedged into the fuller.
b. The shank. The long part of the nail is thinner than the head and goes straight down to the point.
c. The bevel of point. The bevel of point of the nail is flattened on one side, so that it turns towards the outside as it is driven into the horny wall. The end tip of the nail is called the point.

THE NAIL

The horseshoe nail ensures that the shoe stays attached to the hoof capsule. It must fit exactly into the horseshoe.

A horseshoe nail consists of several parts:
1. **The head.** The head fits exactly into the fuller. In new shoes, the nail head stands slightly proud of the ground surface of the shoe, and the nail is driven firmly into the fuller.
2. **The shank.** The shank is the long part of the nail. This part is slightly thinner than the head of the nail in order that the wall of the hoof is damaged as little as possible during shoeing. The shank must fit precisely into the square hole in the foot surface of the shoe; there must be no play.
3. **The bevel of point.** The end tenth or so of the nail, known as the bevel of point, is bevelled on one side so that it turns outwards when the nail is driven into the tough horny wall. The end tip of the nail is called the point.

The horseshoe nail is driven into the white line of the hoof and comes out via the horny wall. Then the nail is 'clenched up': the part that protrudes from the wall is bent over so that it fits into the little indentation that the farrier has created with a clench groover.

The nail shank lies extremely close to the hoof corium. This increases the possibility of nail binding if the horseshoe does not fit well. One talks of nail binding if the nail is driven against or in the hoof corium.

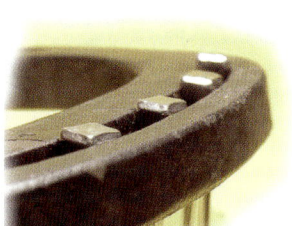

The top of the nail stands a fraction proud of the ground surface. When a horse puts weight on its hooves, it thoroughly fixes the nail in the horseshoe so that the nail does not move.

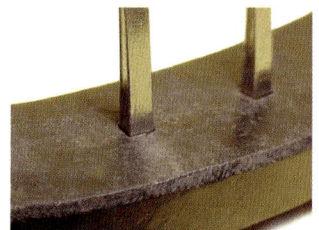

The upper side of the shank must fit exactly into the square holes in the foot surface of the horseshoe so that there is no play. This prevents tearing of the horny wall.

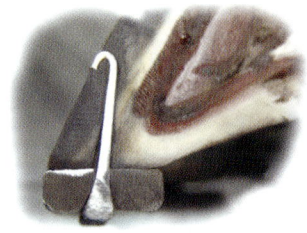

The nail shank is placed extremely close to the hoof corium. If the nail is driven in incorrectly, the chance of nail binding (driving a nail into the hoof corium) is great — with all the consequences of that.

ADVANTAGES OF SHOEING
1. The protection of the weightbearing edge from too much wear.
2. Careful shoeing can enhance the conformation and the gaits of a horse. The horseshoe contributes to the maintenance and furtherance of this correct conformation and good movement.
3. Fixing studs into the shoes helps against losing footing on slippery going such as on wet ground in outdoor competitions or slipperiness due to ice or snow.
4. By fitting special shoes, hoof problems can be ameliorated or even cured so that a horse can continue to be ridden.

HORSESHOES ALSO HAVE SOME DISADVANTAGES
1. It is unnatural: a strange object is nailed to the hoof.
2. It will always somewhat limit the normal movement of the hoof capsule.
3. The nails damage the horny wall.
4. The hoof dries out more quickly.
5. The horseshoe reduces natural shock absorption.
7. Horses with shoes are more likely to slip than those without.
8. Due to the fact that the front half of the hoof is nailed, and the heel part is not and flexes on the shoe, the weightbearing edge in the toe part hardly wears out but in the heel part it does. After several weeks, this causes changes in the hoof shape and thus the foot axis.

The disadvantages of horseshoes are greatly reduced by forging shoes of good quality, by avoiding the unnecessary use of nails, and by not nailing too far back. In general horseshoes are, for many horses under many conditions, the correct solution as long as they are properly put on, properly looked after and repositioned or renewed in good time.

Briefly, good farriery is a blessing and an indispensable part of the correct care of a horse in general and of the hoof in particular.

Trimming and Shoeing

The basis of good shoeing is the same for nearly all horses and the following information applies to all kinds of shoes.

TRIMMING
Correct shoeing begins with the correct trimming of the hoof. The limb conformation and the foot axis of the horse should be studied carefully first. The hooves are trimmed depending on the way the animal stands and moves.

The trimming or paring of the hoof has a particular sequence:
1. First, the frog is trimmed and cleaned. As little as possible of the frog is removed as it has an extremely important function as a shock absorber and thus should remain as complete as possible.
2. Next, the sole is trimmed and checked for stones or irregularities.

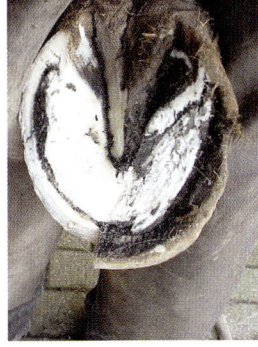

The frog is pared and cleaned. As little as possible of the frog is removed as it has an extremely important function and must remain as large as possible. The sole is trimmed and checked for stones and irregularities.

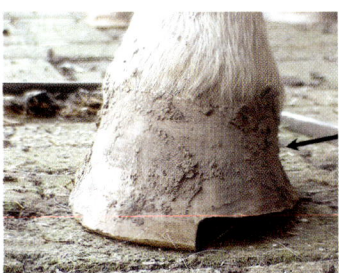

The weightbearing edge is trimmed last because it is only then that the farrier knows by how much the wall must be trimmed. The wall is filed neatly.

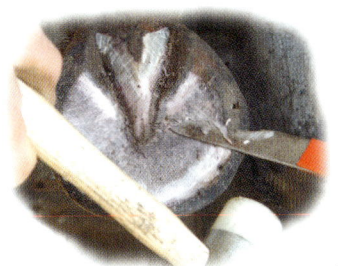

The weightbearing edge, the sole and the frog are pared with a knife, taking the limb conformation into account.

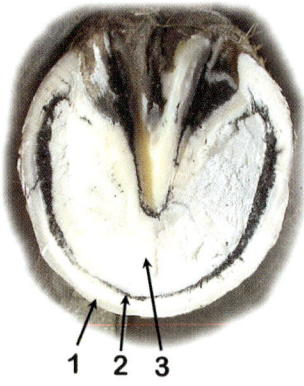

In most hooves, the weightbearing edge, the white line and a small part of the sole may stand on the horseshoe.
1. Horny wall. 2. White line. 3. Sole.

3. The weightbearing edge is trimmed last, as the farrier can now see by how much the wall must be cut back.
4. Finally, the horny wall is firmly filed straight so that the weightbearing edge is of equal thickness in all parts. The farrier should take care not to trim too much away. A too-short hoof is deleterious for the movement because the horse then treads sensitively. A good farrier removes only that which should be removed.

MEASURING

All hooves have the shape that matches the rounding of the underside of the pedal bone. The horn grows down from the coronary band next to the pedal bone, towards the ground. The hoof capsule takes the shape of the pedal bone and is beautifully rounded, thus the horseshoe will also follow this shape. In other words, the shape of the coronary band determines the shape of the horseshoe.

After trimming, the farrier decides the size of the horseshoe. The horseshoe must conform to certain requirements. The shoe must be sufficiently roomy and long so that the horse has maximum support and even after eight weeks will still be standing properly on its shoes. Usually, the farrier assumes that a horseshoe should be long enough to ensure that the branches extend to a point as far out as a vertical line dropped from the bulbs of the heel to the ground. This varies with different hoof positions; upright hooves take much shorter branches than hooves that are low or stand flat on the heels.

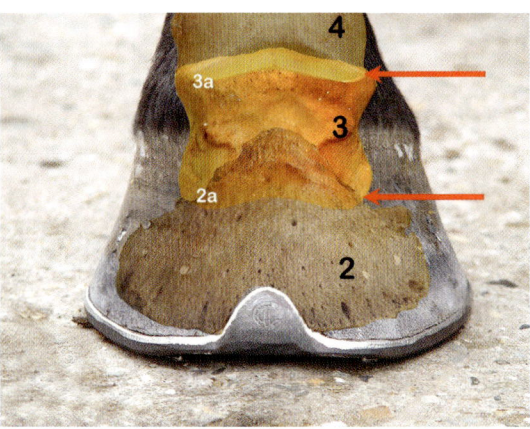

Seen from the front, the farrier must trim so that the joints stand straight on top of each other.
2. Pedal bone
2 a. Hoof joint
3. Short pastern bone
3 a. Coronary joint
4. Long pastern bone

After trimming the hoof, the size of the horseshoe is decided. The horseshoe should be roomy enough and long enough for the hoof to have maximum support. Usually the farrier proceeds from the view that a horseshoe must be as long as is needed for the ends of the branches to extend as far as a line dropped vertically from the bulbs of the heel down to the ground.

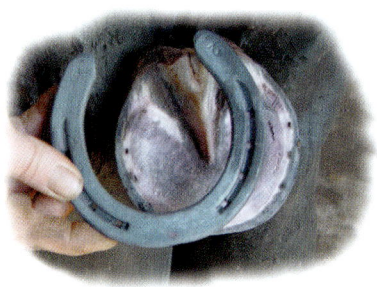

FORGING

When the farrier has decided on the exact size required, the horseshoe is heated. When the shoe is hot enough, a clip is drawn in the middle at the toe, which will ensure that the shoe does not shift in wear. The clip is drawn to fit the trimmed hoof. In a fore shoe, a rocker toe – a rounding up of the toe of the horseshoe – is forged in the front part; it is by this that the horse can easily breakover at the toe. After forging the hot horseshoe, the farrier checks the hot shoe against the hoof to see if it fits. The horseshoe should not be held so long against the hoof that the hoof surface catches fire, which causes immense clouds of smoke. A skilled farrier has already trimmed the hoof flat before fitting the shoe, so prolonged burning is not necessary.

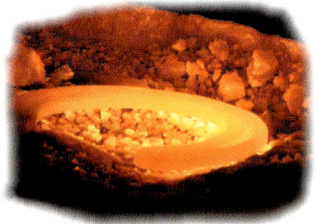

When the size has been determined, the horseshoe is heated . There has always been controversy about which is better; hot setting or cold setting. If one wants a good fit then it is necessary to remodel the shoe , and this cannot be achieved with cold setting.

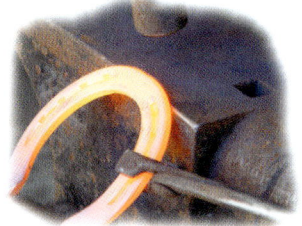

When the shoe is hot enough, a clip is drawn in the middle of the horseshoe at the toe. This will prevent the horseshoe from slipping.

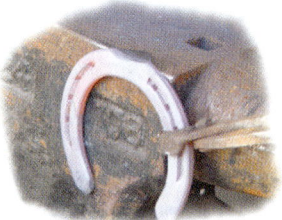

A clip is drawn in the fore shoe; extra clips would hinder the hoof mechanism, which would lead to problems.

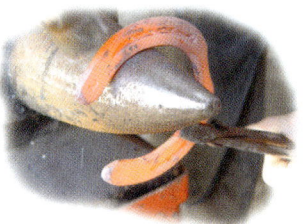

The shoe should be forged exactly to the shape of the hoof.

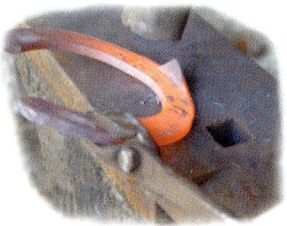

A so-called rocker toe – a rounding up of the toe of the horseshoe – is forged into the fore shoe at the toe part; thus the horse 'rolls' easily over the toe.

Hoof Care and Horseshoes

FITTING

When fitting the shoe, the farrier should take the white line into account as this is where the nails that fix the shoe in place are driven. It is important that the horseshoe fits well, otherwise the nails are not driven into the white line but outside it.

If a farrier fits the shoe too narrowly, the nails will be driven too close to the inside of the hoof and the nails will pass too close to the wall corium – the sensitive part of the hoof. This is called driving the nails 'too coarsely': nail binding or pricking can be caused by this. If this happens, the horse may tread in a sensitive way or even become seriously lame.

If the shoe is fitted too broadly, the nail will be driven not into the white line but outside and thus into the horny wall. When the nailing is outside the white line, the nail tears out more easily from the hoof; in this way the horseshoe is less secure and the horny wall will split at the nails. As the horny wall consists of horny tubules, these are easily split – thus causing horny wall cracks. This is also called nailing 'too finely'. If nails are consistently driven too finely then the horny wall will break and there will be little strong horny wall left. A good farrier can quickly improve this, but prevention is always better than cure.

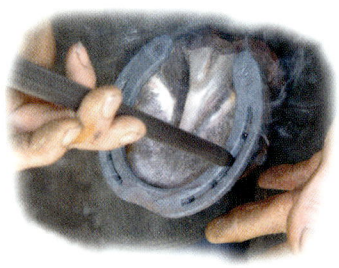

After forging the horseshoe, the hot shoe is pressed against the hoof to see if it fits. The shoe should not be held so long against the hoof that it burns or that immense clouds of smoke ensue.

NAILING ON

After the shoe has been made to fit well, it must be finished by removing the sharp edges – the burr – of the shoe. After this, the shoe is ready to be applied. This is called 'nailing on' and is achieved with as few nails as possible, as each nail slightly damages the wall. As a rule, six nails are enough, although this depends on individual cases. When seven nails are used, it is usual that there are four on the outer side of the hoof and three on the inner side. The nails should be driven into the wall in such away that, as far as is possible, they protrude from the hoof in one line about one-third up from the weightbearing edge. As well as giving a neater look, it also has the advantage that the nails can be driven in more easily in the future.

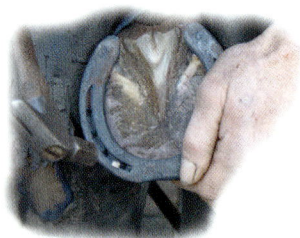

The horseshoe is ready to be nailed to the hoof. This is called 'nailing on' and is done with as few nails as possible because each nail slightly damages the wall. Usually six nails are enough but each situation is different.

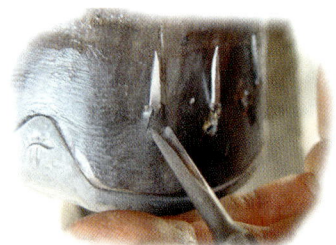

A little indentation is made with a clench groover under the nails where they protrude from the wall.

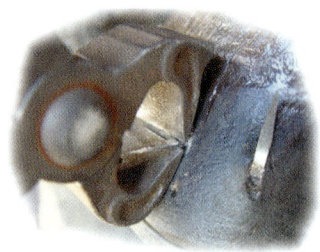

The nail that protrudes from the horny wall is clenched up and clipped off with tongs – so that only the 'clench' remains.

FINISHING

With the clench groover a small indentation is made below the protruding nail. The nail end is then clipped off, leaving a tiny piece protruding. This tiny end – the 'clench' – is 'clenched up' into the small indentation with a special hammer. After this, the farrier completes the finishing so that the whole wall is smooth and the horse cannot injure itself.

THE LENGTH OF THE BRANCHES

A well-fitting horseshoe has branches that are wide enough and have enough extension. That is to say that the shoe protrudes back from the heels and its width is generous enough on both sides so that, as time goes by, the shoe remains under the heels. The outer branch is wider than the inner branch, as a normal hoof is wider on the outer wall.

From the broadest part of the hoof, the shoe continues to widen out as it goes toward the back, so that the heels stand roughly in the middle of the branches. In this way the hoof mechanism can do its work. If the

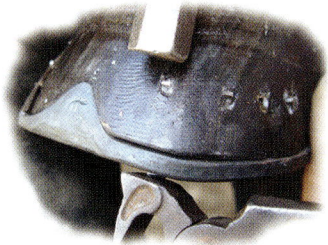

Supported by the tongs that are placed against the nail head, the farrier hammers the clench into the tiny indentation. Thus the nail is kept firmly in the horny wall.

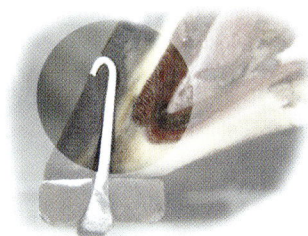

This cross-section shows how the nail is positioned in the horny wall.

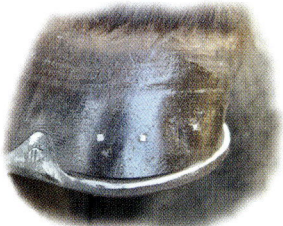

The hoof is finished neatly.

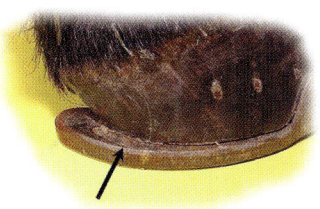

A clear example of a wide branch. The heels are well supported and the hoof mechanism can function fully without the hoof extending over the edge the horseshoe.

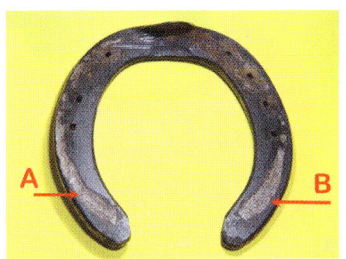

Both these branches, inner (A) and outer (B), show where they have been worn by the hoof mechanism.

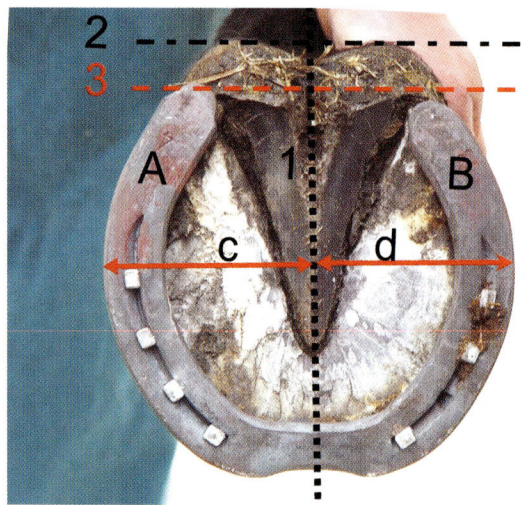

For convenience, the hoof is divided into a horizontal (2) and a vertical (1) line. The vertical line (1) divides the hoof exactly in two, from the central groove of the frog to the point of the frog. The horizontal line (2), parallel to the bulbs of the heel, crosses the vertical line (1) at right angles.

1. *The outside half of the hoof (c) is bigger than the inside half (d). This is completely normal.*
2. *There is a clear difference in length between the horseshoe branches (A and B): the outer branch (A) is always a little longer than the inner branch (B) because the outside half of the hoof is bigger (3).*

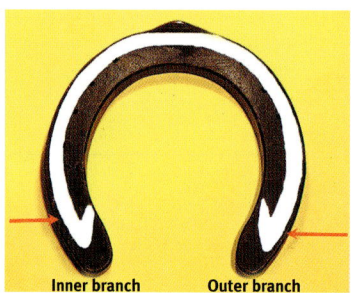

The picture shows how (viewed as from above) the hoof capsule is placed on the horseshoe. A well-fitting horseshoe has outer and inner branches that are long enough with enough extension and width. The branches extend beyond the heels, and on both sides have sufficient extra width so that the horseshoe, as time goes by, does not come to be under the heels. The outer branch is larger than the inner branch because a normal hoof has an outside wall that is a little wider than the inside wall.

branches are too short, then the heels will very soon extend beyond the branches. This would cause the foot axis to collapse, which would put extra weight on the flexor tendons, which can result in serious damage to the horny wall. Sometimes a horse has not much heel, so that even with a well-fitting shoe its foot axis collapses. This can be helped by broadened branches and extended branches.

Sometimes the branches of the fore shoes are made too short because people believe that they will be too easily trodden off. This fear is unfounded. Even when the branches are left long, they are still protected by the heel bulbs. Only when the horse seriously over-reaches and strikes the heel bulbs does even a correctly fitted shoe come into the danger zone. This problem is mostly the result of the way a horse is ridden – for example, by being ridden too roughly or with a martingale – but can also arise by shoes coming loose in deep ground.

To keep the consequences of over-reaching to a minimum, the farrier may shoe the hind hooves with so-called 'brushing' shoes. A fore shoe has one clip in the middle front of the toe part. The toe part of a 'brushing' hind shoe lies slightly underneath and the two clips are at the sides instead of the front. Furthermore, a hind shoe differs from a fore shoe in that it has no rocker toe and the toe section of the hoof capsule stands a little forward over the horseshoe. In this way the horse has a firm grip on the ground.

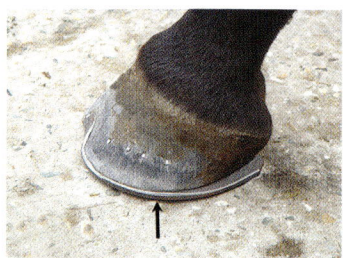

From the broadest part of the hoof, the horseshoe gets wider the further back it reaches, so that the heels have plenty of space to stand on the shoe branch. In this way, the hoof mechanism can do its work.

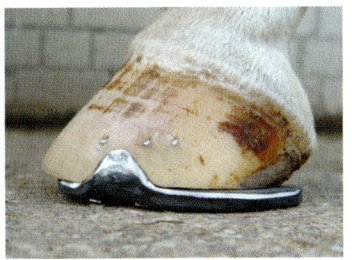

In order to prevent over-reaching, the hind hoof is given a 'brushing' shoe. The shoe, with two side clips, is fitted slightly back. Thus the horse cannot so readily strike the fore shoes (over-reach) and damage itself.

DUMPING

The farrier should not fit the hoof to the shoe in a way that places the horseshoe under the foot. The horseshoe should be adjusted to the hoof, not the other way round. It is therefore important that the farrier forges the horseshoe to the shape of the hoof, and this can only happen if the horseshoe is made to measure – if it is hot set.

The manner of trimming has a direct influence on the foot axis. The foot axis can be changed by paring more or paring less of the toe or the heel; what is more, the sideways balance can also be influenced. When this happens, the hoof and the joints of the whole limb are forced into an unnatural conformation. It is therefore of the greatest importance that the farrier can correctly judge the way of going and the way the hoof is placed on the ground.

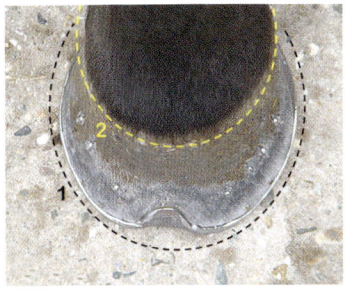

All hooves have a shape that mirrors the curve of the underside of the pedal bone. The horn grows down from the coronary band (2). The hoof capsule has assumed the shape of the pedal bone, thus is beautifully rounded (1). The horseshoe must reflect this shape. In other words, the coronet indicates the shape of the horseshoe.

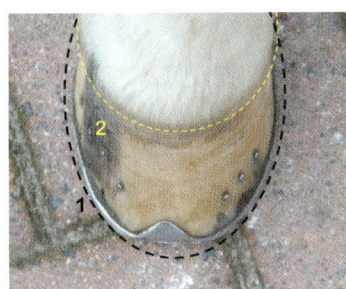

A clear example of how it should not be. The coronet (2) is round, but the underside (1) of the hoof and the horseshoe shape are a narrow oval. The farrier has not trimmed the hoof well.

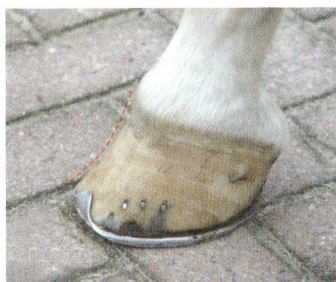

The same hoof, seen from the side. The wall surface (red dotted line) is concave but should, according to the growth of the horny tubules, be straight down. Here, the farrier has not taken note of the thickness of the wall and has left the toe too long. This will hinder the horse's going.

If a horse is forced into what for it is an unnatural conformation or way of going, by changes to its foot axis, then the remedy is mostly worse than the problem. Tendons and ligaments are put under stress, which produces wear. The effect of lateral changes to the foot axis can be compared to renewing worn heels on our own shoes: we have more trouble with the new heels than the old – we only feel comfortable after the heels have been worn in.

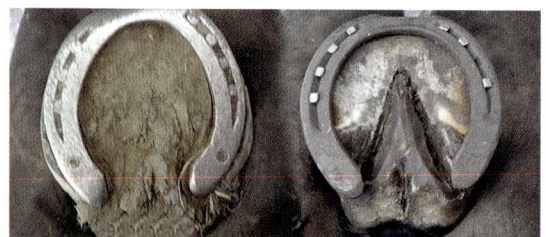

The natural shape of the hoof is often disrespected, and the farrier applies a shoe that fits badly and where the heels are outside the branches with a too narrow, pointed horseshoe. On the right, the same hoof with a properly fitted shoe.

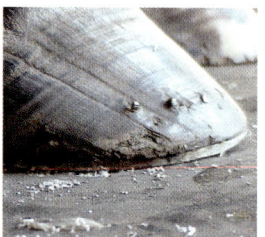

If the horseshoe is not fitted to the hoof, the horny wall breaks, and the hoof extends over the edge of the shoe and the horseshoe becomes loose.

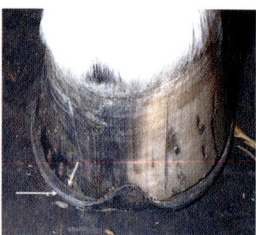

A horseshoe that is too broad can also cause problems for the hoof. The nails have been driven not into the white line but next to it, which causes tearing in the horny wall.

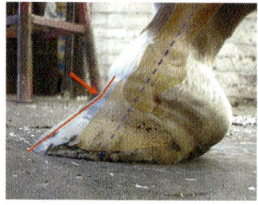

If a hoof is not trimmed correctly, the toe can become too long, which causes too much pressure on the heels. The red arrow indicates the point where the hoof is slanting forward too much and not following the foot axis.

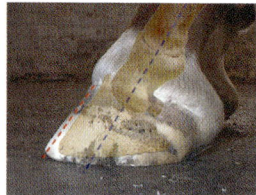

A properly trimmed hoof with a correct foot axis (blue dotted line). The line of the wall is parallel with the foot axis.

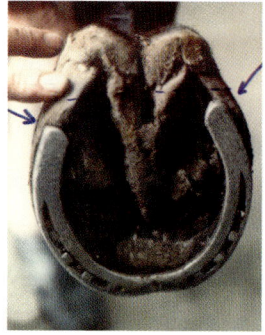

In horseshoes where both branches are too short, great problems are caused in the hoof capsule.

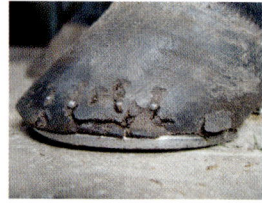

A too short and too narrowly fitted shoe where the wall has been filed away. Above all, the nails have been put in too low down. All this adds up to a horny wall that breaks up.

BAD SHOEING

It is very rare that horses are born with bad hooves. Those who work with horses know that the smallest injury is often sufficient to put such a big and apparently strong animal out of action for longer or shorter periods of time: it is often the hooves that are the weakest link. The majority of horses are not born with bad hooves but the opposite – most horses come into the world with extremely strong and good hooves. That horses have bad hooves is due to inadequate hoof care and bad shoeing.

Horses that can move about freely when young have fewer problems with bad horn quality or other problems such as hollow walls or white line disease. These problems only arise when they begin a new lifestyle: that is to say, being stabled for long periods and moving infrequently. Of course, there are many horses that are stabled all the time, are not even shod, and that have no problems. Horses that cannot do without shoes are competition horses and horses that need shoes because of deviant limb conformation, or horses that have a disease of a hoof or hooves.

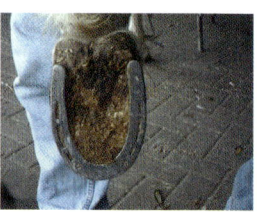

A horseshoe that shows the farrier has not followed the shape of the hoof. This can hinder the gaits.

Part 1 – The Hoof

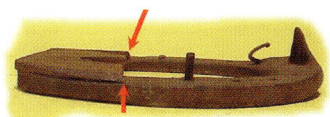

'Therapeutic horseshoes' can damage hooves disastrously. This farrier has welded the bar not between the shoe branches but on the foot surface of the shoe. It caused the horse to become lame.

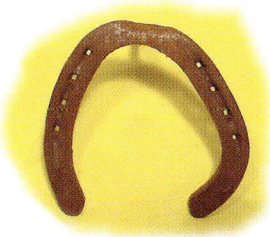

Many horseshoes do not match the form of the hoof.

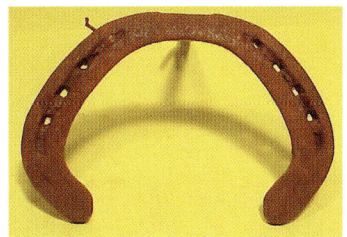

A broad shoe with branches severely bent inwards: this can never reflect the shape of the hoof.

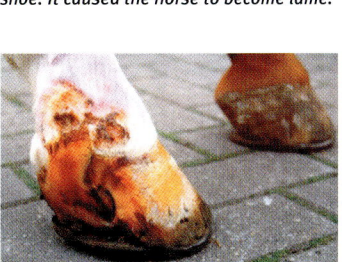

A nasty wound on the outside of the coronet. In order to prevent the horse from striking the infected wound, the farrier had the bright idea of building something around it, forgetting that the horse cannot move like this. This is outright animal abuse. The lame horse's wound was treated again and the hoof was fitted with a normal shoe.

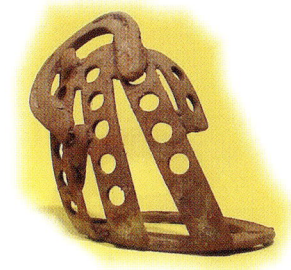 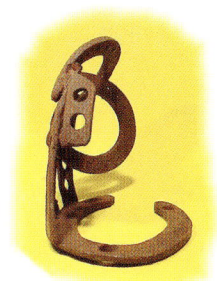

This horseshoe is constructed from heavy strips of iron and smaller horseshoes: unfortunately these 'works of art' are still to be found.

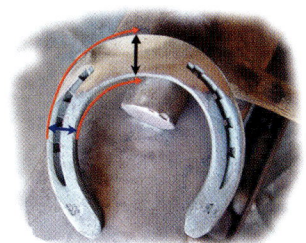

The newly-designed Hoofcare® breakover horseshoe gives many horses with hoof problems a fresh start.

Problems like separating walls, seedy toe, white line disease, cracks in the hoof wall and so on can develop if shoes are badly fitted. Mostly, the problems arising from faulty shoeing cannot be seen from the outside, and all the while the problem can be brewing on the inside for months. If a hoof is put constantly in the wrong position, the horse can suffer lameness or faulty weightbearing of the hoof, or it can move crookedly or have back problems.

A common error is for the standing position of the hoof to be 'corrected' by the farrier. This is very strongly to be discouraged in horses of three years and older, as by this age the growth plates in the bones have stabilised and there should be no further changes to conformation.

Hoof Care and Horseshoes

THE WEIGHT OF THE HORSESHOE

Besides shape, it is also the weight of the horseshoe and how that weight is distributed that is of importance, because of the great influence this has on the movement of the horse. The horse's limb moves like a pendulum, going back and forth. Every gram of weight on the end of a pendulum affects the movement: as the speed increases, this influence becomes greater (kinetic energy). It is for this reason in the shoeing of trotters and race horses, in particular, various distributions of weight in or on the shoes are used to achieve certain effects. But extra weight on the branches – such as steel wedges, egg bars or too heavy bars – is taxing for the tendons and ligaments.

CONCLUSION

As a rule of thumb, the farrier should trim and shoe in such a way that the horse can be brought to the most natural conformation possible and natural for itself – even when, in our eyes, that does not appear ideal. This means that each hoof should be examined and trimmed individually and that each hoof should have its own, fitted shoe made.

CASE HISTORY 1: PHOTOS BELOW

A lame horse that was brought to the clinic had been continually losing its shoes. The farrier who had shod the horse thought that he had solved this by making both shoe branches curve into the heel. It wasn't long

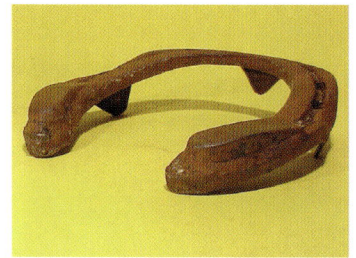

It is not only the shape of the shoe that is important but also the weight. The manner in which the weight is distributed can also be of great importance to the horse's way of going. The limb moves back and forth like a pendulum; a small weight on the end of the pendulum has a great influence on the movement. As the speed increases, thus the effect is increased (kinetic energy).

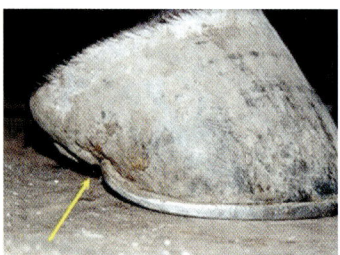 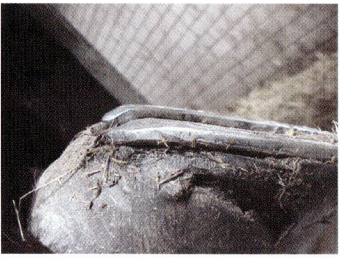

This horse continually lost its shoe. The farrier that shod the horse thought he could prevent this by bending both branches into the heels. After a while the horse became lame due to the great stress on the heels.

before the horse became really lame; the pressure on the heel area had become too great, causing the horny wall to break down. The problem became clear when the hoof was studied from the side view; the toe had been left far too long when trimming and instead of being straight was hollowed out. This meant that the fore hooves could not be picked up quickly enough before the hind hooves were upon them: this explained why the horse kept losing its shoes. This problem would not have arisen if the farrier had trimmed the hooves correctly and had made the wall of the toe straight. The action of this horse was adversely influenced by the shoeing.

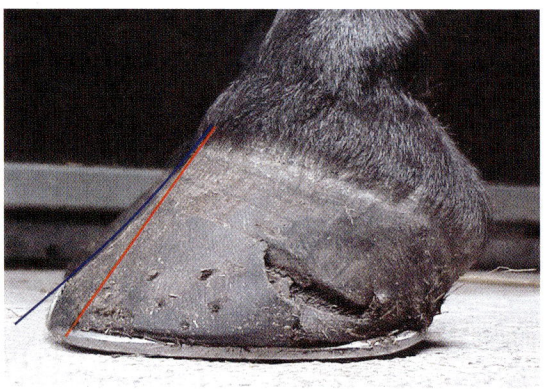

The farrier had not trimmed and finished the toe; the horseshoe was also too narrow.

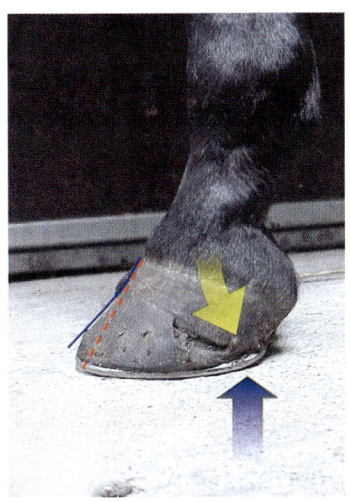

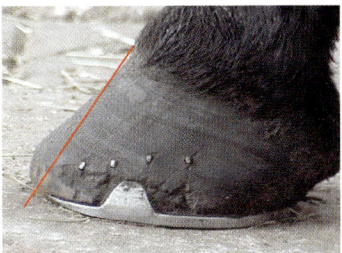

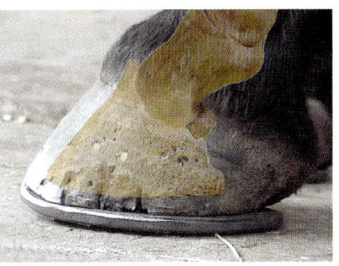

The toe was left too long at trimming, and instead of being made straight was made concave. Thus the fore hooves could not be lifted away before the hind hooves moved forward. This explained why the horse kept treading off its shoes. What is more, at this position (yellow arrow) the heels suffer extra stress.

When trimming the farrier had not pared the toe back enough which meant it became too long. This was the reason the farrier added two side clips to the fore shoes. The two clips had completely destroyed the wall where the hoof mechanism had operated.

The horse was shod with a normal horseshoe whereby the hoof mechanism could move freely. The part where the clips had been was indeed damaged but healed again quickly.

CASE HISTORY 2: PHOTOS ABOVE

A horse that was brought to the clinic had a clip on either side of the fore shoes. The farrier had not trimmed the toe sufficiently and it was left too long, so the farrier drew two side clips into the horseshoe. The two clips had completely destroyed the wall, because of the counteraction of the hoof mechanism. The horse was re-shod with normal horseshoes which allowed the hoof mechanism free movement. Although in rather poor shape, fortunately the part where the clips had been healed quickly.

The Hoofcare® Breakover Horseshoe
(Patented 2003)

The Hoofcare® Breakover horseshoe is a new horseshoe which I and my twin brother have developed and on which we have worked intensively for about five years. How did we arrive at this design? The answer is simple: by looking at the movement of hooves, and observing how the horse actually wants to move.

In nature, there are rarely any problems with horses' hooves; horses have a strong hoof capsule, a thick sole and an extremely well-developed digital cushion. There has already been much research into how hooves develop. It has been determined that hooves show wear both at the toe and along both sides, showing how horses like to move.

Sadly, many horse folk are of the opinion that hooves must be 'corrected' and that the position should be adjusted. However, such adjustments would, in the end, only lead to extra stress on the joints and then to greater wear and tear. Most horse people would also like to see a horse bring its hooves forward perfectly but both animals and humans have variable feet with variable positions and shapes so that each have their own specific way of moving and we mustn't do anything to change this. Think of the toe-in conformation, or of a horse with the toe-out conformation; these horses roll their hooves over to the outside or to the inside – a movement which a traditional horseshoe would block.

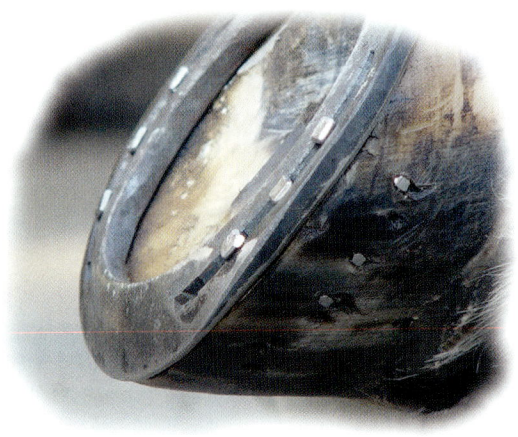

A first look at a Hoofcare® Breakover horseshoe.

The Hoofcare® Breakover horseshoe gives the horse the freedom to decide for itself the moment and the manner of the movement of the hoof. In this way, a horse can find its own balance. As the shoe has been given an extra rolling shape, the stress that is normally placed on the front of the hooves in the area of the wall, wall corium and white line is totally eliminated. When trimming the horny wall, the farrier must ensure that the thickness of the hoof capsule remains even all round so that there is an equal ground pressure. In this way, the hoof wears down evenly.

In horses that we have shod with Hoofcare® Breakover horseshoes, the hoof capsule retains its original shape and the horseshoes remain in place. This can be considered a sign that this horseshoe imitates nature and protects the hoof against wear and tear. It also appears that the horny wall becomes stronger and that the heels are supported for a longer period. Moreover, after even ten weeks, the foot axis is still intact. The shoes allowed the hooves to remain stable on the ground surface, so the horse could easily relax.

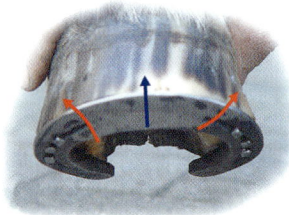 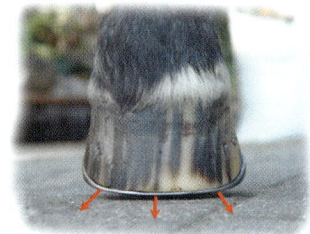 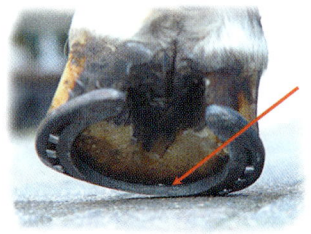

As the Hoofcare® Breakover horseshoe is forged with a rocker at the toe and sides, extra rolling is created not only at the front but also on the inner and outer sides of the shoe. In this way, the horse can choose how it rolls its hoof over. In particular, horses with deviant limb conformation can benefit from this.

THE ROCKER TOE

The rocker toe has an important role in the Hoofcare®Breakover horseshoe. A rocker toe is a curve in the front of the shoe that the farrier forges into the iron. The aim is to allow the hoof to roll over easily.

These days a farrier can get ready-made horseshoes which all have clips. As less and less needs to be done to the horseshoe to make it fit well, more and more hoof and limb problems are emerging among horses. The rocker toe is crucial for the movement of the horse.

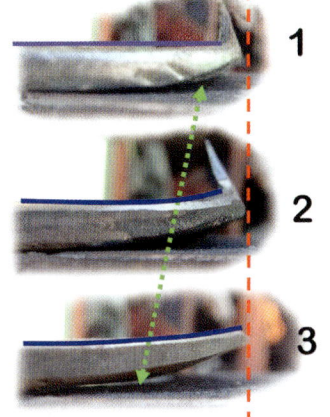

1. A horseshoe without a rocker toe. The surface where the hoof is placed is completely flat (blue line). The horse will itself create a curve at the toe by wear. This will need more pressure; the green line shows the curve.

2. A horseshoe where the farrier has not only created a rocker toe in the shoe but also in the hoof. Thus the horse can roll its hoof over better and needs less energy in order to do so.

3. In the Hoofcare® Breakover horseshoe a rocker toe is created both in the hoof and in the shoe. The rocker toe in this shoe has extra curving which enhances the roll of the hoof.

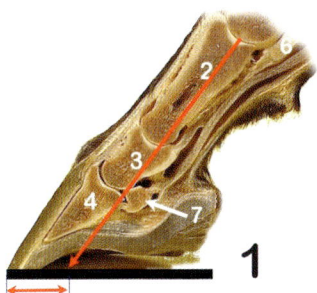 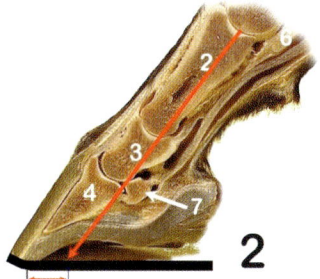 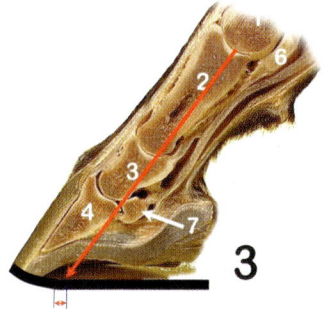

1. A shoe without a rocker toe. The horse needs more energy to breakover the toe (red arrow) which hinders the movement of the hoof.
2. Long pastern bone; 3. Short pastern bone; 4. Pedal bone; 6. Sesamoid bone; 7. Navicular bone

2. A shoe with a rocker toe. The hoof can roll more easily because the breakover moment (the point where the hoof rolls) is somewhat further under the hoof; the energy needed is rather less.

3. The Hoofcare® Breakover horseshoe. Considering the spot where the red arrow is, the hoof needs very little energy to breakover.

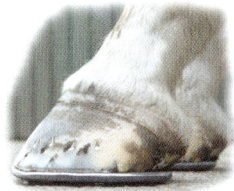 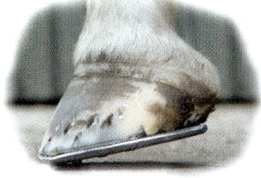 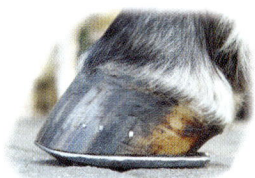 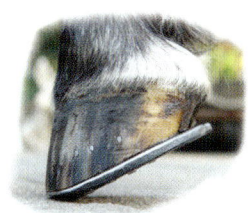

This picture shows the function of a rocker toe: the horse is assisted in the rolling over of its hoof.

With the Hoofcare® Breakover horseshoe, because the breakover moment is placed further back, the horse can roll its hoof over more easily.

Hoof Care and Horseshoes

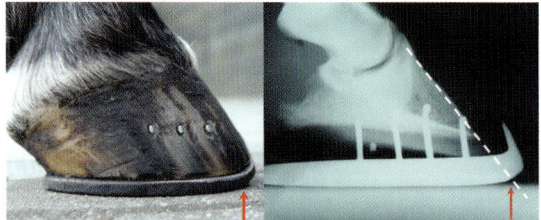

A normal rocker toe on an X-ray. It is clear to see that the line of the front of the pedal bone (white dotted line) meets the breakover moment of the horseshoe (red arrow). The stress will be greatest at the point of the pedal bone and the wall corium.

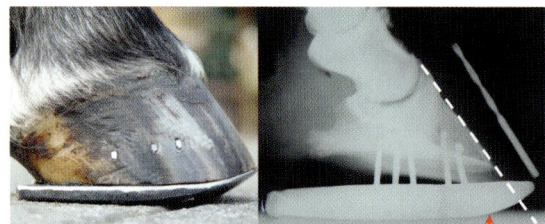

With a Hoofcare® Breakover horseshoe the line of the front of the pedal bone is in front of the breakover moment, which means that the stress in this area is reduced to a minimum.

THE 'BREAKOVER MOMENT'

The breakover moment of a horseshoe is the point where, in the forward movement of the limb, the hoof rolls over.

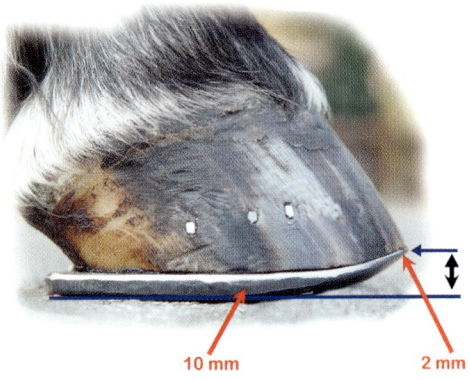

A well trimmed hoof with a correct foot axis. The line of the wall runs parallel with that of the foot axis.

What are the advantages of the Hoofcare® Breakover horseshoe?

1. **The whole hoof capsule is supported.** First and most importantly, the horseshoe should support the whole hoof capsule, because a horse does not stand on its hooves but hangs in the hoof capsule. The pedal bone is firmly bound to the hoof capsule by laminae, therefore the full weight of the horse is carried by the horny wall. This stress is spread over the whole of the hoof capsule. If we only partly support the hoof capsule – allowing the horny wall to be over the shoe – part of the horny wall will not be supported and the part of the wall that is supported will receive more pressure and therefore more wear and/or damage. Many shoes that have been designed to allow the hoofs to roll over sooner have been put on in such a way that part of the hoof capsule is not supported – in the belief that this will not cause problems! It is not for nothing that nature has designed the hoof capsule the way it is.

2. **Easier and better breaking over of the toe.** The hoof is able to breakover better, more easily and in a more controlled way when sudden movement is practically eliminated. Where the shoes are applied straight under the hoof, it is always possible that a horseshoe can tilt suddenly, which is not good for the movement of the horse. The Hoofcare® Breakover horseshoe ensures that, during breakover, the pressure from the ground does not directly impinge on the point of the toe but will instead remain longer under the hoof and thereby will give a controlled breakover.

3. **The breakover moment of the hoof is brought further back.** In a normal shoe, the line of the front of the pedal bone meets at the breakover moment of the horseshoe; the stress is greatest at the point of the pedal bone and the wall corium. In a Hoofcare® Breakover

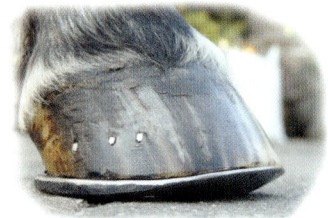

The shoe should support the whole hoof, because the horse does not stand on its hooves but hangs in the hoof capsule. The hoof should not extend over the shoe.

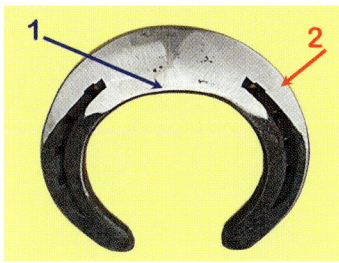

As the shoe is forged to curve up at the sides (2) as well, breakover can occur separately both in the front and at the sides without forcing the hoof. The breakover moment is far back under the hoof.

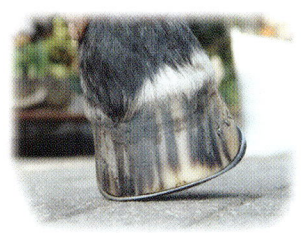

As the Hoofcare® Breakover horseshoe is also hollowed out on the foot surface, the carrying of weight on the solar surface is prevented (during weightbearing, the sole can spring downwards). This avoids too much stress, and a greater part of the solar surface is protected from ground pressure.

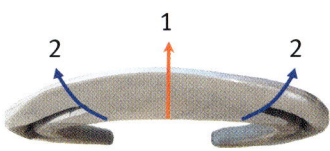

The toe part is forged up to one and a half times the width of the branches to a thickness of 2mm. The sole surface is hollowed out so that the solar surface does not rest on the shoe. By forging the shoe in this way, the breakover moment (1) in the toe is brought back under hoof and the energy needed to move the hoof forward is reduced.

horseshoe the line of the front of the pedal bone will be in front of the breakover moment, reducing the stress in this area to a minimum.

4. **Roundness in toe and sides; breakover can also be sideways.** As the Hoofcare® Breakover horseshoe is markedly rolled in the toe and sides, this allows for extra breakover not only in the front but also on the inner and outer side of the horseshoe. The shoe is, on both front quarters, curved up in such a way that the horse may also breakover sideways if necessary. Thus a horseshoe has been created that permits a horse to choose for itself how it will roll its hooves over. The Hoofcare® Breakover horseshoe will, above all, enhance the horse's way of going and give it the freedom to decide the moment when it moves its hooves. In this way a horse can find its balance. It is, above all, horses with deviant limb and hoof conformation that benefit.

5. **The solar surface is unburdened.** When the hoof is bearing weight, the sole will bounce down slightly; as the foot surface of the Hoofcare® Breakover horseshoe is concave, the horny sole area is prevented from being borne by the shoe. In this way undue pressure is avoided and a good part of the solar surface will be protected from ground pressure.

6. **Increased rocker toe without damage to the hoof.** To create a better rocker toe, a normal rocker toe is brought into the hoof – just as is done with all horseshoes. The extra rocker toe or rolled toe that is forged into the shoe is achieved by firmly hammering at the toe to form a wedge going from 10mm to 2mm. This results in an extra rocker toe of at least 8mm; and as we also work the horseshoe at the sides, the rolling occurs not only at the front but towards the outside as well.

WHAT DOES THE HOOFCARE® BREAKOVER HORSESHOE LOOK LIKE?

The toe section is hammered out to one and a half times the width of the side branch, to a thickness of 2mm. The foot surface must be hollowed out so that the solar surface does not rest on the horseshoe.

By hammering out the iron, the breakover moment in the shoe at the toe is brought further under the hoof, so that the energy needed by the limb to bring the hoof forward is less. The breakover moment can easily be varied by hammering out the toe less. As the iron is also rounded up at the side edges, the rolling of the hoof is mostly at the front but also in both sideways directions.

RESULTS

After five years of experimenting, the results of the horseshoe have been amazing.

We have helped many horses with problems of arthrosis, navicular disease, laminitis, sensitive soles, tendon injury, problems of the horny wall and also horses with long toes and low heels. Horses that had to go long distances tired less quickly. Above all, it appeared that the wear of the horseshoe was distributed over the whole ground surface. From this we can conclude that the weightbearing and the breakover of the hoof were correct.

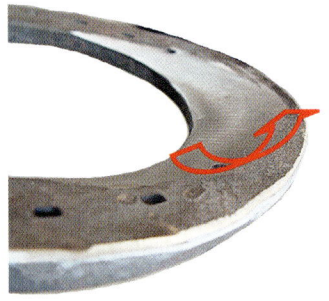 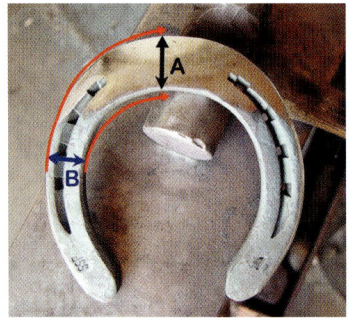

An extremely important feature of the Hoofcare® Breakover horseshoe is that the foot surface is hollowed out so that the sole area cannot be pressed on to the shoe.

The Hoofcare® Breakover horseshoe is wider at the toe (A) than at the branches (B). The toe is wedge-shaped and hollowed out, to unburden the sole and to bring the breakover moment further under the hoof.

CONCLUSION

TheHoofcare® Breakover horseshoe must be applied broadly and with length in order that the maximum hoof mechanism is achieved with the accompanying maximum blood circulation. The Hoofcare® Breakover horseshoe does not solve all hoof and limb problems, but in many cases it has a positive effect and allows the horse to function better.

If the shoe is not fitted correctly the horse can suffer. This has already been seen in practice so we therefore once again advise that this horseshoe, for maximum results, is fitted in the way described here. This shoe is also not suited to every horse: each horse must be individually assessed.

This horseshoe has been developed and patented by:
J.R. van Nassau, Middenstraat 15 in Oud Gastel, Netherlands
A.E. van Nassau, Middenstraat 17 in Oud Gastel, Netherlands

Part 2

Disorders of the limbs and hooves in relation to hoof care and horseshoes

1 THE LIMB

Arthrosis

Arthrosis is a form of degeneration of a joint. This chronic condition in horses can be compared to rheumatism in humans. A horse with arthrosis has formed new bone on the edge of the joints after the joint

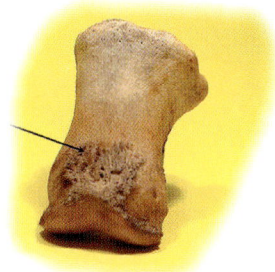
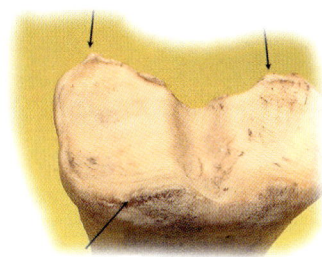
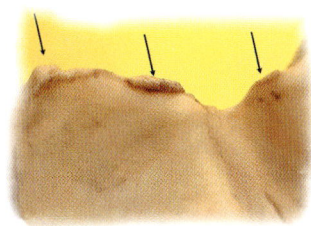

The pictures show a long pastern bone with some bone proliferation on the front underside (left). On the edges of the pastern ginglymus joint (centre and right) there is also proliferation of bone growth. This bone proliferation – or arthrosis – prevents the pastern from moving properly.

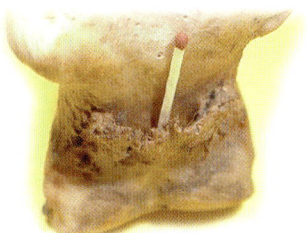
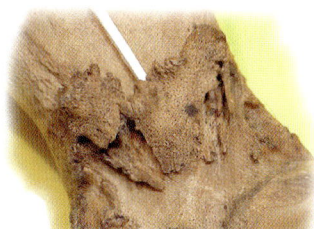
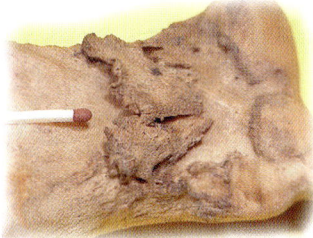

At the rear of this long pastern bone aggressive bone proliferation is visible. The deep digital flexor tendon and the superficial flexor tendon run over the rear side.

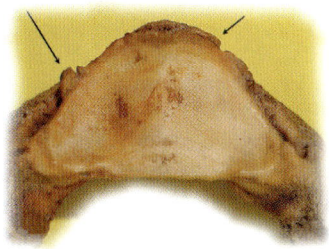

Arthrosis on the sides of the joint surfaces of the pedal bone – the surface on which the bones move.

cartilage and/or bone has been damaged or eroded. Arthrosis is often inherited, although it can also occur without being inherited. This mostly occurs among horses that have been taxed too much when young or who have had damage to the bones.

SYMPTOMS

Arthrosis usually begins with a light, varying irregularity that can degenerate into permanent lameness. The condition usually develops slowly, although sometimes horses can become suddenly very seriously lame. Horses with arthrosis generally have shortened gaits.

Examples of arthrosis are low and high ring-bone, which can occur in the fore and hind limbs in, respectively, the coronary joint and the hoof joint. Another form of arthrosis is bone spavin that occurs in the hind limb on the inner front side of the hock.

DIAGNOSIS

Arthrosis can be detected by X-rays. In this way, the extent and the seriousness of the condition can be established. Arthrosis can be discovered at the time of a veterinary examination, for example when having flexion tests, even if the horse has never been lame. It is thus apparent that the extent of the arthrosis is not always connected to the extent of lameness.

An established arthrosis is impossible to cure. There are, however, various possibilities for keeping the horse in a working condition. It is of great importance that the horse is shod well and appropriately. The use of horseshoes with leather pads can be helpful here in order to reduce the level of concussion. The application of adapted shoes can also afford the horse some relief and slow the development of the condition; in some cases this can even bring the arthrosis to a halt. The horseshoes should be fitted in such a way that the horse can move freely in the way it chooses naturally.

Arthrosis can be so serious that the flexing of the joints is really

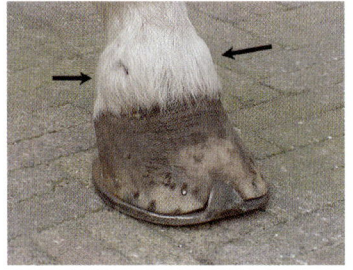

Arthrosis on the front and side of the short pastern bone. This is also called low ring-bone; this seriously hinders the movement of the horse.

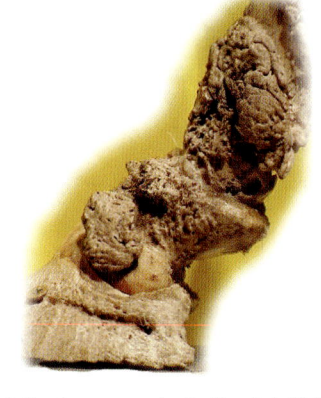

A disastrous example of arthrosis is high ring-bone. For many horses this means the end, because the arthrosis develops extremely rapidly and nothing more can be done about it.

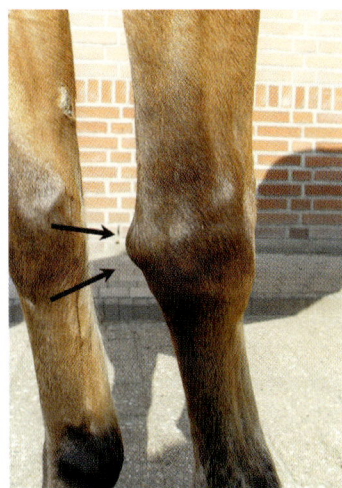

Arthrosis occurs in many bones and joints. This picture shows visible bone proliferation on the inside of the left fore knee. In the long run this will cause lameness.

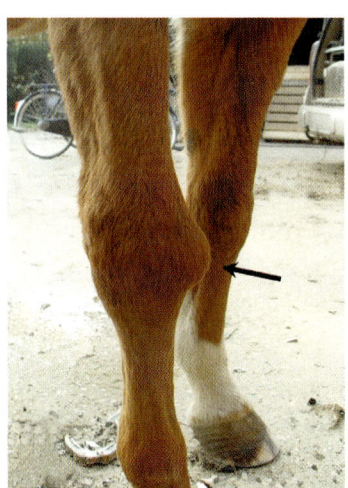

An extremely serious form – as big as a tennis ball – on the inside of the fore knee; this severely limits flexion.

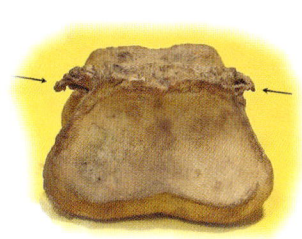 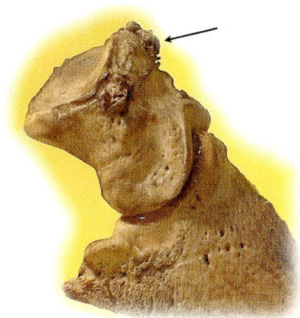

Left: side view of a short pastern bone. Right: top view of a short pastern bone. Enormous spurs on both sides of the short pastern bone will clearly limit the movement because of interference with tendons and ligaments.

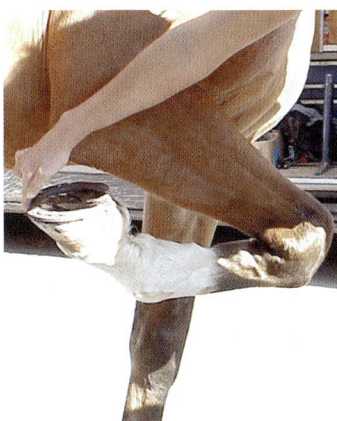 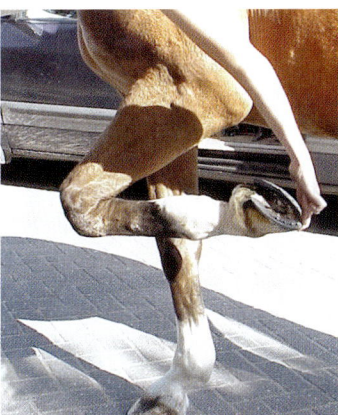 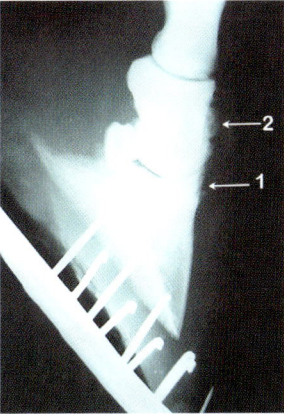

A clear example of pastern arthrosis; the flexion of the right fore limb is limited to half and it can only flex 45 degrees on the horizontal line.

There is an even bigger problem in the left fore limb; flexion is no longer possible.

This X-ray shows clearly the development of the arthrosis on the front of the short pastern bone (2) and the epiphysis (1); the top front of the pedal bone.

limited, which causes problems for the movement of the horse. A healthy horse can easily flex its lower foot to an angle of 90 degrees. A horse with arthrosis can sometimes flex its hoof only to 45 degrees and in the worst cases not at all: nevertheless, horses with a serious form of arthrosis can often still move reasonably well because they have learned how to cope with their limitations.

HORSESHOES

Various forms of arthrosis need various forms of horseshoe, and in this each horse is different. It is important to shoe the horse in such a way that it can move more easily.

Wire Wounds

It happens every summer: horses get caught up in smooth fencing wire, wire mesh or barbed wire because they have been alarmed by something or they have kicked out because of flies. Serious to extremely serious wounds can be the result. It can happen to any horse. Wire injuries occur on the lower foot up to the hock and can cause irregularities of movement or permanent lameness.

In serious wire injuries, the wire has cut away a great part of the tough outer skin of the lower foot – the skin above the coronet – and cut off the side of the hoof and the whole coronary corium and periople corium have disappeared. If the underlying bone and the cartilage – the pedal bone and hoof cartilage – have not been too damaged, even serious wire injuries can heal quickly and well.

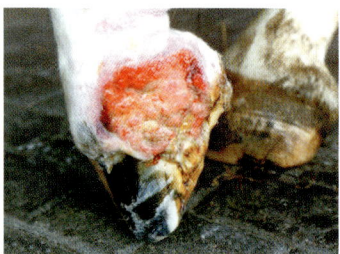

This horse has a wire injury where a part of the coronary band, the heel wall and the solar surface have been sliced off.

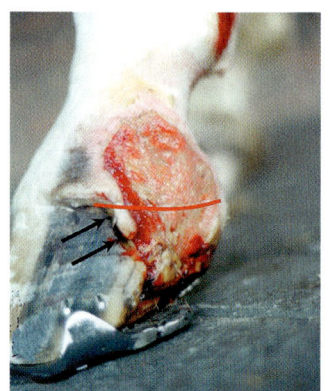

The black arrows show where there is a piece of the coronary band with the perioplic ring pulled loose. When bandaging the wound, the coronary band and the perioplic ring must be carefully put back in place (in accordance with the red line).

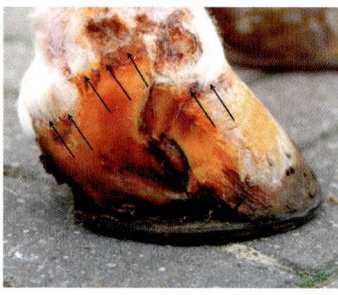

In this wound, the perioplic ring has fixed itself above the normal coronary band. The germinating layer will start new horn growth from here. It doesn't look very nice but the defective horn does protect the interior of the hoof.

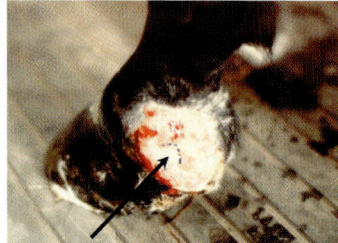

In this wire injury a part of the cartilage is visible above the pedal bone lateral cartilages (blue arrow). This does not have consequences for the horse or for the healing of the wound.

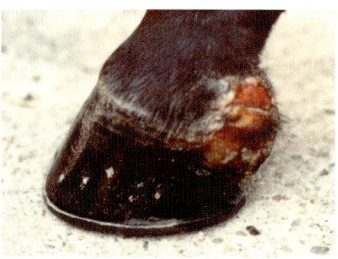

After three months the wound is nearly healed, with barely any defective horn growth.

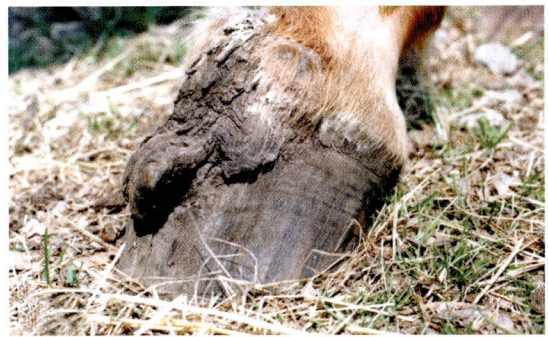
This defect in the hoof will cause problems for the horse because the growth of the new horn is above the hoof joint.

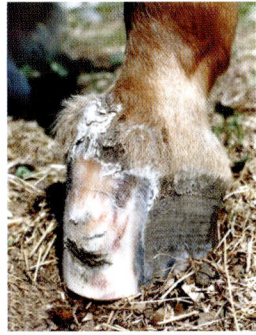
This growth proliferation must be completely removed and the hoof capsule must be given its normal shape. The horn above the original coronary band must be pared as thinly as possible so that the horse's movement is limited as little as possible .

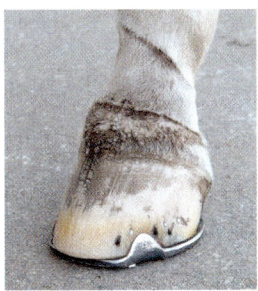
A wire has left its trace around the lower limb.

TREATMENT
Wire injuries must be treated carefully. To keep the wound clean and to staunch the flow of blood, a Betadine (iodine) compress is applied. It is important that the horse is vaccinated against tetanus. The wound should be bandaged for several weeks after the treatment so that dirt and bacteria cannot hinder the healing process.

If wire injuries of the coronary band remain untreated, proliferation of the growth of the horn can occur – this proliferation obstructs the horse's movement: there will be a difference in the lengths of stride – that is to say, in the length of the step the horse makes.

HORSESHOES
A horse with a serious wire injury must be fitted with horseshoes that do not cause any pressure to the wound. When there is injury to the heel, by applying a three-quarter shoe with a bar, the heel area is not burdened. A three-quarter shoe with a bar is a shoe where the branches have been removed. When the hoof is weightbearing, the painful part can move freely without having to touch horseshoe branches, otherwise the wound would be under pressure, which would result in lameness.

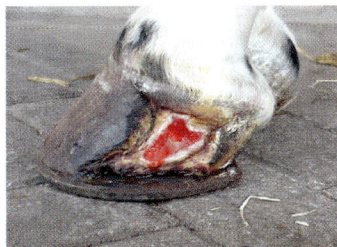 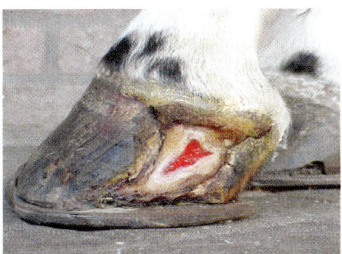
With good treatment, the pulled off side piece of this hoof capsule will heal rapidly. A white edge is visible around the wound; this indicates healthy, rapid healing.

Stringhalt and Spasms

Stringhalt and spasms are conditions of the hind limb. Both problems are similar but reveal themselves with different movements.

SYMPTOMS

When having a spasm, the horse picks up its hind leg excessively high, the leg quivers and it is then dropped suddenly. In stringhalt, the same leg is brought up high when stepping forward. Stringhalt is most clearly seen at walk. As soon as the horse is put under pressure to work the condition can no longer be seen clearly. A horse that has stringhalt or spasms is not lame but when coming from the stable moves stiffly.

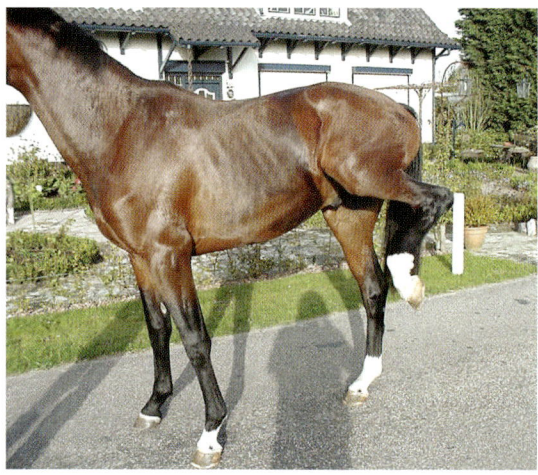

TREATMENT

The disorders as described above have been operated upon in the hope that this would help, but results are questionable. The cause of stringhalt and spasms is actually rooted in the nervous system. The nerves send an exaggerated signal from the spinal cord for lifting up and putting down the limb. Disorders of the nervous system can rarely or never be treated – but that does not matter as stringhalt and spasms do not prevent the horse from being ridden.

TRIMMING AND SHOEING

Stringhalt and spasms are rather problematical for the farrier. Horses with such disorders lift their legs extremely high at every touch, and in the worst cases collapse to the ground. Symptoms get worse when trimming and shoeing, particularly when the nails are being driven home. The movements can be so exaggerated that the horse falls down and hurts itself. The horse has no control over this and does not do it on purpose. To make it easier for the horse, the veterinary surgeon can give a tranquilliser.

It is very difficult for a farrier to put shoes on well on a horse with stringhalt and/or spasms. What is important is:
- NEVER get angry. The horse has no control over its exaggerated movements
- Work calmly and make the horse feel confident and praise it repeatedly for every movement it makes – even if it is not the correct movement
- Ensure that the horse is standing in a quiet spot, so that it can give the farrier all of its attention

To help the horse, it can be stood next to a wall, so that when its foot is being lifted up it can lean against the wall. The biggest problem with these horses is their anxiety because they have been roughly treated. Rough treatment is always counterproductive. The farrier must teach the horse that it will not have a spasm if, when lifting its foot, it keeps it low – that is, about 20cm from the ground. After a little practice the horse will calm down and understand what is meant. A horse that has been handled properly and with confidence suppresses its anxiety and after a while regains its trust in those who are treating it.

2 THE LOWER LIMB

Splint

A splint is a thickening of the limb or building up of bone on the cannon bone of the fore or hind limb of a horse.

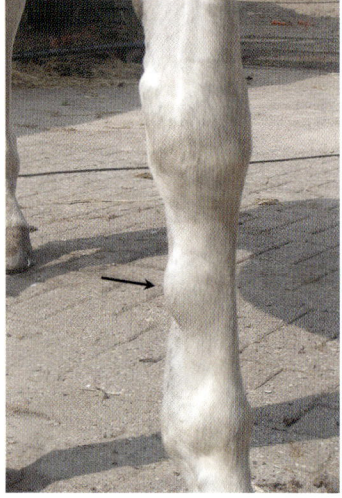

A splint on the fore limb on the inner side of the cannon bone (black arrow). A splint at this spot does not usually directly cause lameness.

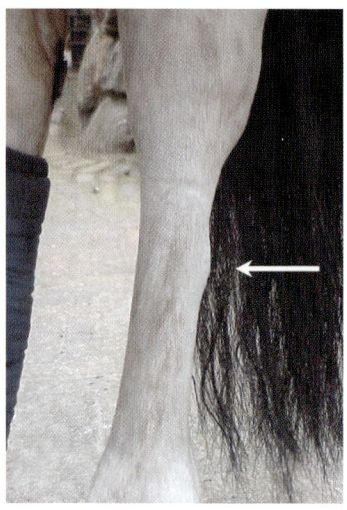

A splint on the outer side of the hind limb. Here too, it does not cause problems.

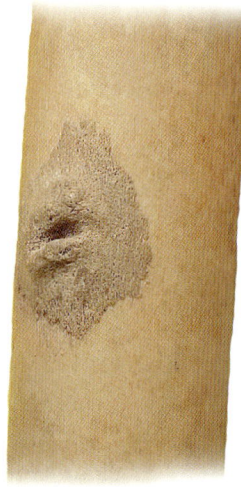

An example of a splint on the cannon bone.

CAUSE

Splints are often seen in young horses, in horses that have a deviant conformation and way of going, and in untrained horses and horses that strike themselves – in the latter, horseshoes can play a role. Splints are most frequently seen among horses that are out at grass with other horses. The splint originates from a blow, for example if a horse strikes its own fore limb with its other fore hoof, or if it kicks or bangs its leg against something. This stimulates the periosteum and sets up a reaction which causes new bone to be formed. This reaction can be accompanied by pain and much swelling where the horse displays – sometimes very serious – lameness.

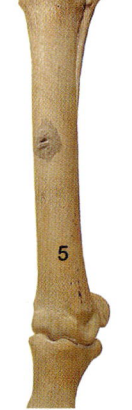

A splint on the front of the cannon bone (5) can cause lameness because the extensor tendons pass here.

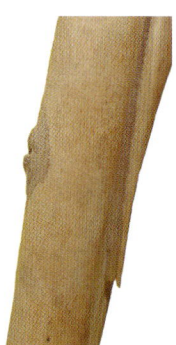

A splint seen from the side. The extensor tendon which passes over here becomes irritated by the raw surface. This splint can be removed by operation.

Part 2 – Disorders of the Limbs and Hooves

A horse need not always be lame if a splint develops – this depends on the spot and how hard the blow was. Splints on the side of the cannon bone generally do not result in lameness. Splints on the front or back of the cannon bone and near the flexor and extensor tendons increase the possibility of lameness. Lameness that is caused by a splint can spontaneously disappear after a few weeks.

For example, the swelling that is caused by a blow gradually hardens because it has formed new bone. Small metacarpal bone fractures can also develop extra bone. If the splint or build-up of bone develops on the inner side of the small metacarpal bone, between where the flexor tendons lie, then it can hinder the working of the tendons. If a horse is troubled by this bone build-up, it can be removed by an operation.

TREATMENT

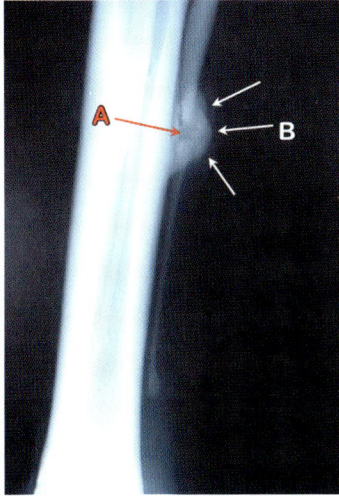

An X-ray of a small metacarpal bone fracture (A) with extra bone growth around the fracture (B).

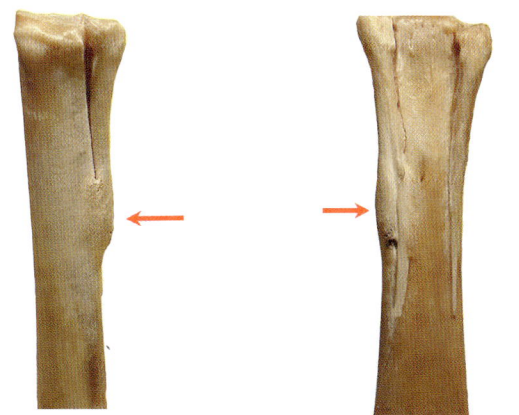

Left: a splint on the side of the cannon bone and the small metacarpal bone, possibly as a result of a small metacarpal bone fracture.
Right: The back of the cannon bone with small metacarpal bone. The splint is partly embedded in the cannon bone, which can cause problems as flexor tendons pass here.

In the acute phase of this disorder the treatment consists of cooling the spot where the splint is, or giving medication. In some cases, splints disappear by themselves but this is not the rule.

Bone Spavin

Bone spavin is a serious arthrosis disorder that appears only in the hock joint.

CAUSE

In order to understand the cause of bone spavin, it is necessary to know something about joints. The hock joint is a combination joint made up of three different joints. The bending and stretching of the hock joint takes

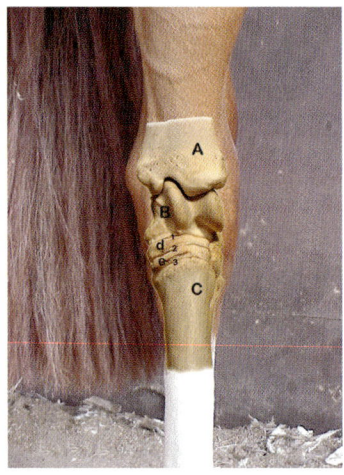 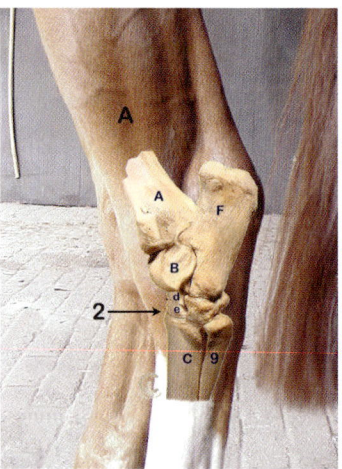 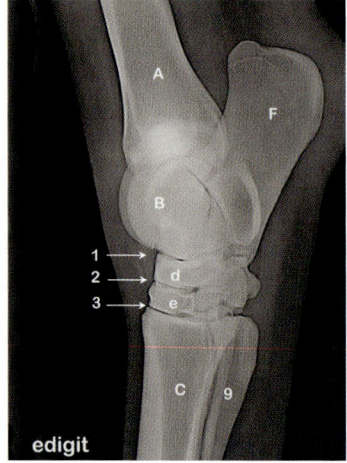

The near hind leg of a horse as seen from the front:
A. Tibia
B. Talus
C. Cannon bone (third metatarsal)
d. Central tarsal bone
e. Third tarsal bone
1, 2 and 3. Lower joints

The near hind leg of a horse as seen from the outside:
A. Tibia
B. Talus
C. Cannon bone (third metatarsal)
d. Central tarsal bone
e. Third tarsal bone
F. Os calcis
2. Area of inflammation
9. Fourth metatarsal bone

This X-ray shows a beautiful hock joint; it is possible to look through the joint crevices (1, 2, 3).

place only in the top joint – the joint between the tibia bone and the talus bone. The lower joints, the central hock joint bones and the lowest row of the hock joint bones are, because of the joint ligaments, so tightly connected that they hardly move. Bone spavin is chronic inflammation of the lowest articulation (joints) of the hock joint and is mostly found in the

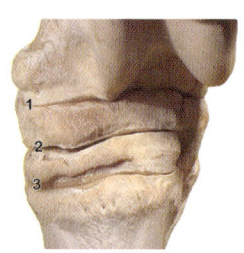

A normal hock joint. The joint crevices (1, 2, 3) are open and without a build-up of bone (arthrosis).

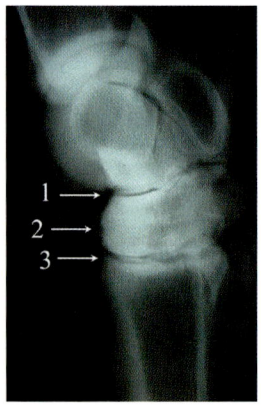 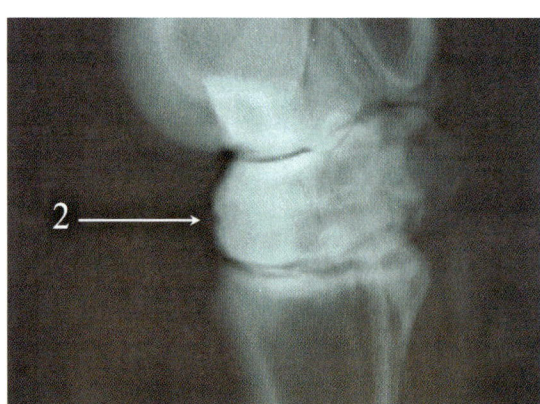

The right-hand picture is an enlargement of the left-hand picture. 1, 2 and 3 show the joint crevices. The X-ray shows a classic bone spavin. The joint (2) is completely fixed and can thus no longer function. The horse, however, can still be ridden because the joints 1 and 2 still work, although the horse will display some stiffness.

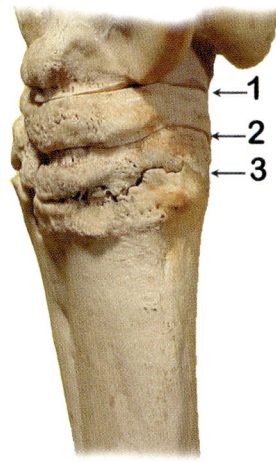

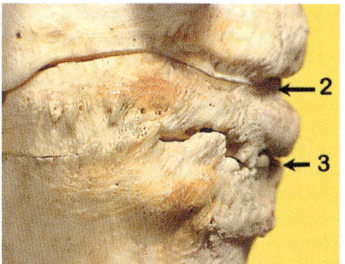

The lower hock joint bones have been merged into the cannon bone by the prolific bone growth.

Aggressive bone proliferation occurring on the edges of the joints 2 and 3. The joint crevices can hardly be seen.

central hock joint bones and the lowest row of the hock joint bones. This chronic inflammation mostly occurs on the front and inside of this area. The chronic inflammation is accompanied by an inflammation of the joint cartilage and an aggressive growth proliferation of bone on the joint edges of the lowest articulation. In serious cases of bone spavin the growth proliferation of bone is so great that the separate crevices of the joint can no longer be discerned.

Bone spavin is a serious limb defect that can provoke serious lameness and sometimes extremely serious lameness. Moreover, bone spavin is both a lameness of movement as well as weightbearing lameness. Bone spavin can gradually evolve over months or it can suddenly and aggressively appear within a couple of weeks.

Horses with bone spavin show light lameness and will recover within a couple of days. Then, after a while, the lameness returns. The periods of alternating lameness and recovery become more frequent. Horses that like to lie down display lameness earlier and have more and more difficulty getting up, which makes the situation worse. These animals have difficulty getting started in the morning: their paces are then very short. As the horse moves about, the paces improve. As time goes on, the

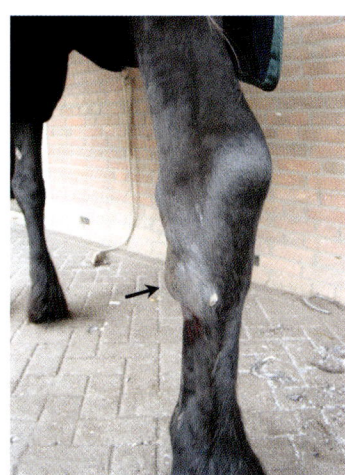

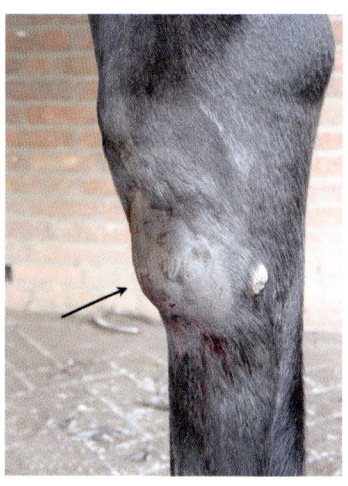

The extra bone growth can be clearly seen on the inner side of the hock joint. There is much thickening on the spot where the bone spavin is. When the bone spavin is active, this spot can feel warm.

A normal area for bone spavin (black arrow) with a nice even line.

The Lower Limb

length of step of the hind limb becomes shorter and shorter because the horse does not want to put weight on the painful leg or legs. By contrast, the horse puts more weight on the toe and tries to take the weight off the heel area.

When a veterinary surgeon talks of a 'classic bone spavin', then the arthrosis is limited to the joint of the central and lower rows of small bones in the hock joint. The arthrosis has completely blocked the joint which can no longer function. A horse with a 'classic bone spavin' can still be ridden; the animal displays a light stiffness in the first few steps but this disappears again of its own accord.

Bone spavin can arise from a faulty conformation in the limbs such as an undershot position, sickle hocks and cow hocks; this then causes stress in the hock joint. Conformation correction can also be a cause of bone spavin. A horse which makes a twisting movement of the hocks should never be hindered by horseshoes.

DIAGNOSIS

Bone spavin can be confirmed by X-rays. After diagnosis, treatment can begin. These days Tildren® is available for horses with bone spavin. It ensures that the arthrosis is checked or even completely stopped. This medication has been a breakthrough in the treatment of bone spavin. When using it, special horseshoes for bone spavin are recommended.

HORSESHOES

Usually, horses with bone spavin are given shoes with a wedge added to the outer branch of the horseshoe; this is called setting the hoof 'front to the inside'. Equestrian specialists have contradictory opinions about this treatment: in Holland, the hoof of a horse with bone spavin is set 'front to the inside', and in Germany with 'front to the outside'. Above all, these ways of shoeing throw up various problems.

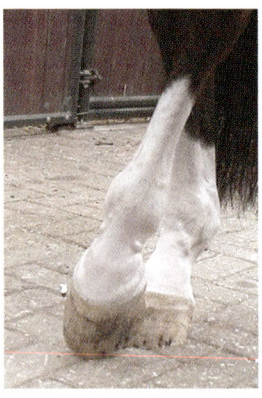

A horse with bone spavin stands in a particular way: it puts the toe of one hoof in front of or crossing its other hoof in order to let it rest. Subsequently, the horse puts the hind limb in front of or crossing its other hind limb.

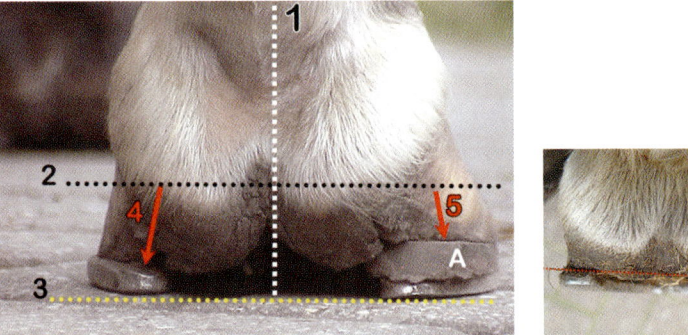

The horse will always seek to have its foot axis (1) straight, to keep in balance (black dotted line 2). The yellow dotted line 3 indicates the ground. People think that by fitting a synthetic wedge (A) on the outer side of the hoof they can give height, but the opposite occurs. The horse will put more weight on the side with the wedge to seek a normal foot axis and thus will push in the heel wall. The outer heel wall (5) will be pushed in further than the inner heel wall (4). The wedge will not be accepted by the hoof.

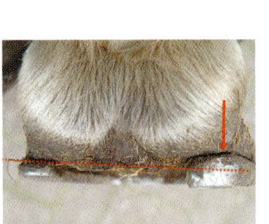

A horseshoe with steel wedges which have also been put on crookedly: this has a negative effect on the hoof and does not solve the problem.

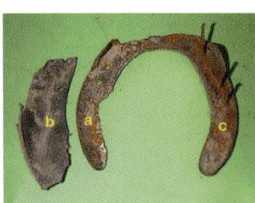

Sometimes a horse is so disturbed by a wedge that the heightened branch with the wedge (a, b) is extremely worn away as the horse seeks its normal position.

Part 2 – Disorders of the Limbs and Hooves

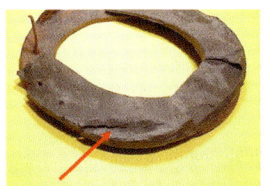

Horseshoes with wedges are, in nearly all cases, not recommended. Wedges lead to more pressure on the heels and therefore cause great problems.

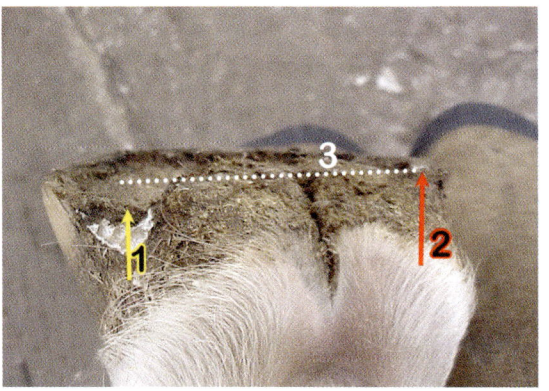

The outer part of the heel area (yellow arrow 1) has been completely pushed away by a horseshoe with a wedge (according to the line of balance, the white dotted line 3). The red arrow (2) shows where the heels should be.

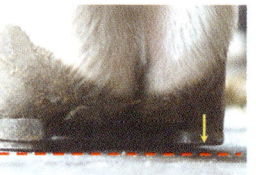

One of the big mistakes made frequently is to put a wedge on the outer branch and not have the inner branch (yellow arrow) touching the ground. This horse is constantly wobbling on its horseshoe.

In recent years, together with my twin brother, I have researched the development, weightbearing and stress on the hoof with horseshoes with wedges. It has been proved that a horse wants to keep its hoof to the foot axis – and this also applies when it has problems of bone spavin. It could be theoretically correct to place the position of the hoof in a way that reduces the stress on the place with bone spavin, but it is quite different in practice.

Suppose for example, a horse with bone spavin is shod with horseshoes with a wedge on the outer branch. The horse has a ginglymus joint and wants to put even pressure on it despite the problems it has. Thus the horse will put more weight on the side with the wedge so that the wedge pushes the heels away; a case of the remedy being worse than the disease. Even a horse that is always ridden on soft going will push the branch with the wedge more into the ground so that the development of the hoof is counteracted. Changing the position of a horse's hoof is not easy to achieve. Above all, if the natural conformation is adapted, the hoof breaks down.

CONCLUSION

The conformation of a hoof cannot be changed arbitrarily. It is important to allow each horse to stand and move in its own way. A horse with bone spavin also needs to determine its conformation. The farrier's task is to keep in line with this conformation as much as possible when shoeing.

For years, my twin brother and I have tried to change the bone spavin horseshoes with wedges, or tried shoes where the hoof is set 'to the inside' or 'to the outside' because with these 'theoretical' shoes problems have arisen more and more and horses' hooves have thus grown worse. Thirty years of experience has shown that a change in foot conformation continued to throw up more problems. Again and again, it could be seen that a horse with 'front to the inside' bone spavin horseshoes with a wedge will set the hooves a little to the outside so that the whole hoof can bear pressure. It is only on soft going that a horse puts its hoof down normally – which is very logical seeing that it can then

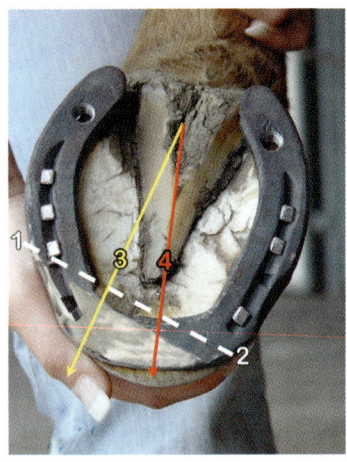

In the back 'brushing' shoe the toe extends a bit beyond the shoe. The rocker toe is slanted across the inner quarter (line between 1 and 2). The horse would normally roll its hoof forward (4) but with this slanted rocker toe it can also roll its hoof to the inside (3).

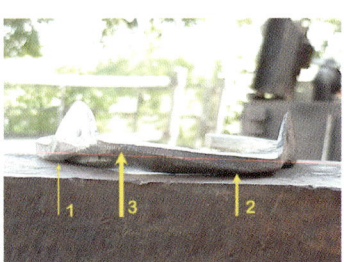

When forging the shoe of a back 'brushing' shoe, a rocker toe is brought in at the toe in the inner quarter (between 1 and 2).

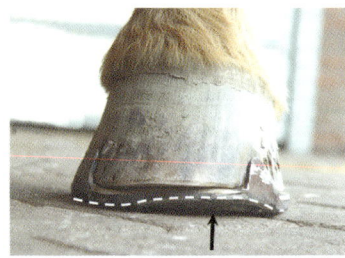

At the front, the rocker toe can be clearly seen in the horseshoe and hoof which will help the horse with its problems.

easily push the outer branch of the shoe into the ground. A horse at rest appears not to have any problems from bone spavin as it can adjust its own conformation. The problems only arise when the horse moves.

Meanwhile we have developed a shoe that ensures that the hoof capsule no longer breaks down, while the unrolling of the hoof is guided toward 'front to the inside' or 'front to the outside'. The results are the same as a horseshoe with wedges. Our spavin shoe is a normal 'brushing' horseshoe that is placed far back under the hoof – the toe of the hoof extends over the shoe – and it has, in the inside front quarter, a rocker toe. The rocker toe is strengthened by forging a rounding of the inner front toe part. As soon as the horse moves, the hoof rolls over to the inside. The advantage of this shoe is that the horse, when at rest, can put weight on its whole hoof so that it can relax normally. Extremely good results have been had from this horseshoe.

3 THE LOWER FOOT: OUTSIDE

Over-reaching

Over-reaching is the striking or catching of both bulbs of the fore hoof with the toe of the hind hoof. An ugly injury of the bulbs of the fore hoof can result from over-reaching, which has nasty consequences for the horse. These consequences depend upon the place and extent of the injury and the possibilities for recovery. Over-reaching can be very

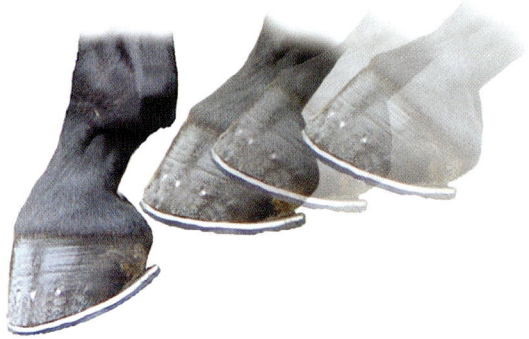

A horse without shoes does less damage when over-reaching. When the horse is shod, the consequences are serious and can be very serious.

serious because the coronary band – the coronary corium – can also be sliced off, which will interfere with the subsequent growth of the hoof capsule at that spot. Over-reaching that does not result in an outwardly visible wound results in painful bruising.

CAUSES

There are various causes of over-reaching. One cause is the horseshoes or the manner of trimming. Normally, a farrier will look at the foot axis and trim in such a way that the foot axis remains intact. Unfortunately, in practice, this is not always the case. The result can be that the horse 'strikes' so that the hind horseshoe catches the end of the branches of the fore horseshoe. The horse can also strike itself in the heel bulbs of the fore hoof and thereby seriously damage itself.

A second cause is the irregular trotting of a horse. When a horse has toes that are too long it can be hindered in its movement. If too much has been trimmed away from the heels of the fore hoof the hoof sinks back and it becomes slow moving: the horse then takes too much time to bring

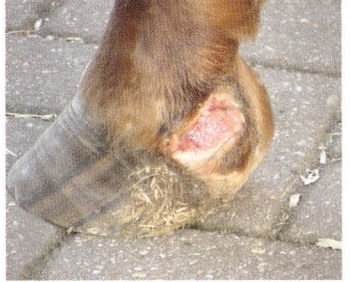

Over-reach heel bulb damage with a nice healthy wound.

the hoof forward. A third cause is deep and muddy going. Horses that are regularly ridden in deep mud can over-reach due to being hindered in their going. Horses that are always stabled and are suddenly put in a field can also strike their heel bulbs by sudden or odd movements. A fourth cause is strain: a tired or overstrained horse can have over-reach problems. A final cause is lameness; when a horse is lame it moves unevenly, which could lead to over-reaching.

TREATMENT

Damage to bulbs by over-reaching is easily diagnosed. The wound on the bulb or bulbs of the fore hoof is evident. As soon as over-reach damage has been established, the wound should be thoroughly cleaned. This is best done by hosing with water and then applying Betadine (iodine). Other remedies are not advised as a wound cleaned with Betadine (iodine) can always be cleaned up later – that is to say, it can be treated by a veterinary surgeon at a later date who can also stitch it if necessary.

Place a piece of gauze on a bulb wound that is bleeding a lot and close the wound up with pressure from a bandage without binding the hoof. Subsequently, a veterinary surgeon should treat the wound. The injured parts must be carefully cleaned and, if necessary, loose parts removed. The coronary band – which develops the hoof capsule – has to be placed back with great care so that it can, in the future, continue to develop healthy horn. This is an extremely delicate task that should only be carried out by a farrier or veterinary surgeon. The whole wound is then firmly bound so that the bulbs regain their normal shape. When the

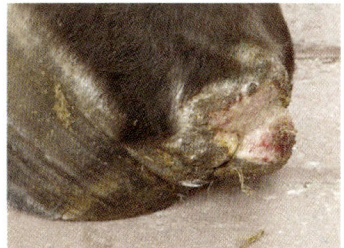
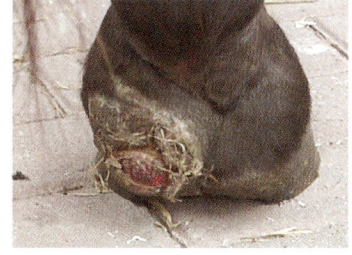

An over-reach wound where the damage has not been properly treated. It should be treated again: the loose parts should be removed to obtain a normal heel bulb.

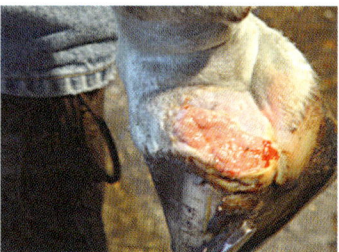

This wound should be properly treated because it is close to the coronary suture, which could influence the growth of new horn.

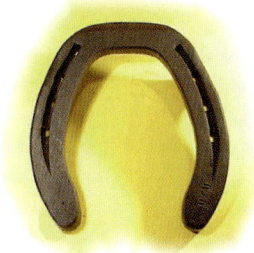

The correct shape of a hind 'brushing' shoe with a straight front at the toe.

wound is healed, the horse will suffer no adverse consequences.

To prevent over-reach damage or to enhance healing, it is important that a horse is well shod. The hind hoof is trimmed in accordance with the foot axis and the horse is shod with a hind 'brushing' shoe. With this shoe, the toe of the hind hoof extends over the front of the shoe so that if the bulbs are struck, it is only by the hoof and damage is limited.

Deformed Hooves

A deformed hoof is a hoof where the shape is permanently changed by damage to the coronal suture or to parts of the horny wall together with interior parts.

CAUSES

The growth of the horny tubules takes place at the coronal suture or the coronary corium. The horny tubules grow straight down from the coronet and are connected to each other by sensitive laminae. If the coronary corium is slightly displaced – for example, by being struck or pinched or by another trauma – then horny tubules are produced in the wrong place. The hoof subsequently changes form by the abnormal downward growth. In reaction to the damage that moved the coronary corium, the hoof develops as much horn as possible; the extra horn forces the hoof into another direction and this can be a nuisance to the horse.

A deformed hoof can cause serious lameness. This is due to the fact

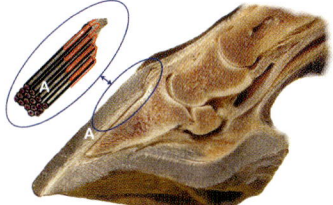

The outside horny wall consists of horny tubules (a). These are bound together by secondary laminae and grow straight down from the coronary band.
The extra horny growth is removed and the hoof regains its former shape.

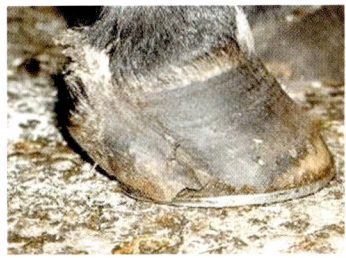

An example of a deformed hoof.

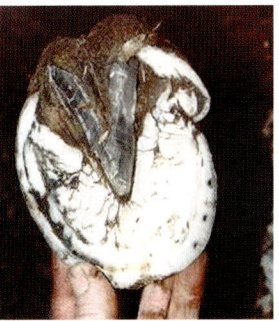

The same hoof as in the left picture: the wall has been pushed outwards by the prolific horn growth.

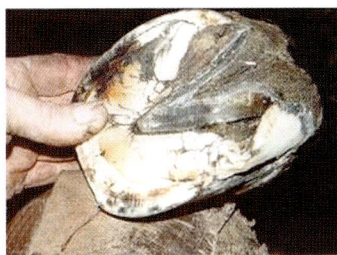

The extra horn growth is removed and the hoof regains its normal shape.

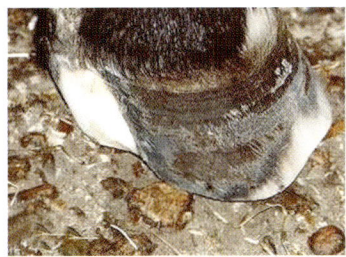

The extra horn growth on the bulbs is removed so that the epidermis can move freely.

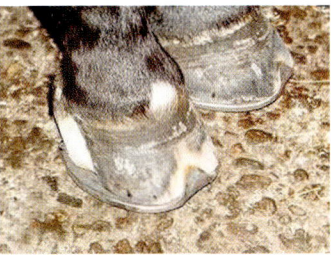

The hoof has to be shod very generously taking the removed horn into account.

The Lower Foot: Outside

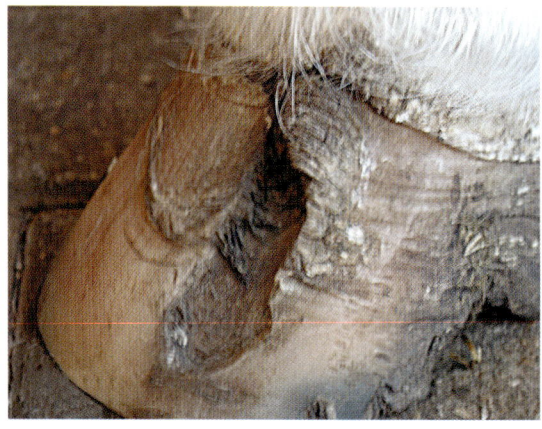

An inflammation of the coronary suture that is not properly treated can lead to permanent lameness.

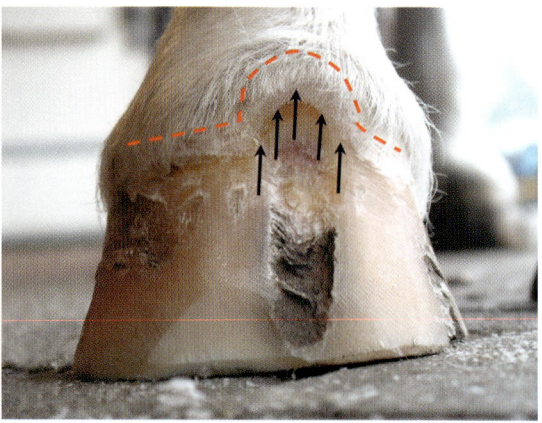

The inflammation was so serious that the coronary corium was displaced to a much higher position.

that the pressure on the hoof capsule changes, whereby the sensitive corium develops unwanted horny growth.

Severe inflammation of the coronary suture can even cause the coronary corium – which is responsible for the making of the horny tubules – to be displaced. The coronary corium will just start making horny tubules again but the results of this can lead to restricting the movement of the horse.

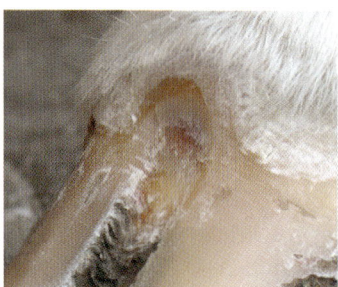

The whole wall and corium has been cleaned and thinned down so that normal horn growth can resume.

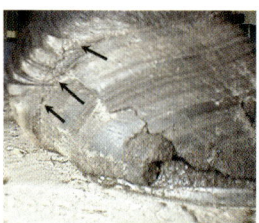

The horny tubules have been completely pulled apart because the pressure here was too great. The heel area has completely 'collapsed' (arrows).

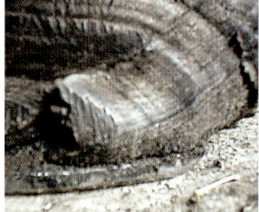

Here the hoof is not supported by the horseshoe as it is meant to be. The whole heel area must be removed in order to regain a healthy hoof. This deformity cannot heal without aid.

HORSESHOES

Nothing much can be done about a deformed hoof. A skilled farrier, who gives continuous correct handling, can reasonably adjust the hoof or get the horse functioning well despite the deformed hoof. When a horse has a deformed hoof, this should be shod with a normal and generous shoe with a sufficient rocker toe – the curve at the toe which allows easier movement. A light bar can be forged between the branches of the shoe so that movement or friction of the horseshoe is reduced. In serious cases the deformed parts should be removed, as necessary, to achieve as normal a hoof as possible.

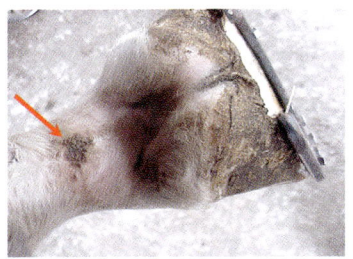

Greasy heel in the pastern cavity – a small wound can have enormous consequences.

Greasy Heel

Greasy heel is the umbrella term for skin problems such as eczema in the pastern cavity of the horse.

CAUSE

There are various causes that irritate the skin surface, creating greasy heel:

1. Damp, mud, filth and urine.
2. Sensitivity to certain irritating substances such as caring or cleaning products.
3. A wound in the pastern cavity.
4. Skin parasites such as mange mites.
5. Dirty stables or sawdust as bedding. Sawdust is indeed clean but it does not absorb moisture, thus urine fumes that irritate the pastern cavity remain present and provide the conditions for greasy heel. Straw is better bedding because the stalks absorb the urine by capillary action. The ideal bedding is deep litter: by continually adding a top layer of straw, the under layer dries out in the warmth and the stable remains dry.
6. Fields and arena surfaces where there are many droppings; places which are used by many horses.
7. Close shaving of the hair in the pastern cavity.
8. Oversensitivity to ultraviolet light.

SYMPTOMS

Greasy heel comes in many forms:

1. **Simple form.** Redness in the pastern cavity; thickening of the skin, together with itching.
2. **Scaly eczema.** The peeling of the skin is rapid and abnormal.
3. **Moist eczema.** The pastern cavity is moist and the hairs stand upright.
4. **Serious form.** Little bulges appear, that develop into blisters. When the blisters break, fluid is released. Subsequently scabs are formed and fissures develop that cause irritation in the area. This form of greasy heel is the result of neglect where too little attention has been paid to the cleaning of the stables and the care of the horse.

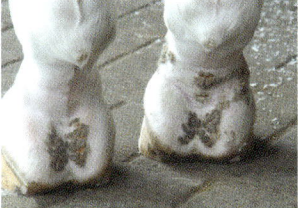

Greasy heel usually appears in more than one limb; horses with white limbs are particularly vulnerable.

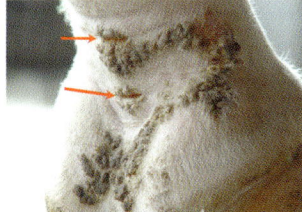

When fissures, arising from greasy heel, appear in the mobile part of the pastern cavity, the horse can become seriously lame (arrows).

The Lower Foot: Outside

Inflammation of the skin in the area of the lower foot, the pastern joint and the cannon bone often leads to swollen legs and water retention in the lower limb. Swollen legs can continue after the skin inflammation has already healed; it should be treated by a veterinary surgeon. Bandaging of the limbs is not advised as this can restrict blood circulation. Horses with a serious form of greasy heel can display lameness.

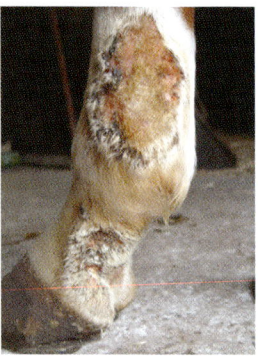

With the wrong treatment or neglect, greasy heel can take on serious forms.

TREATMENT

A horse with a greasy heel should be put into a clean, dry stable. Keep the limb clean and the greasy heel disinfected. In cases of very mucky infection, the area must be well washed; for this, use Betadine (iodine) scrub shampoo.

If a fissure due to greasy heel has developed in an area that moves a lot – for example, in the pastern cavity – then it is important that the

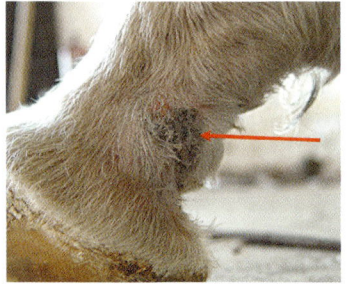
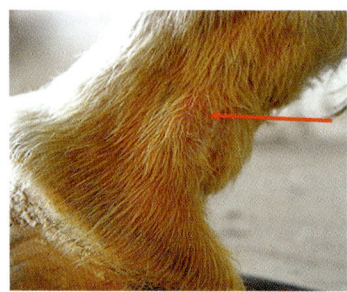

When there are scabs, they can be covered for a day with a greasy ointment such as Vaseline. This makes the scabs soft, and they can be removed more easily without harming the horse.

The limb should be thoroughly cleaned with Betadine (iodine) scrub shampoo to remove all the scabs. Afterwards, the wound can be rubbed with a soothing, anti-bacterial product.

horse gets a few days rest so that the fissure has time to heal. Don't scrub the cavity out every day – this will just make things worse as it will cause wounding.

Greasy heel can be treated with zinc ointment. The ointment softens the fissures and has a soothing effect. In cases where there are serious scabs, the greasy heel can be covered with a greasy ointment such as Vaseline. This softens the scabs so that they can be removed easily without disturbing the horse.

CONCLUSION

A horse with greasy heel should never be neglected. If it is neglected the greasy heel can lead to serious infection and even blood poisoning or swelling of the limbs. It is therefore advisable to call in the veterinary surgeon if the greasy heel does not heal rapidly.

Over at the Pastern: Moving and Standing

Going or standing 'over at the pastern' are both defects that evolve from a stiff conformation. These defects are generally inherited but also arise out of long-term lameness. In these positions the pulling power of the deep and superficial flexor tendons is extremely high.

'Going over at the pastern' is a conformation where the foot axis is only just in front of the vertical of the cannon bone. The horse goes over the pastern when it moves forward. When the horse stands still, it can hold its joints in their place. 'Standing over at the pastern' is a

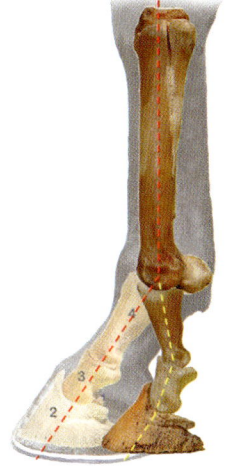

In a normal conformation, the foot axis is on a line of about 45 to 50 degrees (red dotted line). This line deviates strongly in a horse that is over at the pastern (yellow dotted line). In both conformations the horse has a correct position to the fetlock.

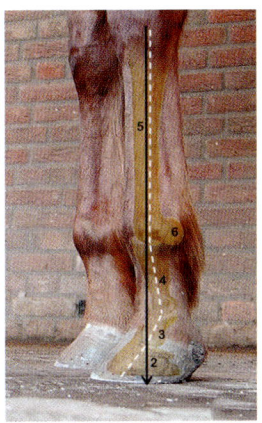

'Going over at the pastern' is a conformation whereby the foot axis is just over the vertical line of the cannon one. The horse goes over at the pastern when it begins to move forward. When the horse is standing still it manages to keep its joints in place.

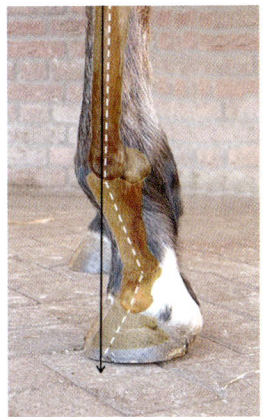

'Over at the pastern' is a position where the foot axis is behind the vertical of the cannon bone. This horse is always over at the pastern and cannot keep the pastern joint straight.

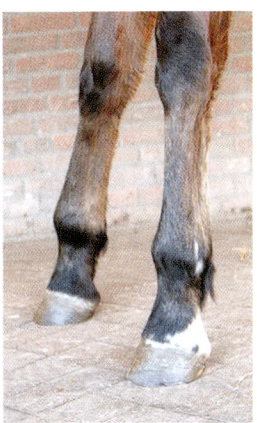

Horses that are over at the pastern have the characteristic of standing with both fore limbs far out in front, to bring the fetlocks behind.

conformation where the foot axis is behind the vertical line of the cannon bone. These horses always stand over at the pastern and cannot keep the pastern joint upright. They have the characteristic of spreading both fore limbs widely in front of themselves to bring the pasterns behind. In both conformations the horse has an upright stance of the limbs with an upright or even vertical foot axis.

SYMPTOMS

Horses that move over at the pastern often stumble, causing them to become more and more frightened of moving. Moreover, the joints and joint ligaments can become irritated, which can lead to inflammation in the joints and joint ligaments.

TREATMENT AND HORSESHOES

To ease the horse's movement it needs more support in the toe area. For this, a horseshoe can be used where an extension is made on the front so

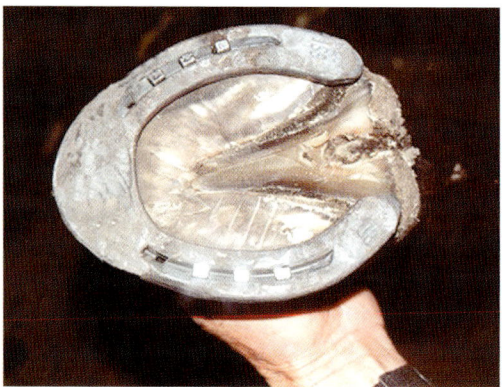

A toe extension shoe will give extra support.

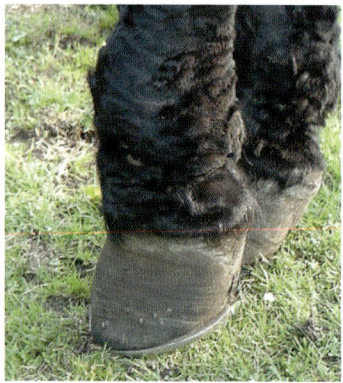

A Belgian cart horse with mange. For a long time, the horse would not set its hoof down because of pain, and stood over at the pastern. The limb was shaved and treated.

that the toe becomes longer (lever). This is called a 'toe extension' horseshoe. The shoe ensures that the hoof loads at the heels and gives the horse more support in standing. When trimming horses with these defective conformations it is of importance that the heels are kept as low as possible. If necessary, the foot axis in the hoof joint is broken toward the back.

It is above all with foals that one must intervene at an early stage with the placing of 'toe extension' shoes or the placing of synthetic extensions which will improve the chances of repair.

CASE HISTORY 1, PHOTO ABOVE RIGHT AND CENTRE

A Belgian cart horse was presented at the clinic and mange was detected. The whole limb was infected. The horse went over at the pastern because of the pain and, due to lying down a lot because it had a lot of pain, the tendons in the limb had shortened. The heels of the hoof were barely loaded. To treat this condition, a strong iron extension was made on the toe so that the horse had to load its heels. In this way, going over at the pastern was improved.

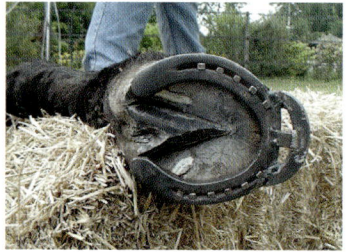

A strong iron toe extension was forged onto the toe of the horseshoe so that the horse was forced to load the heels of the hoof.

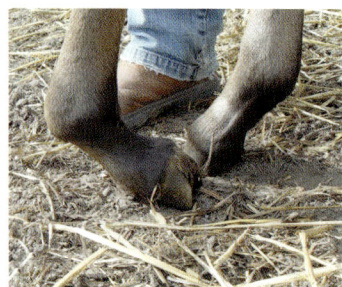

This foal of three weeks old could not straighten its lower foot and moved using the fetlock – the flexor tendon is seriously stretched.

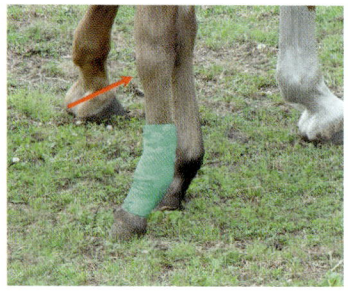

The lower limb was completely bandaged in plaster so that the flexor tendon could heal. The thickening of the fore knee can clearly be seen.

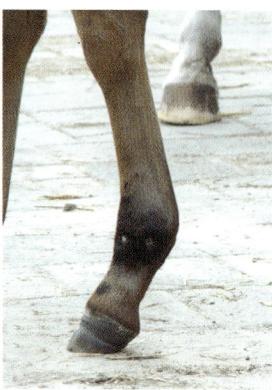

After three weeks, the foal could use its hoof normally. This will not affect its sports career.

Part 2 – Disorders of the Limbs and Hooves

CASE HISTORY 2, PHOTOS FOOT OF PREVIOUS PAGE

A foal of three weeks could no longer put its hooves down properly. The extensor tendon was stretched so much that the lower foot could no longer be brought forward. A plaster cast was immediately put on the whole lower limb so that the extensor tendon could heal; after three weeks, the foal could bring its hoof forward normally. The swelling quickly disappeared and the foal suffered no unpleasant after effects.

CONCLUSION

Going over at the pastern and standing over at the pastern are serious disorders: the prognosis is mostly unfavourable.

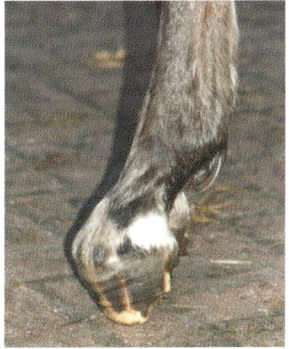

Pes equinus is the result of a shortening of the deep and superficial flexor tendons and a deviation in the joints. The horse moves on its toe and cannot load the heels.

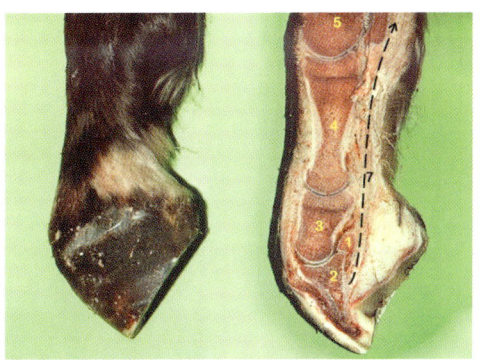

Left: an example of pes equinus (outside). Right: the same hoof in cross-section. The black line (7) shows the too-short deep flexor tendon.
1. Navicular bone; 2. Pedal bone; 3. Short pastern bone; 4. Long pastern bone; 5. Cannon bone.

Pes Equinus and Club Foot

Pes equinus is an upright limb conformation where the long pastern bone is an extension of the cannon bone or where this disorder is a result of a club foot. Horses with these disorders cannot put their heels on the ground and they walk on their toes.

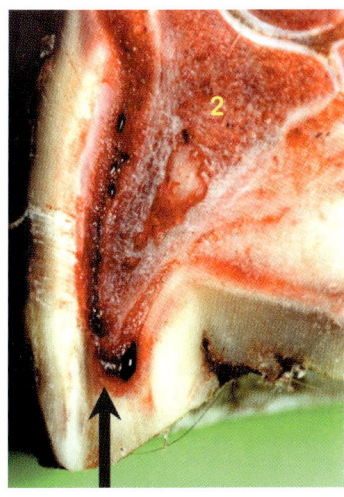

The pressure on the toe from the ground is so great that the pedal bone (2) changes shape.

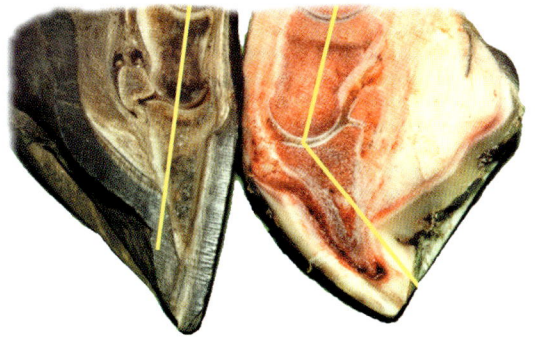

A clear difference between the position of the pedal bone of a normal hoof (left) with a straight foot axis, and pes equinus (right) with a broken foot axis.

CAUSE

A club foot arises from hoof problems. A foal can get a club foot by too much wear, cutting away of the toe area, or being left too long at the heels. A club foot is always accompanied by a permanent bending of the hoof joint although the horse can load the whole hoof. A club foot can also arise from a long-term painful disorder in the back half of the hoof; an undesirable upright limb conformation – pes equinus – is the result.

There are various causes of club foot:
1. An aberrant position in the womb.
2. An inherited condition.
3. Too hard or too soft going.
4. Lack of hoof care.
5. Waiting too long for trimming.
6. A painful disorder of the joints.

Pes equinus is a too-upright limb conformation arising from faulty weightbearing of the hoof or a congenital (inherited) condition where there are disturbances in the growth and the development of bones, tendons and ligaments. Pes equinus arises from a too-short deep flexor tendon and support tendon or from a defective joint functioning in the lower foot. The prognosis for pes equinus is very poor. From the point of view of movement, a limb conformation that is too upright will give an undesirable gait. An upright limb conformation can be the cause of too much stress on the joints and tendons in the lower foot.

Defective limb conformation in foals or young horses can be corrected, as a maximum, until three years old. The methods of correction depend on the cause of the defect and the age of the animal. The farrier plays a crucial role in the treatment.

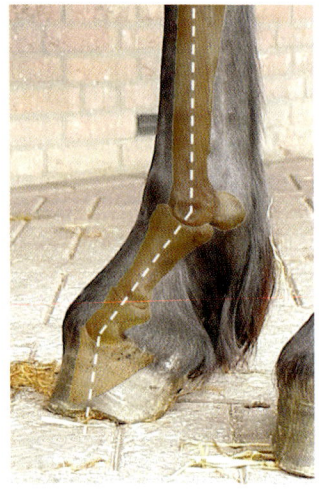

A club foot is an upright hoof with an extreme angle at the toe of 70 to 90 degrees. The heels are high but the whole hoof is loaded. The foot axis is broken forward in the hoof joint.

TREATMENT

Pes equinus that arises from too short flexor tendons requires intensive treatment. The aim of the treatment is to allow the foal's limb to bend more in the lower foot. The hoof correction is the same as that for club foot. To bring more bending in the lower foot, a toe extension (lever) is added to the shoe. This shoe forces the horse to use the back part of the hoof and thus load the heels. On the underside of the horseshoe branches calkins are placed that are regularly shortened. By walking the foal regularly, the flexor tendons are stretched. Gradually the limb conformation and the hoof shape will adapt to the 'toe extension' shoe by becoming a normal shape and a normal hoof position results.

A second method of treatment that is used with young foals is to stretch the flexor tendons under anaesthetic. Here, the support ligament of the deep flexor tendon – the strengthening ligament of the deep flexor that is attached to the back of the topside of the cannon bone – is cut through. This ligament plays an important role in the passive (that is, without using energy) use of the limb in standing and bearing weight. The operation also ensures that the transition to the muscles is stretched as well as the deep flexor tendon. In this method, the stretching is rapid – a muscle is easier to stretch than a tendon. After the operation, the limb is put in plaster.

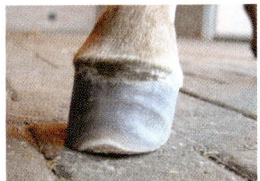
If a farrier can no longer put nails in the hoof – the white line can be seen at the toe – then the placing of a synthetic extension is a very good alternative. First the horny wall is thoroughly cleaned.

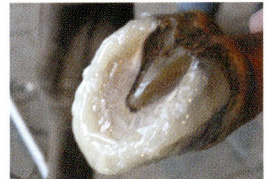
Equi-Thane Hoof Pak® is put under the hoof at the weightbearing edge whereby the toe becomes thicker than the heel area. After this, a layer is put on the front of the horny wall.

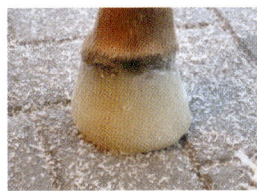
Equi-Thane Hoof Pak® can be worked after 1 minute and can always be applied at the desired thickness and height.

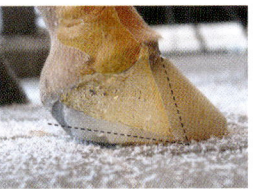
An upright hoof (black dotted line) of a foal can also be helped with this method.

A third method is by cleaving (cutting along its length) the tendon of the deep flexor in combination with a toe extension shoe to correct the limb conformation. This remedy is in some cases worse than the cure and will stand in the way of a good sports career for the horse, as the cleaved deep flexor tendon weakens.

The club foot is treated by protecting the toe. By adding a synthetic or metal protector under the toe part against excessive wear, the club foot can be prevented or cured. This is not to say, however, that this goes for all foals. Lifting up the foal's hoof is a necessary daily procedure when training the foal. In this way, a traumatic experience with a farrier or veterinary surgeon is avoided.

It is important for all foals that from an early age their hooves are checked and if necessary corrected. Correct and timely treatment can usually prevent a too-upright conformation caused by club foot or pes equinus.

CONCLUSION
A toe extension shoe is the ideal solution for pes equinus or club foot.

CASE HISTORY 1, PHOTO PAGE 96
A horse was presented that had too-upright hooves. As treatment, the horse was fitted with toe extension shoes and around the hoof capsule a cast– a strong synthetic bandage – was put on. This disorder can appear on one or both fore hooves. After three months, the hooves had grown enough and the cast could be removed. In this period, the hooves were supported by the extension so that their position was reinstated to a normal foot axis. The subsequent horseshoes consisted similarly of an extension shoe but with a somewhat shorter extension. The horseshoes had to be replaced a number of times for the hoof to regain a normal

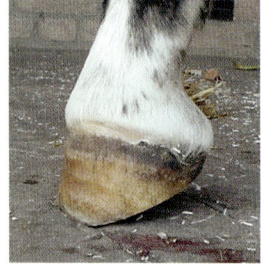
The hoof can no longer take weight on the heels and becomes increasingly upright; the pressure on the toe increases and the hoof is well on the way to having pes equinus.

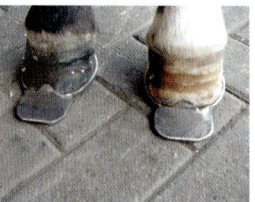
Both hooves have been given shoes with an iron toe extension so that the foal can no longer stand on its toes.

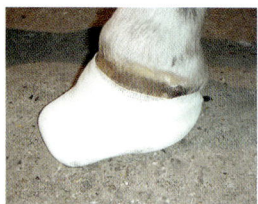
After shoeing, the hooves are set in a synthetic cast to give extra strength and to prevent the horseshoe being pulled off.

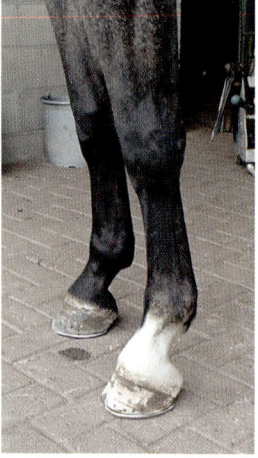
With careful guidance the farrier can ensure that the young horse can regain good limb conformation.

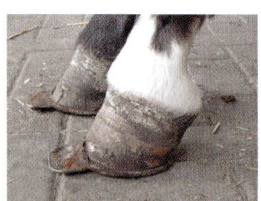
After three months, the hooves have grown sufficiently, the toe extension has done its work and the foot axis is nearly normal.

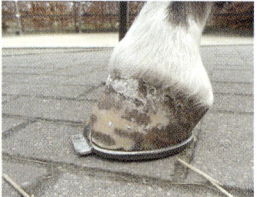
The hoof is re-shod but with a much shorter toe extension to ensure that the foot position is retained.

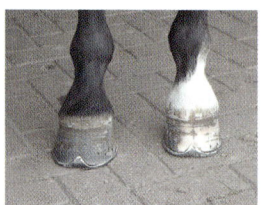
After two months the hooves are fully recovered and the traction of the deep and superficial flexor tendons is normal again.

position. After having shod the hoof several times in this way, the position was so changed that the foot axis was back to normal and the extension could be left off the shoe. In order to maintain the conformation the horse had always to be shod in good time. The traction or pulling power of the flexor tendon was reduced after a while; the position was thus kept correct, even without shoes. The hooves began to resemble each other in circumference and size. With the guidance of a good farrier this horse could enter competitions without problems.

3 THE LOWER FOOT: INSIDE

Cyst

It is generally accepted that the structure in the bones of horses is compact and close-knit and has a normal blood circulation. There is a bone membrane around the horse's bones. When there is loss of structure in a bone, commencing at the outer edge and travelling to the centre, then this is as a result of osteolyse (destruction of bone) and/or osteoporosis (bone disintegration). The cavity that appears as a result is called a cyst. Cysts can be very small – the size of a pin head – or very

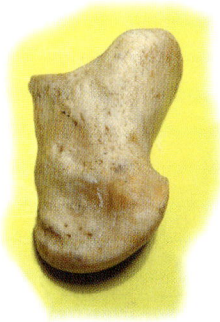

A healthy bone.

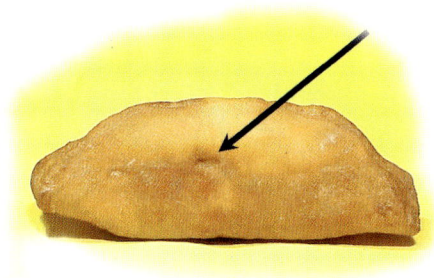

An example from the navicular bone. The black arrow shows a cyst at an early stage and which is just coming through to the joint surface; the deep flexor tendon slides over here.

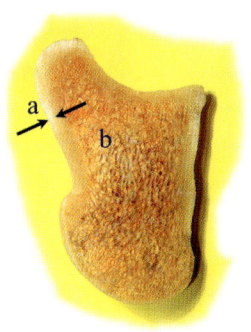

A cross-section in the length of a healthy bone. The outside is thin and hard (a). Toward the centre the structure becomes more weak and soft (b).

large, the size of a marble. A cyst is not detectable on the outside of a horse's limb, but when the cysts are big they can clearly been seen on X-rays.

CAUSE

A cyst can develop when there has been overtaxing or a trauma or a constant disturbance through disease. Trauma or overtaxing, especially among young horses, causes a disturbance in the supply of nutrients to the bone part concerned. Thus the bone part will die off, and destruction starts in the bone structure in the form of a cavity or cyst.

Horses that are troubled with one or more cysts display sporadic lameness. This lameness can appear suddenly, and then after a day completely disappear. People then think, incorrectly, that it is an inflammation of the hoof. However, lameness from hoof inflammation has a particular pattern, while that of a cyst does not.

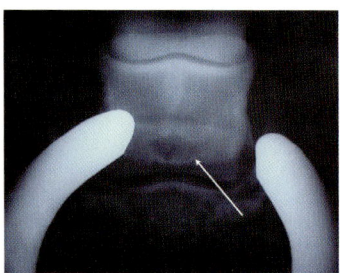
An X-ray of a navicular bone with a cyst on the gliding surface.

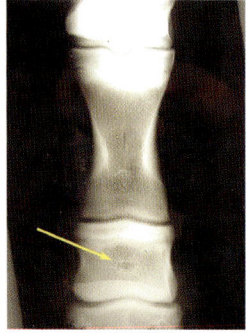
The yellow arrow on the X-ray shows a cyst in the short pastern bone of a horse. This cyst will not necessarily cause problems because it is in the centre of the bone.

DIAGNOSIS

Presence of a cyst can only be established with the help of X-ray photographs; on an X-ray of a horse with a cyst, small black flecks can be seen clearly. The black fleck indicates a cavity in the bone.

The degree of seriousness depends on the position of the cyst. Cysts under the joint cartilage surface are considered to be extremely serious because they lead to damage to the sliding surface of the joint. Cysts on the gliding surface of the joint always cause sporadic or serious lameness. For example, a navicular bone consists of practically only joint surfaces. A cyst at this spot will always cause lameness. When cysts lie deeper in the bone, they usually do not cause lameness and rarely create problems.

Cysts are quite common, mostly in small bone parts such as the hoof, coronary, pastern and navicular bones and the sesamoid bones. Horses with cysts are likely to be declared unfit at a veterinary examination yet they may possibly never have problems. They could, perhaps, nevertheless be approved but then there must be an examination to establish exactly where the cyst or cysts are. The exact spot of a cyst is difficult to pinpoint. X-rays must be taken from all sides so that the cyst's position can be established as accurately as possible.

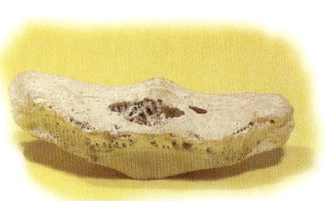
A sample of a navicular bone. The cavity (cyst) is clearly visible.

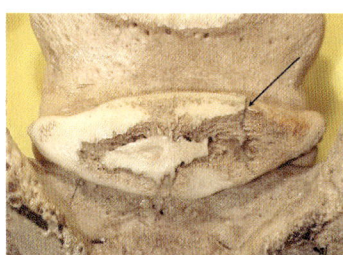
A navicular bone where the whole gliding surface is dissolved. As well as this, the bone is so weakened that a fracture has developed on the side.

TREATMENT

Cysts are extremely difficult to treat. When there is a cyst in the joint, the joint is often injected with hyaluronic acid at the spot where the cyst is. Hyaluronic acid is a fluid made by the body itself that can restore the cartilage of the gliding surface. In some cases an operation is helpful.

HORSESHOES

Horses with cysts are usually shod with a leather pad placed between the hoof and the shoe, to absorb concussion. Despite these horseshoes the prognosis can only be called moderate to poor.

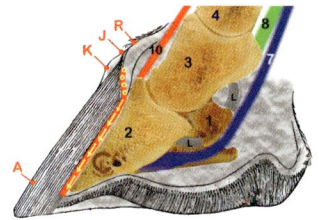

The horny wall is formed by the germinating layer of the coronary corium. This coronary corium (j) can, through trauma from outside, develop an abnormal cylindrical horny growth or a broad horny growth on the inside of the hoof capsule (red line with white arrows).

Keratoma

A keratoma is a new piece of horn tissue that grows from the coronary corium down the length of the hoof capsule internally; it grows down between the horny tubules and the wall corium. A keratoma is difficult to identify: there is mostly nothing to be seen on the hoof and sometimes it resembles harmless cracks in the horn at the coronary band.

CAUSE

Keratoma can form at any place in the hoof capsule. The cause is nearly always an inflammation, injury or a blow from outside, for example when a horse bangs its hoof against a pole when jumping or because it kicks against a stable door. The horny wall is formed by the germinating layer of the coronary corium. The damage causes the coronary corium to form an abnormal, internal, extra piece of horn growth. A keratoma runs the whole internal length of the horny wall next to the pedal bone. The keratoma presses on the corium against the pedal bone so that a groove develops even in the pedal bone and the horse becomes chronically lame.

A keratoma can also start in the middle of the horny wall. It is assumed that the interlaminar horn, formed by the wall corium laminae (insensitive laminae), receive a stimulus that causes a keratoma to commence. There are various kinds of keratoma that can each have different causes. A horse that constantly kicks against a door with its fore hoof can develop a wide or fan-shaped keratoma. A deep crack in the hoof capsule that has not been properly treated can also be the cause of a keratoma.

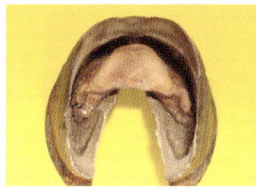

The hoof capsule seen from above, with the pedal bone inside.

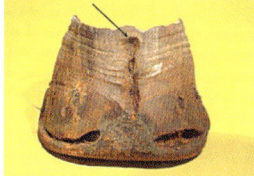

The full thickness horny wall crack is generally seen with coronary band injuries (striking of the coronet). The coronary corium can be so damaged that the hoof capsule can no longer heal properly.

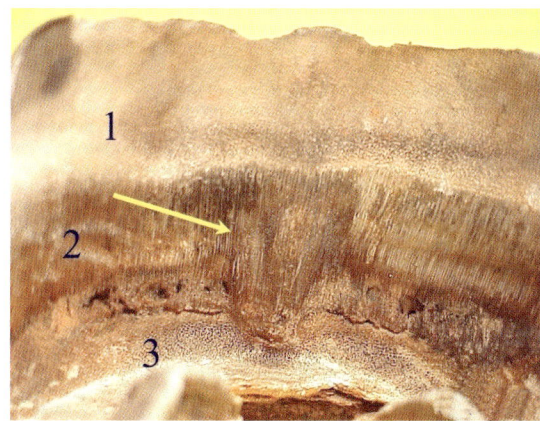

The internal horn growth of a keratoma: 1. Coronary corium. 2. Wall corium with laminae. 3. Sole. 4 The yellow arrow shows the keratoma.

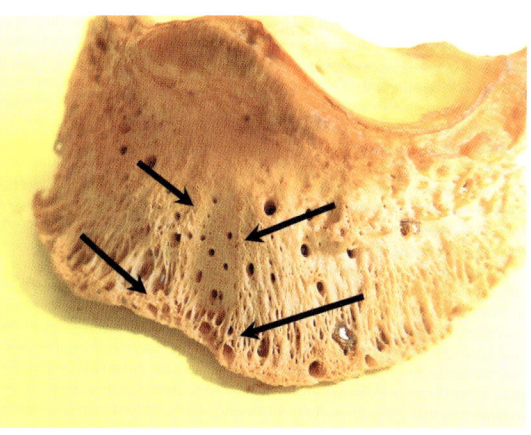

A groove develops in the pedal bone caused by the pressure of the keratoma; this leads to serious lameness.

The Lower Foot: Inside

DIAGNOSIS

A keratoma is extremely difficult to identify as it is very difficult to see on an X-ray. Sometimes it can be identified by little cracks under the coronary band that bleed every now and then; this indicates an infected keratoma. In some cases the white line reveals that there is a keratoma: the white line runs inwards in a crescent shape.

TREATMENT

A horse with a keratoma need not necessarily become lame, but if the horse does have difficulties then it must be operated upon and the keratoma must be removed in its entirety.

HORSESHOES

The shoes must be fitted before the operation. This prevents the hoof being drained of blood for an unnecessary length of time. This disorder requires a bar shoe – a horseshoe with a flat piece of steel welded between the ends of the branches – for stability of the shoe so that the hoof can function well. It is important to have the hooves shod in good time.

FAN-SHAPED KERATOMA

A fan-shaped keratoma is a new, fan-shaped piece of horny tissue formed by the germinating layer of the coronary corium; it grows down internally the length of the hoof capsule. Fan-shaped keratoma usually develop because the coronary band is constantly irritated, for example by being banged against a door. As well as this, a fan-shaped keratoma can result from an inflammation under the hoof that grows upward, toward the germinating layer, via a number of insensitive laminae.

A horse with a fan-shaped keratoma is not necessarily always lame as there is no pressure on the pedal bone. If the horse is lame, the fan-shaped keratoma must be removed. If the horse is not bothered by it, it need not be removed. It is difficult to identify a fan-shaped keratoma as it starts narrow and fans out, which often cannot always be seen on an X-ray.

CASE HISTORY: PHOTOS RIGHT AND OPPOSITE

A horse was presented with a fan-shaped keratoma; when the horny wall was filed away, a glass-like, viscous mass became visible where normally neatly joined together insensitive laminae should have been. As well as the fan-shaped keratoma, a fungal infection was discovered. This fungus is often present when there is inflammation or injury of the horny parts (see section on white line disease). The fungus was immediately treated, as it could loosen other parts of the hoof capsule.

A small channel was visible at the height of the entrance to the fan-shaped keratoma. This was the hoof inflammation that had caused the fan-shaped keratoma; the inflammation had already reached the germinating layer. Thus the germinating layer of the coronary corium had become irritated and it had developed a horny substance on the inside of

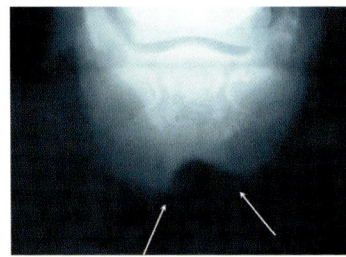

On this X-ray a hollowing out of the pedal bone can be seen, which indicates a keratoma. A keratoma that does not cause lameness need not be removed.

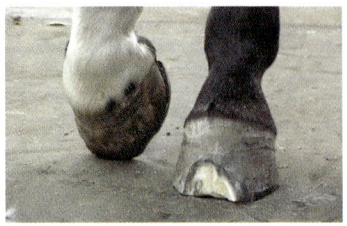

The horny wall must be removed to reach the keratoma.

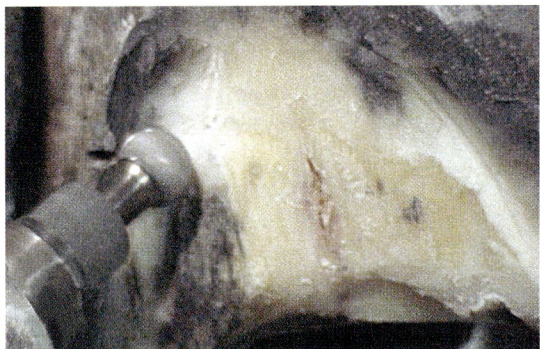

The affected part is laid bare to see if this keratoma will be troublesome.

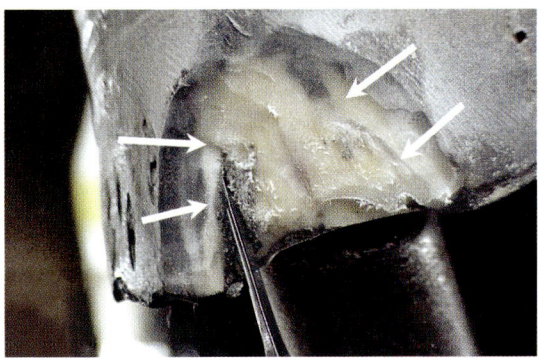

Next to the fan-shaped keratoma, a fungus is visible (white arrows).

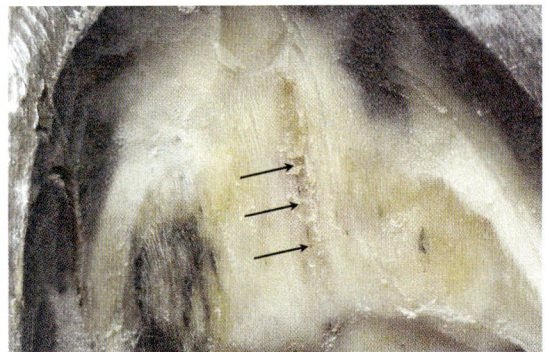

In the centre of the keratoma, a channel is visible. It is in this channel that the inflammation of the hoof could develop that was the cause of this fan-shaped keratoma.

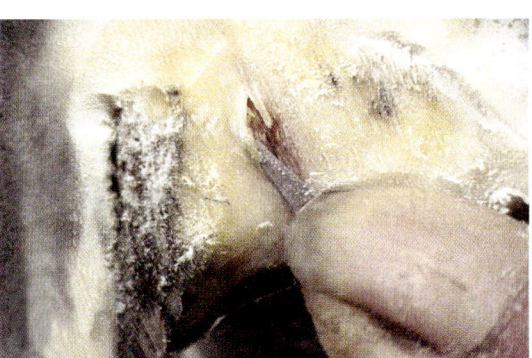

When opening up the channel, the insensitive and sensitive laminae can be separated from each other. Next to them, a glass-like, deviant tissue is visible.

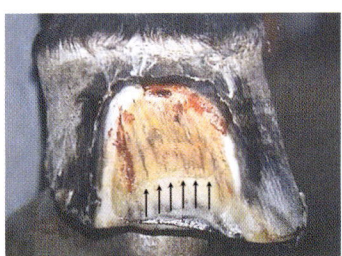

The fan-shaped keratoma is loosened from underneath, in the direction of the arrows.

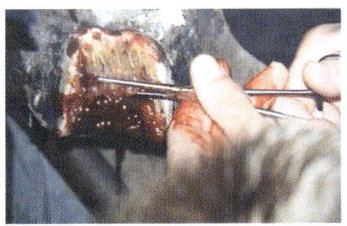

The whole shaft is pulled away from the hoof corium instead of being cut away, so that the tissues are sure to be removed.

the horny wall that subsequently grew down in a fan shape. After the channel had been opened up, the insensitive laminae could be separated from the sensitive laminae. As the horse was slightly lame, the fan-shaped keratoma was removed.

TOE KERATOMA

A toe keratoma is one in the toe part of the hoof. The cause of the development of a toe keratoma is nearly always an inflammation or injury on the coronary band or an inflammation of the white line that breaks out in the coronary band above. This causes the growth of a rather defective horny substance that forms a toe keratoma. As the toe keratoma presses on the wall corium and the pedal bone, a groove-shaped indentation can be created in the pedal bone, although this does not always occur. If such a groove-shaped indentation does occur this usually results in a permanently lame horse.

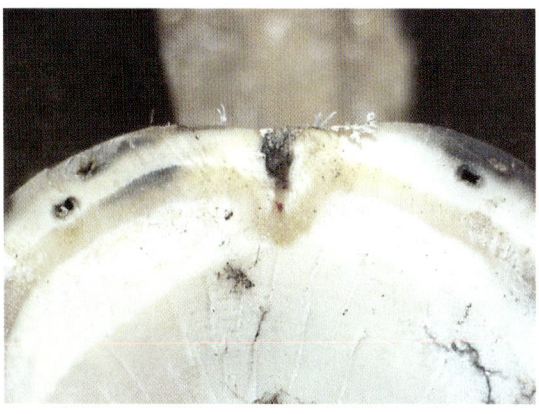

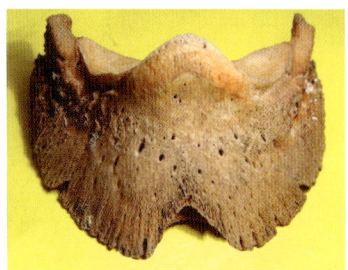

The toe keratoma has made a crescent-shaped indentation in the pedal bone.

On the sole side, a crescent-shaped curve in the white line is visible. This can be from damage coming from outside if, for example, the horse steps on a sharp object. In this way, dirt and small stones can get forced into the hoof and cause an inflammation. If the inflammation is treated too late, there is a chance that it will migrate upwards and break out at the coronary band. The keratoma causes the white line to be malformed.

DIAGNOSIS

The toe keratoma can be identified with X-rays. The X-ray shows the presence of a crescent-shaped or groove-shaped indentation in the pedal bone.

TREATMENT

If an indentation is present the keratoma must be removed in its entirety. It must be loosened from the hoof capsule and pulled away from the hoof corium. It is a very painful situation and of course it is done under anaesthesia of the lower foot and with draining of blood (by ligature).

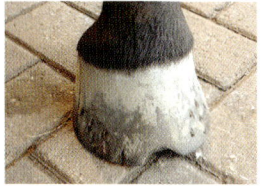

This horse stepped onto the clip of the horseshoe and was lame for months afterwards.

CASE HISTORY 2, PHOTOS HERE AND OPPOSITE

The owner reported that his horse had kicked off a shoe and had stepped onto the horseshoe clip. After that, the horse had irregular paces for months on end. Under the hoof it appeared that the white line displayed an extreme inward curve which seemed to indicate a keratoma. An X-ray examination showed that there was indeed a groove, which suggested a keratoma on the front of the pedal bone.

During treatment, the horny wall was filed out. The corium had a yellowish, glass-like structure and at the place where the inflammation had arisen – between the insensitive and sensitive laminae – a channel was visible. After the lower foot had been bound to restrict the blood flow, the keratoma under the hoof was cut away and pulled away from the wall corium in its entirety to ensure that all bad tissue was removed. This created a concavity in the horny wall

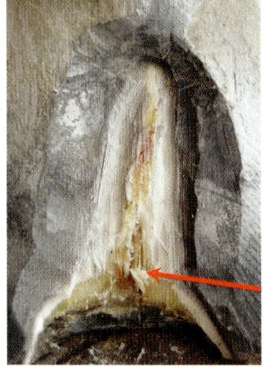

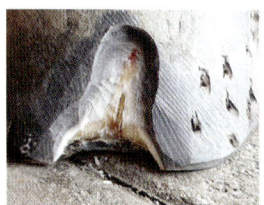

After the horny wall has been filed out, a yellowish corium and a channel between the insensitive laminae is visible where the inflammation can migrate upwards.

Part 2 – Disorders of the Limbs and Hooves

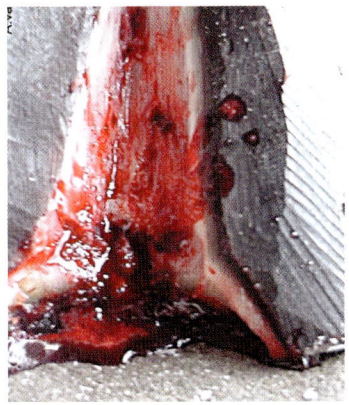
The toe keratoma is removed from the hoof capsule.

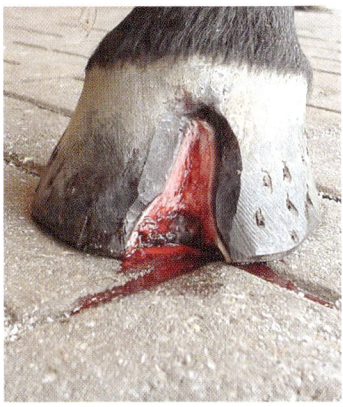
After removal of the toe keratoma, there is a cavity in the hoof as far as the pedal bone.

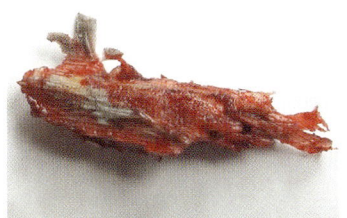
The keratoma after removal: it was between the pedal bone and the horny wall.

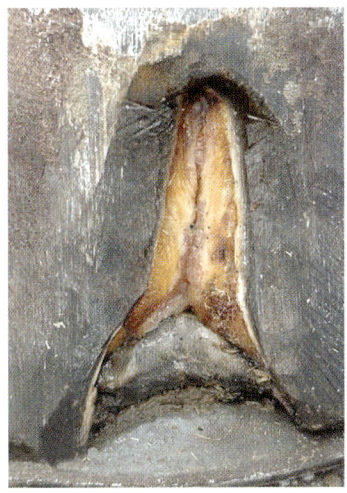
After two weeks the wound is dry. The corium has been compressed for two weeks and must now dry out.

reaching to the pedal bone. This concavity or wound was dressed with a compress so that the corium could not bulge out.

The farrier put the hoof on a horseshoe with two side clips to prevent the hoof capsule – of which part had been removed – from moving or collapsing. After the corium had been compressed for two weeks, it had healed and then had to dry out. It is important that such wounds are never closed with filler or paste because the corium would run the risk of infection. After about ten weeks, the hoof was shod with a normal horseshoe to stimulate the blood circulation of the hoof. The horse could begin gentle exercise again to stimulate the growth of the hoof. Indeed, movement is circulation, circulation provides nutrients, and nourishment means growth.

CASE HISTORY 3, PHOTOS HERE AND ON PAGE 104 (TOP)

A horse with a toe keratoma had its hoof unnecessarily damaged by the treatment given. The horseshoe was put on back to front in an attempt to reduce the pressure on the sole at the toe part. However, this had the

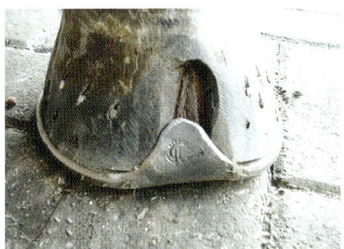
After ten weeks, the wound has hardened. The horse must begin gentle exercise to stimulate growth in the hoof.

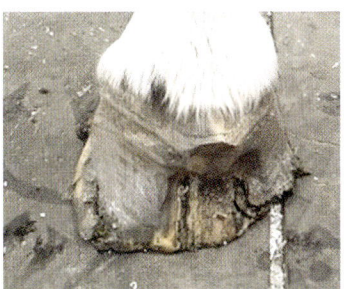
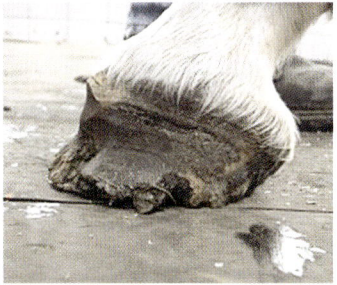
In this hoof, a keratoma has been removed; an example of unprofessional treatment. The coronary band has collapsed and has caused a deformed hoof. Such harrowing situations always lead to serious lameness.

The Lower Foot: Inside

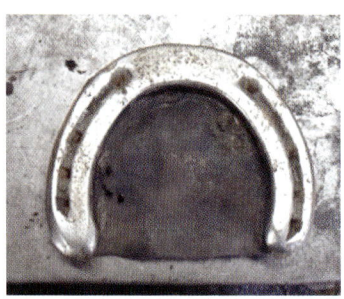

The horseshoe was placed back to front to reduce pressure in the area of the keratoma; this had an adverse effect because support in the toe area is actually extremely important.

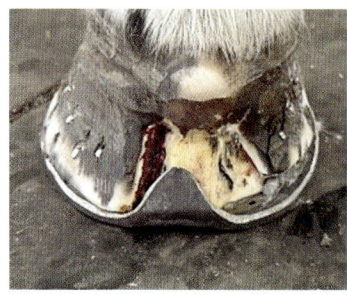

A normal horseshoe with a bar has been fitted under the hoof. The shoe has a toe clip to protect the area and thus it can be easily bandaged.

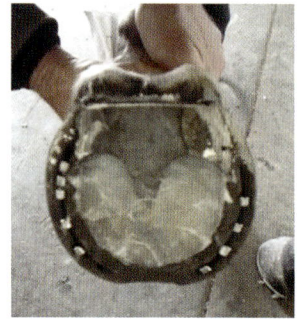

The horseshoe has been given a bar to prevent movement in the branches. Equi-Thane Hoof Pak® has been applied so that ground pressure is distributed over the whole horny wall and solar surface.

opposite effect because it is extremely important, with a toe keratoma, to support the toe area. The horse did not load the toe area any more, thus it remained lame.

In treating this problem, the hoof was trimmed in a normal way. Afterwards, the area with the toe keratoma was thoroughly cleaned by removing the bad parts. A normal horseshoe with a bar added was put on. The horseshoe had a clip at the toe to protect the area and for ease of bandaging. To relieve the wall, an Equi-Thane Hoof Pak® was put on to spread the pressure from the ground over the horny wall and the sole.

SIDE WALL KERATOMA

Side wall keratoma is distinguished from other types by cracks and distortion in the side of the horny wall or by too great a pressure on the heel area (long toes, low heels) of the hoof capsule. Through these defects of the hoof capsule, the pressure of the ground on the wall can be too great, which means extra pressure on the coronary corium.

An inflammation of the white line or nail line can equally be the cause of the development of a keratoma, but is less frequent. A similar inflammation stimulus causes the growth of a rather defective horny substance that forms a side wall keratoma.

HORSESHOES

Horses with side wall keratoma are shod with a bar shoe, preferably with wide branches and, between both branches, a light bar to prevent movement of the shoe. The walls must not be fixed, because the hoof mechanism on the underside of the hoof would be interfered with. Good shoeing is extremely important for side wall keratoma. The horseshoe must be generous and long so that the hoof capsule, even after eight weeks, rests on the shoe and does not shift from it. After a keratoma operation, nature always has an impulse to produce extra growth whereby the downward growth of the treated hoof can be much more than that of the other hooves.

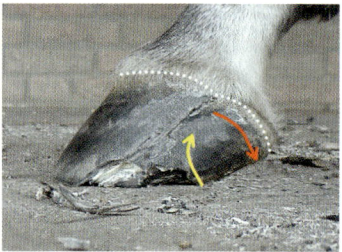

In the defective rounding of this coronary band (dotted line), the hoof capsule was caused to be pulled apart by the extreme ground pressure (yellow arrow). At the wall crack, the two parts of the hoof capsule in the coronary corium could move separately. A wall corium injury can result from this, with bleeding and inflammation.

CASE HISTORY 4, PHOTOS BELOW AND ON PAGE 106 (TOP)

A horse was presented that had a crack in its hoof. The farrier had fitted the shoe and, as protection, had put an extra clip on the crack in the hoof. Afterwards, the horse became lame. The horse had trouble with a continuously inflamed hoof crack. Actually, the crack made the hoof move in two separate parts. The heels of the hoof were extremely flat. The crack was pressed upwards (red arrow) from the ground pressure and the two parts of the hoof could move separately. The line of the coronary band was much too bulbous. If the foot remained in this condition, the crack would continue to bleed because of the movement of the separated parts of the hoof. After filing away part of the hoof capsule, a glass-like horn was visible. The glass-like horn should really be white in the form of laminae lying next to each other just as they are in the surrounding horn. Glass-like horn indicated that the cause of the crack was a side wall keratoma; the crack was sustained and had even split the hoof capsule into two separate parts.

The horse was lame so the side wall keratoma had to be removed. The horny wall was opened up as much as possible in the direction of the horny tubules so that the side wall keratoma was properly visible. The side wall keratoma was loosened underneath and pulled away from the wall corium and the pedal bone. No pieces of the keratoma should be left

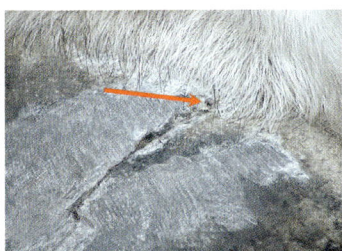

A traumatic horn crack; the horny wall has not closed up again.

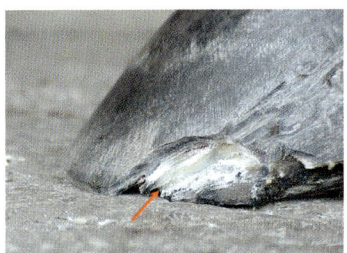

A piece of glass-like, tinted horn is clearly present in the horn (red arrow) that should actually be white just like the surrounding parts.

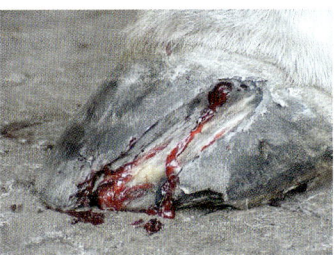

The horny wall is cut away so that the side wall keratoma can be exposed.

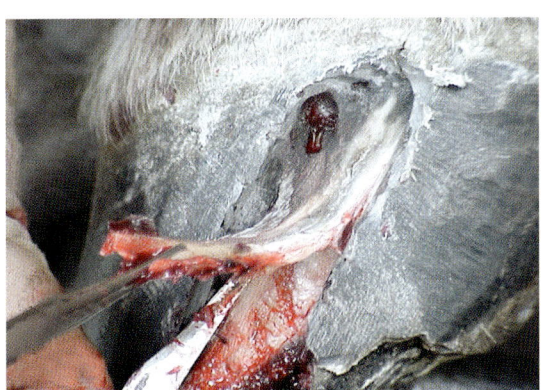

The keratoma is loosened underneath and pulled away from the wall corium and the pedal bone.

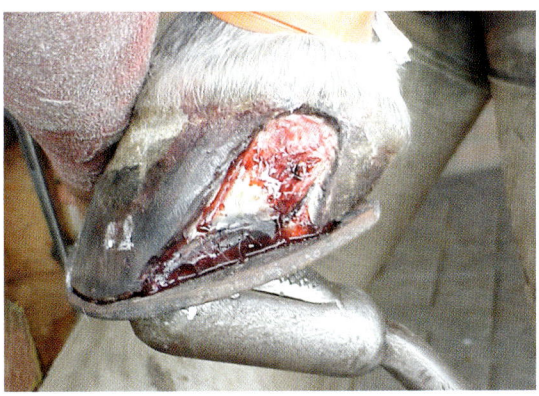

The side wall keratoma has been completely removed. Now a compress must be applied to prevent the corium from bulging out.

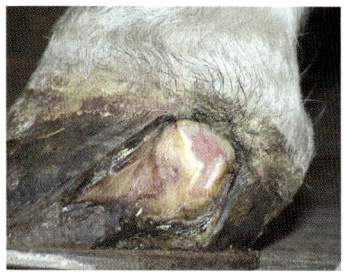
After two months, the wound is nearly healed. Above the wound, healthy horn growth is already present.

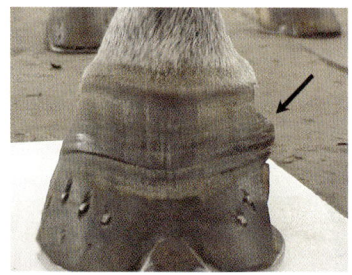
There is a deep, irregular horn growth visible and on the outside a thickening of the horn.

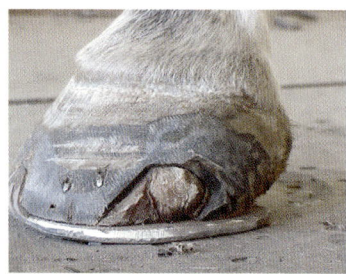
The new horn growth is well on the way, with a hoof of normal shape as a result.

behind. The germinating layer of the coronary corium – where the side wall keratoma had developed – was also thoroughly cleaned. After removing the side wall keratoma a compress was applied so that the corium would not bulge out. After a couple of months, the wound was nicely dry and the horse was no longer lame.

The growth downwards continued steadily because the horse had no more pain; when there is pain in the lower foot, no matter what the cause, the growth of the hoof capsule is reduced. A deep, irregular horny growth became visible and, on the outside, a thickening of the horn. The thickening was caused by a reaction from the coronary corium to the hoof being treated. This thickening acts as a strengthening of the hoof and should remain as long as possible. With the thickened horny wall – which develops because of an impulse from the coronary corium – a collapse of the coronary band can be prevented. The newly thickened horn growth can sometimes grow thickly for months; afterwards, the hoof capsule will resume its normal thickness.

Low and High Ring-bone

Ring-bone is a chronic inflammation process that goes together with bone proliferation. Ring-bone appears in the pastern joint (high ring-bone) and/or in the hoof joint (low ring-bone) or in the bones in the area close to these joints. Ring-bone is a form of arthrosis.

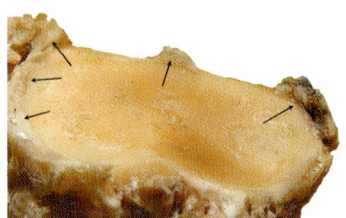
On the joint sides of the short pastern bone, the build-up of bone is clearly present.

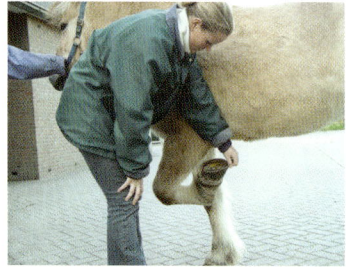
A good example of a flexed lower foot: the fetlock can easily be bent to 90 degrees.

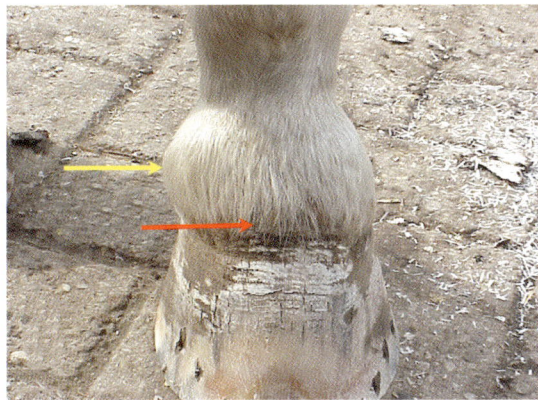

High ring-bone is clearly visible (yellow arrow; the red arrow shows where there is low ring-bone). The germinating layer of the hoof capsule will react with coarse growth of the horny wall.

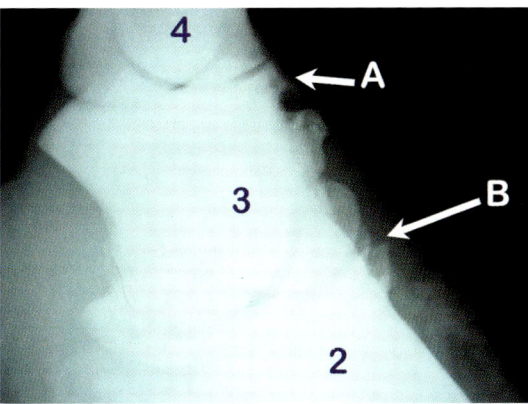

The low ring-bone is partly enclosed in the hoof capsule under the coronary band (B). This will finally lead to a lot of pain when the hoof is moved forward and also result in a thick, swollen edge above the coronary band. In the high ring-bone (A) the joint does not bend sufficiently. This leads to serious lameness that unfortunately is beyond curing.
2. Pedal bone; 3. Short pastern bone; 4. Long pastern bone.

CAUSE

Among other things, ring-bone can be caused by:
1. An inflammation of the joints (arthritis) that has not healed well and which, as a result, has caused extra bone formation.
2. Too much weightbearing of the limbs.
3. A strike or blow in the area of the coronary band, such as can happen in show jumping.

Before continuing further, let us first look at a little of the anatomy of the foot extremity. In the foot extremity the horse has only hinge (ginglymus) joints. The most important flexor tendons lie over these joints in the

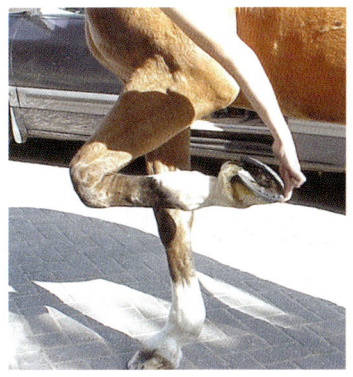

A clear example of high ring-bone; flexing in the lower foot is absent.

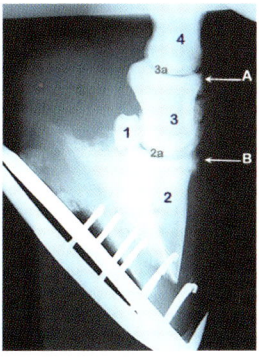

On this X-ray, taken at an angle sideways, ring-bone is clearly visible. A: High ring-bone (at the pastern joint 3a); B: Low ring-bone (at the hoof joint 2a); 2. Pedal bone; 3. Short pastern bone; 4. Long pastern bone.

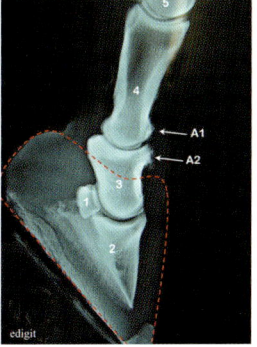

The commencement of high ring-bone. On this X-ray, the top of the short pastern bone (A2) and the bottom of the long pastern bone (A1) clearly have bone proliferation. This horse is already sporadically lame. When moving, the arthrosis will put pressure on the coronary band, which will cause lameness. (Hoof capsule, red dotted line.)

The Lower Foot: Inside

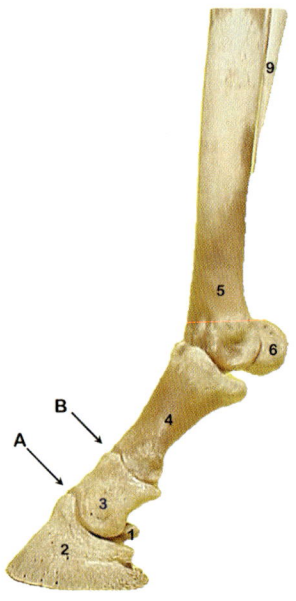

1. Navicular bone
2. Pedal bone
3. Short pastern bone
4. Long pastern bone
5. Cannon bone
6. Sesamoid bone
9. Small metacarpal bone
A. The hoof joint. Low ring-bone can occur here.
B. The coronary joint. High ring-bone can occur here.

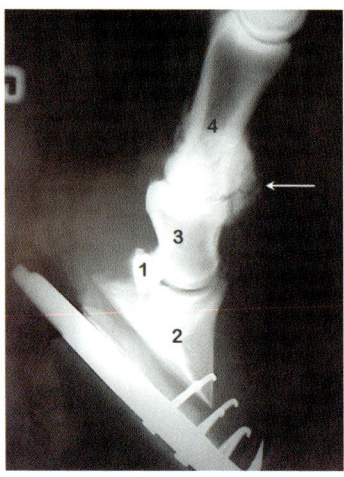

An X-ray taken of the side-view of the lower foot. Ring-bone can be seen clearly on the coronary joint. It can also be seen that this ring-bone is extremely coarse and has spurs; this will have serious consequences for the movement of the horse.

lower leg: the extensor tendon in the front and the deep and superficial flexor tendons at the back. The horse flexes these tendons as the lower leg moves forward. If the tendons move across a place where bone proliferation (arthrosis) has formed, a pain reaction commences. The horse reduces the forward movement of its hooves and picks them up more quickly; the result is a short movement because the horse wants to place its hooves on the ground carefully. More weight is put on the heels of the hooves, thus the toe of the hoof capsule becomes longer.

Ring-bone leads to an insidious lameness that can vary from a slight form to a very serious form. Horses with low ring-bone become lame more quickly than horses with high ring-bone because the pastern joint has much more movement than the hoof joint and is enclosed in the hard hoof capsule.

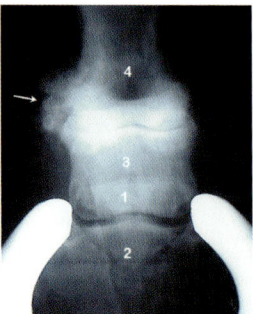

This X-ray was taken from front to back and shows that this high ring-bone also has prolific bone growth on the side of the coronary joint.

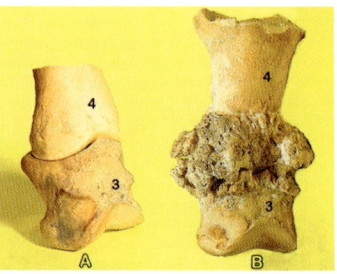

These specimens show again the seriousness of the bone proliferation. The coronary joint as it looks normally (A). On the right, the same joint with extra bone growth (B).

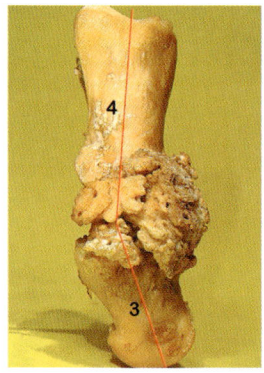

The short pastern and long pastern bones of this specimen look even more serious than that of the X-ray; there is extremely aggressive bone proliferation.
3. Short pastern bone; 4. Long pastern bone

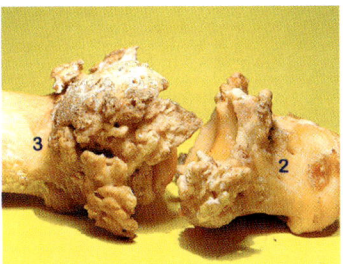

Here, both bones could still move separately, but the bone proliferation was entangled together, which caused the horse much pain and it displayed serious lameness.

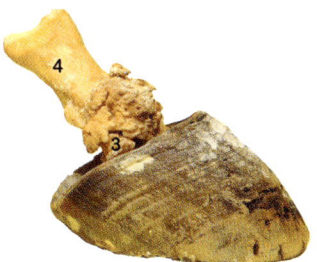

If the short pastern and long pastern bones are placed in the hoof capsule, it is clear to see here that the bones no longer fit and this causes the horse severe pain.

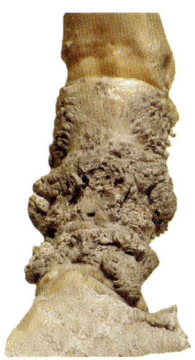
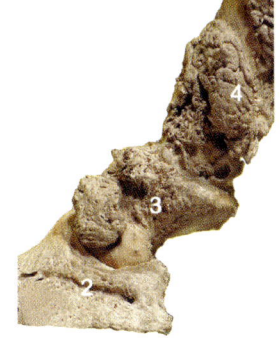

A high and low ring-bone where the joints can no longer be seen. The whole lower foot can no longer move.

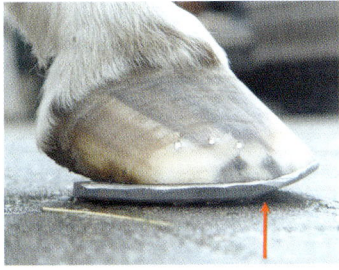

A horse with ring-bone can be really helped with a Hoofcare® Breakover horseshoe. This horseshoe ensures that the horse can, without difficulty, roll its hoof forward (rocker toe). The breakover moment (red arrow) is further back under the hoof as compared to traditional horseshoes. Shoeing in this way means the horse has less difficulty in rolling the hoof over and will thus suffer less pain.

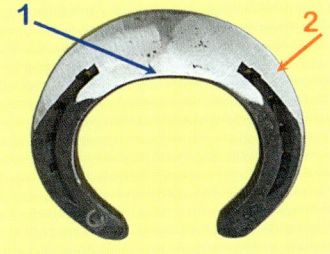
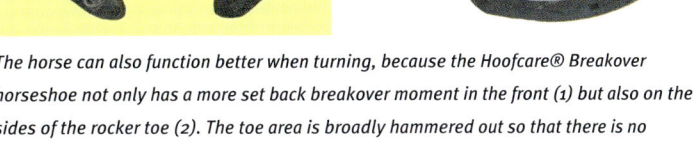

The horse can also function better when turning, because the Hoofcare® Breakover horseshoe not only has a more set back breakover moment in the front (1) but also on the sides of the rocker toe (2). The toe area is broadly hammered out so that there is no pressure on the sole.

HORSESHOES

When fitted with special shoes, a horse that has ring-bone problems can move reasonably to well. The axis of the foot should not be changed because, in so doing, the painful joints would be put into another position: this horse should not have its conformation corrected but must be put under guidance in its existing conformation. A horse with ring-bone will put more pressure on the heels in order to reduce the pain. In this way, the horn wall of the toe has every chance to become longer.

The Lower Foot: Inside

The actual conformation of the horse must be fully respected when shoeing. Indeed, to help the horse to be able to make the correct breakover at the toe, more hoof wall at the toe should be trimmed than is normal. The shoe should be roomy and long and be so forged that the hoof can easily move forward. This can be helped by using a Hoofcare® Breakover horseshoe: the Hoofcare® Breakover horseshoe helps the hoof to breakover smoothly without difficulties. The breakover point should lie 2 to 3 centimetres behind the point of the toe. This can be brought about by hammering the toe at the front of the shoe so that it becomes wedge-shaped. This horseshoe can also improve turns as the sides of the shoe can be designed in the same way.

Ostitis

Ostitis is an inflammation of the bone tissue.

CAUSE
Ostitis can develop when a horse bangs its hoof against something. This causes a reaction, which causes an inflammation of the bone, which instigates a disintegration of the bone.

CASE HISTORY 1, PHOTOS BELOW AND PAGES 111–112
A horse that was presented was extremely lame. In the front of the hoof capsule there was a deep hoof crack. The veterinary surgeon had partly removed it but the horse was still lame. The corium under the hoof capsule was inflamed and dark in colour; when healthy, the corium is creamy white in colour. The hoof crack was filed away at the coronary band to see if there was any healthy tissue. When the horny wall was removed, a rotted corium was discovered, which indicated an inflammation in the hoof capsule. The horny wall was filed out further and the inflamed part removed. It ejected a mass of thick, viscous pus; this indicated an inflamed piece of bone tissue that had been under pressure in the hoof capsule. This had caused lameness in the horse.

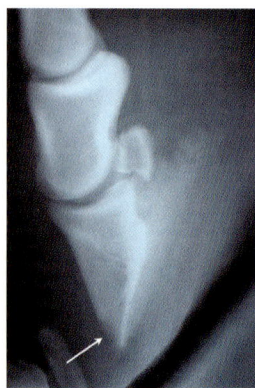

An X-ray of a side-view of the pedal bone clearly showing a cavity.

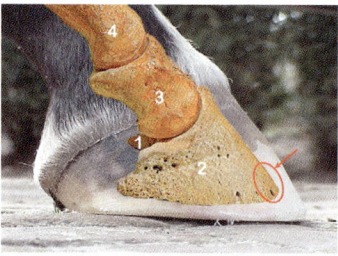

The red circled area shows where the problem lies.
1. Navicular bone; 2. Pedal bone; 3. Short pastern bone; 4. Long pastern bone.

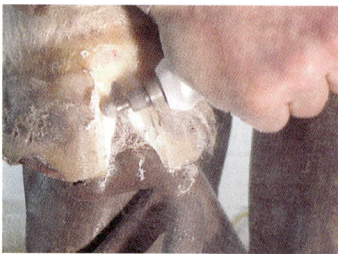

The hoof crack is filed out until a healthy attachment of the horny wall is reached.

After treating the horny wall, the pedal bone was cleaned. The whole treatment took place under full draining of blood whereby the lower foot was temporarily tied off. The hoof was shod and put in a compress. After careful treatment of the wound for three weeks, it appeared that the hoof had healed well. Subsequently, the corium had to dry out so that this could once again give strength to the hoof.

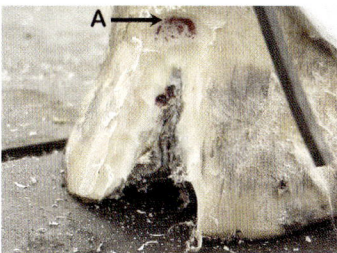

Under the removed horny wall, the rotting corium is clearly visible, which indicates that there is an inflammation in the hoof capsule. (A) The filed-out part of the coronary corium.

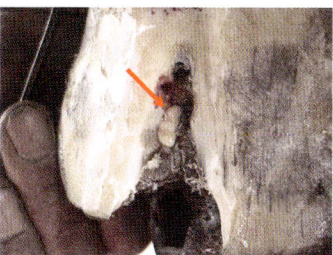

When the horny wall was filed out, a thick viscous substance was made visible; this indicates inflammation in the bone tissue that has been under pressure in the hoof capsule.

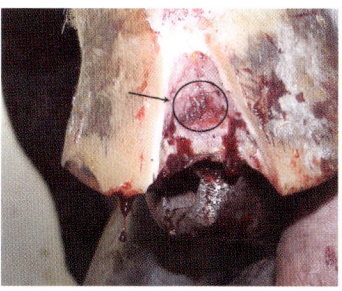

After the horny wall has been further opened out, the pedal bone is drained of blood and cleaned (black circle).

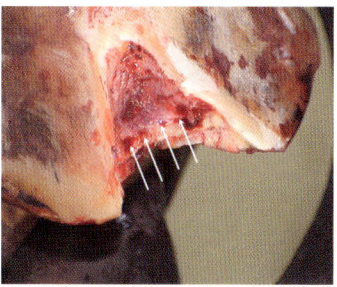

The filed-out pedal bone. The horny wall is thoroughly filed-out so that everything can be seen. Here, the edge of the pedal bone is easier to see (arrows).

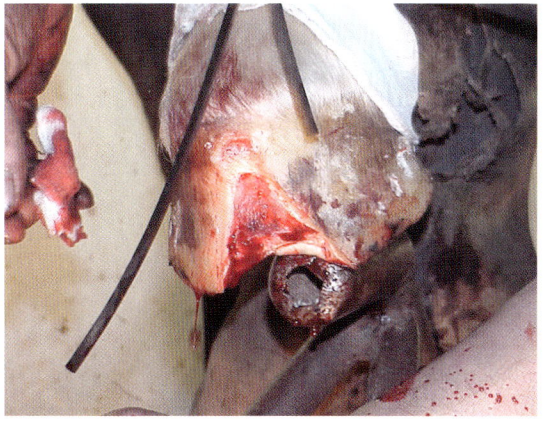

After the area has been treated, a clean wound is visible. The hoof is immediately shod with a shoe with two clips which keep the front part of the hoof 'at rest'.

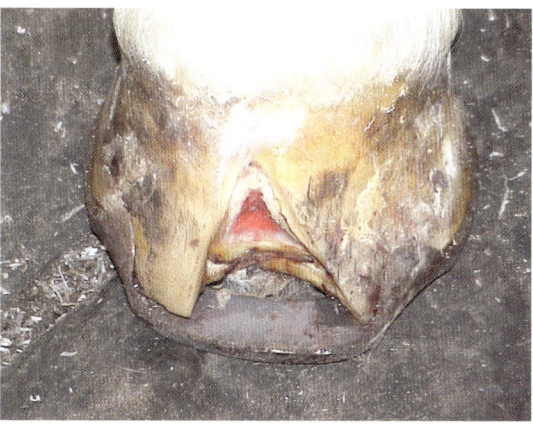

The wound is properly treated for three weeks and thus the horse is quickly and nicely healed.

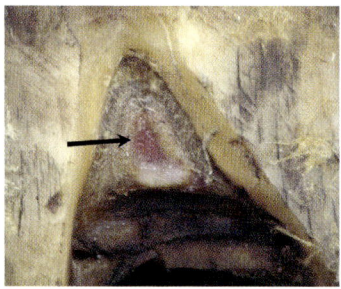
The wound is dry except for a small area; in a couple of days it will close off.

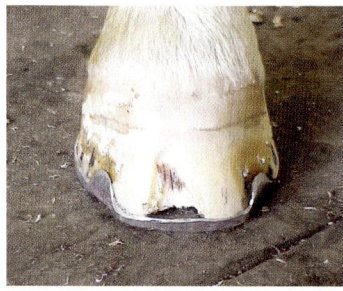
The hoof after five months: the hoof capsule has almost completely grown down. The horse can start gentle exercise.

During treatment the horse was given a horseshoe with two clips so that the affected part could be temporarily 'rested'; the clips ensure that the hoof capsule moves as little as possible. The front of the horseshoe – the part between the two clips – was broadly forged so that the treated area was protected and to prevent ground pressure on the hoof stressing the wound. In this way the hoof could be properly bound.

4 THE HOOF: CORONARY BAND

Irritation of the Coronary Band

This is an irritation of the perioplic ring and/or the coronary corium at the coronary band. It is found in horses that are kept stabled for long periods and where the hooves are looked after intensively on a daily basis.

CAUSE

Irritation of the coronary band can be caused by frequently scrubbing the hooves with a stiff brush, such as a steel brush, and by an excessive use of oils, ointments and irritant products. An irritation of the coronary band under the hairs can be the result of this. The perioplic ring, together with the perioplic corium and the coronary band with the coronary corium, are sometimes even blistered by these products.

By long-term use of irritant products, irritation of the coronary band

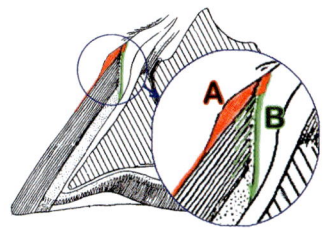

Irritation occurs in the area of the coronary band. The perioplic ring (A) is responsible for the protective layer: the glaze-like layer of the hoof capsule. The coronary band with the coronary corium (B) is responsible for the development of the hoof capsule.

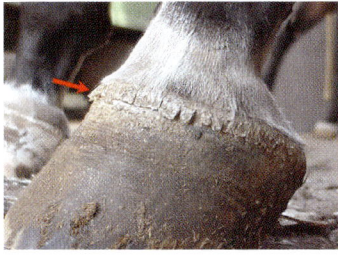 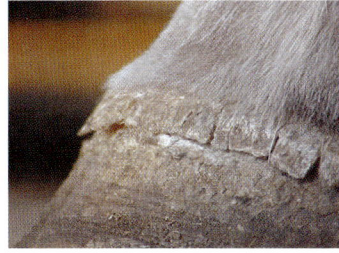

By constant oiling of the coronary band, the perioplic ring can become irritated and sometimes even blister. The perioplic ring on the horse in the picture has become irritated and displays defective horn growth (2). The coronary corium hasn't yet been affected; the problem is limited to the perioplic ring but the horny wall shows no defect.

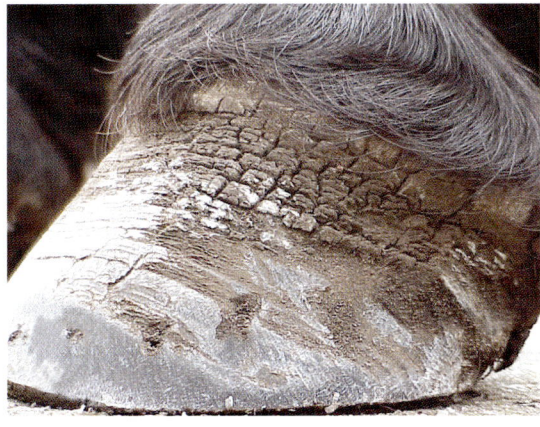

can lead to an inflammation of the perioplic ring, the coronary corium under the perioplic ring, and the bulb corium at the back of the hoof. When there is irritation at the perioplic, coronary and bulb coriums, abnormal horny growth commences, which can lead to a change in the horn structure.

An example of serious irritation; the horny wall changes in structure.

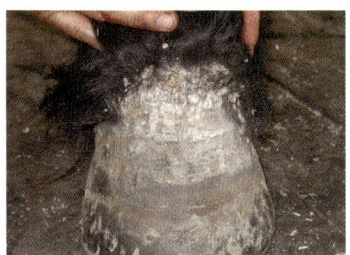

The perioplic ring and the coronary band are irritated and inflamed; this is a frequent problem among horses with a lot of feather.

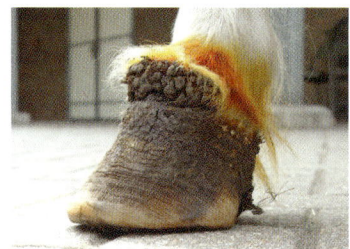

A case of extreme irritation where the coronary corium has produced an explosion of horn so that good growth of the horny wall is no longer possible.

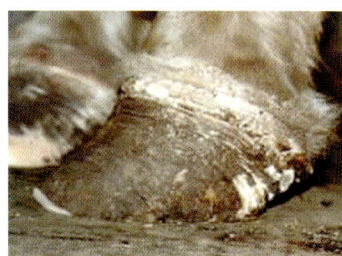

The hairs are standing on end at this perioplic ring and the epidermis is irritated. This irritation can lead to an inflammation of the perioplic ring, the coronary band (under the perioplic ring) and the bulb corium (at the back of the foot). Due to the irritation of the perioplic ring, coronary and bulb corium, the production of abnormal scaly horn with fissures and cracks occurs. This is very painful for the horse.

IRRITATION OF THE PERIOPLIC RING

When there is irritation on the perioplic ring – not on the coronary corium – the protective or varnish-like layer that grows down with the horny wall becomes loose and hardened. The drying-out is extremely painful for the horse. When removing it, there will be heavy bleeding at the coronary band. There are rarely serious complications. However horses can, in the long-term, get an 'explosion of horn' and a painful coronary band or become seriously lame due to the fact that fissures develop in the epidermis which are extremely painful. The horny wall will not display any structural changes.

IRRITATION OF THE CORONARY CORIUM

When there is irritation on the coronary corium the structure of the horny wall does change and there will be an over-production of horn with small horizontal and vertical cracks.

TREATMENT

The treatment of this type of irritation is simple. It is extremely important that the application of oils, ointments and irritant products to the

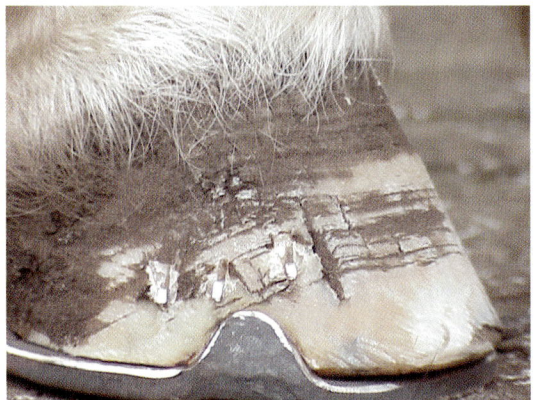

After shoeing and treatment of the hoof capsule, the horizontal and vertical cracks are visible. These continue to develop but lessen when the coronary band has been treated for a time.

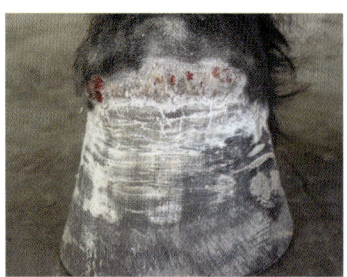

The horny wall and the coronary band area are cleaned. The hair is shaved so that this painful area can be properly treated. After cleaning, a little pure Vaseline or baby ointment is massaged into the irritated skin.

coronary band and the horny wall is stopped immediately. If the hoof is oiled every day, the horny wall and the horn sole are sealed off from moisture and dry out. Many people think this can be avoided by wetting the hoof before oiling so that the water remains under the oil. Oil needs a good base and this is not the case if water is used: the water is pushed off the hoof by the oil and the hoof becomes sealed and can become dried out.

When treating the irritation, wash the hooves with water and soft soap (containing glycerine). Do this with a soft brush or sponge. After washing, it is best to massage the irritated skin with a small amount of pure Vaseline or baby ointment.

HORSESHOES

A horse that is troubled by irritation should have large horseshoes so that the hooves can function to the optimum. To get rid of the irritation, it is necessary to remove the superfluous horn and to clean up. By making the coronary band and perioplic ring wet for a while the superfluous horn softens and can easily be removed. Horses with this type of irritation need constant and intensive treatment.

Damage to the Coronary Band

Coronary band damage is damage or injury that is on and/or around the area of the coronary band.

CAUSE

Damage to the coronet occurs, for example, during transport. While being transported, a horse can lose its balance and can thus step on its own hooves, whereby the coronary band is injured. Coronary band damage

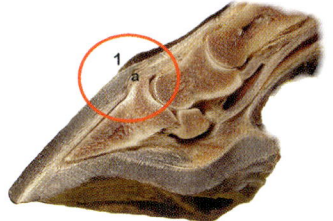

The red circle indicates where the perioplic ring is (1). The perioplic ring ensures that the hoof capsule is protected. The coronary corium (a) produces the horny tubules of the wall.

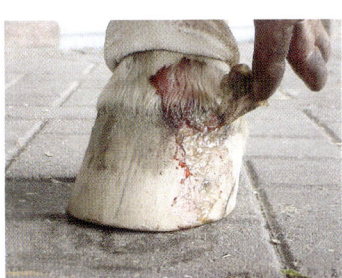

A piece of the coronary band has been kicked off. Fortunately, the coronary band is still reasonably intact. The owner acted quickly and immediately dressed the wound so that no dirt could get in.

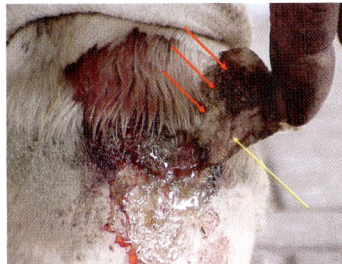

The horn has been torn off from the coronary corium (red arrows) and the wall corium (yellow arrow). The loose piece is removed. The wound is cleaned and a Betadine (iodine) compress is put in to prevent the coronary corium and the wall corium from bulging out.

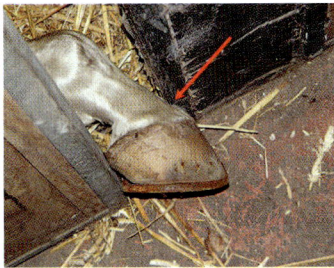

The coronary band can be damaged by all sorts of accidents. In this case the horse caught his hoof while rolling in the stable.

also occurs in equestrian sports such as in eventing or show jumping. In sport, a horse must give its all and it does not always watch where it is putting its hooves; damage easily occurs. Damage also occurs if a horse gets its hoof trapped and injures itself when pulling free. Usually, coronary band injuries occur with great force and the wound is often very serious.

If the coronary band is seriously damaged at the time of wounding, the development of the horn will change. This can lead to a change in the hoof capsule. Permanent cracks can also develop; from these, keratoma and deformed hoof capsules can result. Both can lead to the horse becoming lame.

TREATMENT

A coronary band injury must be treated straight away. Apply a bandage immediately to staunch the blood and to prevent dirt from entering the wound. Call the veterinary surgeon immediately. During healing of the wound, the germinating layer of the coronary band produces an extra thick horny wall. This is a natural reaction of the germinating layer to the serious injury at the coronary band. It is important that the extra layer of horn remains temporarily, because it gives extra support to the coronary band and ensures that the damaged and slowly healing coronary band does not collapse. After the horny wall has grown a couple of centimetres, the coronary corium resumes a normal thickness whereby the hoof capsule once again resumes its original form. The thickening of the horny wall grows down with the hoof capsule and in the end is

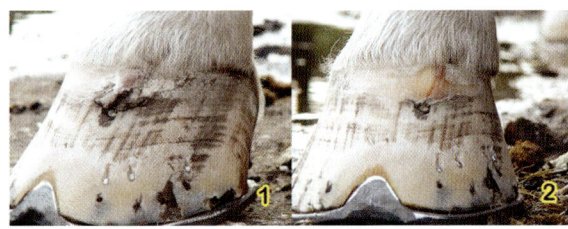

The horny wall will react to damage by thickening (1). After removal of extra horn, the defect is clearly visible (2).

trimmed away by the farrier. A horseshoe should be fitted that supports the whole hoof capsule; a light bar is welded between the two branches to prevent friction from the horseshoe.

CASE HISTORY 1, PHOTOS OPPOSITE

A horse, rolling over in the stable, caught its foot under the door; when rolling, the horse pushed its leg between the sliding doors and then tried to pull it out. Thus the coronary band and epidermis above were bruised. Due to the localised swelling, the coronary corium – which ensures the growth of the hoof capsule – was not able to continue normal hoof capsule growth. This meant a break in the growth process. As long as there is pain in the hoof, the horn growth will be temporarily retarded. It is an extremely difficult task for the farrier to keep such horses functioning.

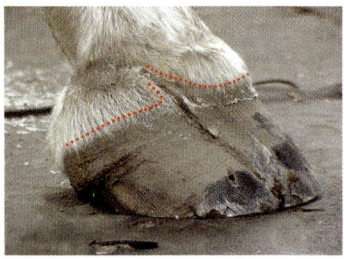

A permanent crack in the horny wall can occur when there is damage to the coronary band. The coronary corium (red dotted line) has attached itself in another spot which results in defective horn growth.

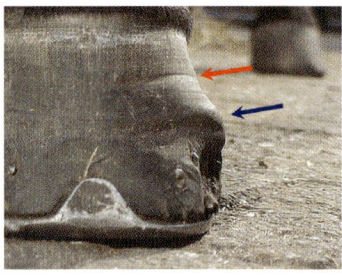

It is important to allow extra horn growth (blue arrow) to remain temporarily as this gives extra support to the coronary band and ensures that the coronary band – which heals slowly – does not collapse. After a time, the coronary corium grows normally (above the red arrow) and the hoof shape will be restored.

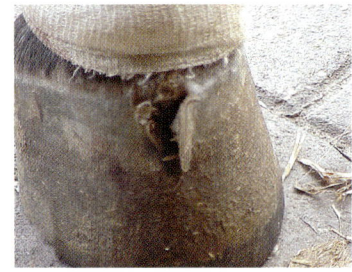

Coronary band damage due to calks in the horseshoe.

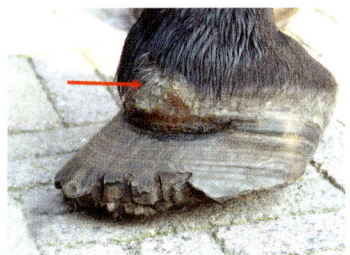 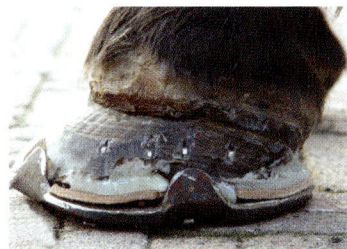 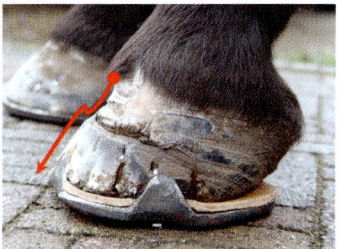

The epidermis and the coronary band are bruised. This has caused swelling in the area, and the coronary corium, responsible for the hoof capsule growth, can no longer produce normal horn growth.

As long as there is pain in the hoof there will be no horn growth. The swelling must subside before the coronary corium can heal. It is however important to shoe the hooves to protect the healthy walls. When the horse tried to free itself, it pulled off both its shoes; a lot of horn was lost, and the farrier had a difficult task because a lot of the weightbearing edge was missing. In this case, the hooves were shod with three clips; between the horseshoe and the sole there is a leather edge enabling the horse to carry more weight on the soles, as well, which is actually not usual (a horse cannot walk on its soles but only on the horny wall).

After two months, the hoof capsule is healing well, once again producing healthy horn that grows down correctly. We try to keep the rest of the wall intact although it is loose. The loose part is left as long as possible as it is needed for the nailing.

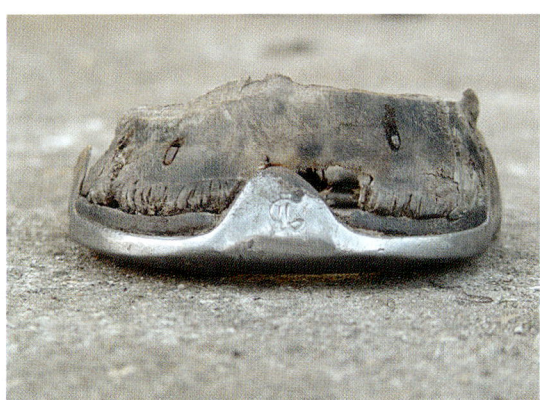 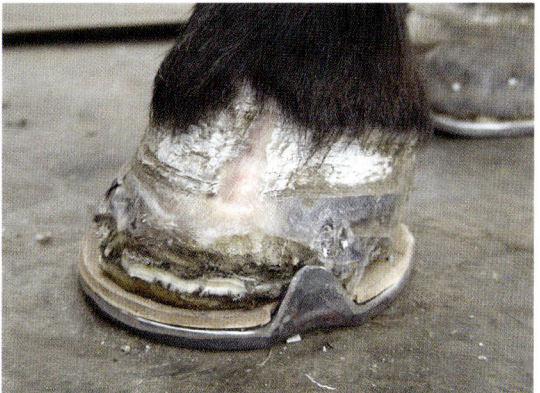

After four months. This shows just how loose the horny capsule was. Nevertheless, it could be used for a while. We can now also see the effects of a serious bruising of the coronary band and the coronary corium.

There is only a small stump of hoof capsule, yet it is of good quality. The hoof will be shod temporarily with two clips. The shoe can only have four nails. The horse had, up until then, been able to produce a very strong, normal hoof without complications. It will take time but, with good guidance and care by the owner, this horse can resume normal work. The stable was repaired so that no more accidents of this sort could happen.

The Hoof – Coronary Band

Sandcrack

Sandcrack is a break in the horny tubules of the horny wall in or around the area of the coronary band. It can be superficial or full thickness – that is to say, through the whole thickness of the wall. These cracks can also be infected.

CAUSE

Sandcracks arise from an outside blow, chronically inflamed laminae inside the hoof capsule, a keratoma or as a consequence of stresses arising from chronic foot imbalance. Sandcracks can also develop from damage to the coronary band. Damage to the coronary band can occur during transport or if, during movement, the horse catches its fore hoof with its hind hoof. Sandcracks that arise from damage to the coronary band always follow the direction of growth of the horny tubules. If a

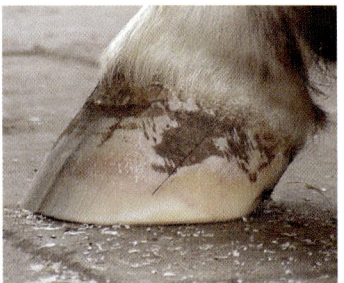

A tiny crack can have huge consequences.

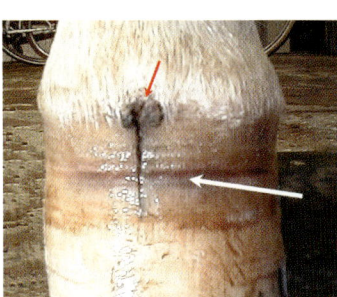

An infected sandcrack (red arrow). The break in the coronary band has been there for about eight weeks (white arrow).

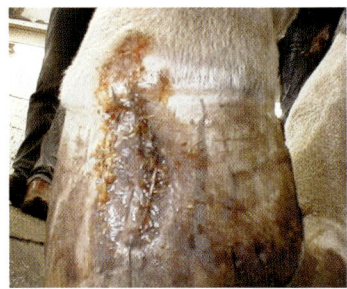

An inflamed sandcrack as a result of an internal keratoma that is infected. If the keratoma is not removed, the coronary band will continue to crack. This causes serious lameness.

sandcrack grows down in a wavy line without following the direction of the horny tubules, it indicates a serious problem. These cracks can even bleed.

Sandcracks can appear gradually but they can also appear suddenly. When there is a sandcrack, the germinating layer of the coronary band, the coronary corium, ensures that the normal horn growth is arrested. Horses with sandcrack can become lame gradually. If nothing is done about the sandcrack, the horse can suffer serious lameness.

TREATMENT

The area around the sandcrack must be thoroughly examined. In so doing, note should be taken of the depth of the crack and the cause of the crack, for example by a blow, trauma or a keratoma.

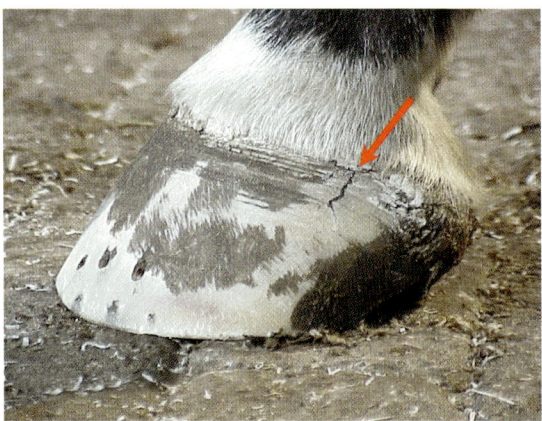

A crack which runs in a wavy line. This indicates the problem: it can be a result of infected insensitive laminae or a keratoma. Both are very serious.

A hoof with a sandcrack is better not shod with clips on the side of the horseshoe: extra pressure could then develop in the coronary band due to the horny wall underneath being immobilised. The horseshoe should be large and long so that the hoof mechanism can function well without hindrance.

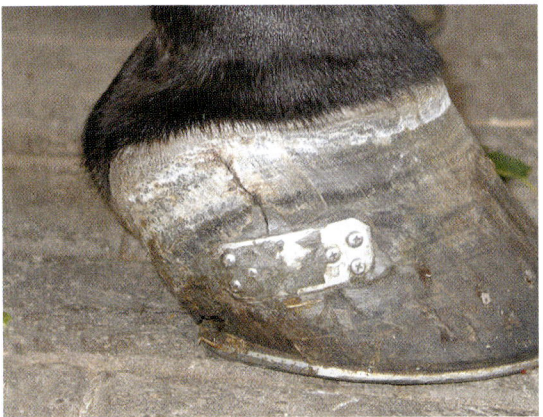

Many farriers think that all cracks in the wall can be fixed by screwing or sticking with metal plates or even with clasps. The saying 'putting the cart before the horse' is appropriate here.

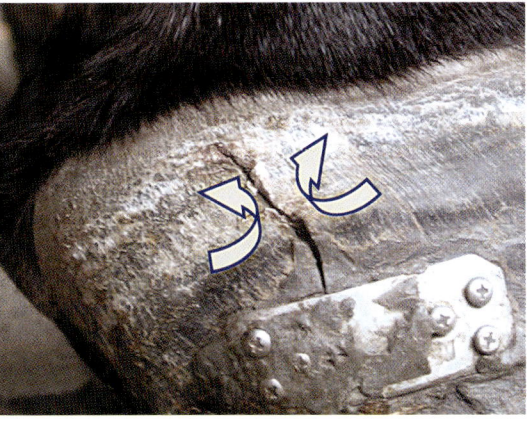

The sandcrack can never heal this way and can even cause more pressure on the coronary corium.

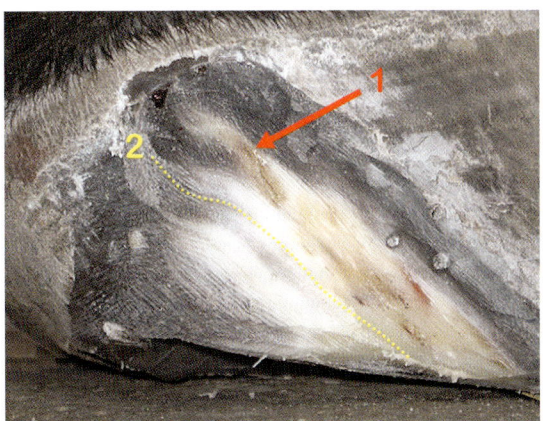

The cleaned out horny wall. The cause is infected insensitive laminae (1) that began below (yellow wall corium) and rose up. The direction of the horny tubules was changed by this (2).

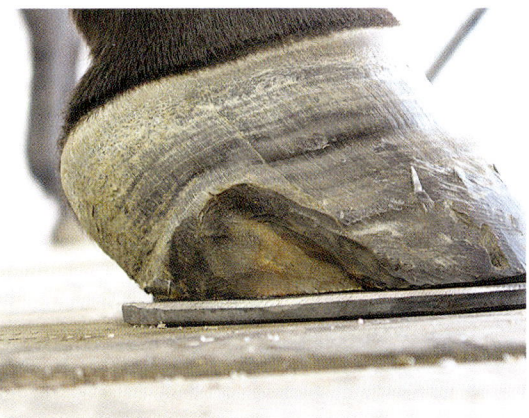

After three months, the hoof capsule healed well.

The horseshoe should have a bar so that there can be no movement in the shoe. The wound must absolutely not be closed with filling material as there is the chance that inflammation could develop again underneath. Moreover, the wound cannot be examined; it will heal better under normal conditions and with the help of oxygen. During the first days, the wound should be dressed with a Betadine (iodine) compress to prevent infection and allow the wound to dry out. This demands thorough checks.

CASE HISTORY 1, PHOTOS BELOW

A horse that was presented had a problem with a sandcrack that bled sporadically. By filing out the sandcrack, it was clear that the cause was the commencement of an inflamed keratoma. The keratoma had to be removed. The coronary corium was carefully filed away (filing away and cleaning of defective tissue) until healthy laminae were reached. Normally, horny tubules grow in a straight line downwards. The tubules in the hoof of this horse actually had a wavy growth pattern. This meant that, within the hoof capsule, something had been wrong for some time. As well as the wavy growth of the horny tubules, there was a glass-like, hard horn which indicated a keratoma. The inflamed keratoma needed a lot of space, which then led to the outside horny wall cracking open. The coronary corium was cleaned carefully. If too much horn is removed, the hoof capsule can no longer develop. The keratoma was loosened and pulled away from the corium. The hoof was dressed with a compress with Betadine (iodine) to prevent the corium from bulging out. After a few days, the wound was dry and the coronary band could grow down as normal. The operation and the aftercare of the horse had been carried out by a team made up of a veterinary surgeon, a farrier and various assistants, which finally produced a satisfactory result.

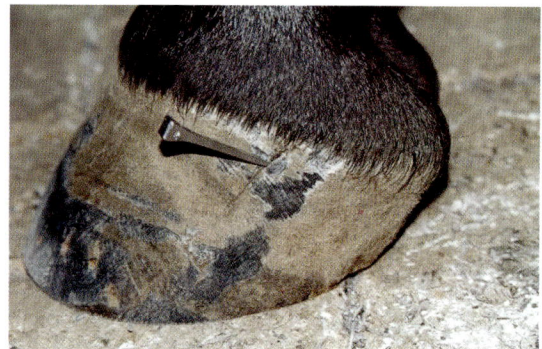

Sandcracks can appear suddenly. The germinating layer of the coronary corium then produces abnormal horn growth. After filing away, it appeared that the cause of the crack was a keratoma.

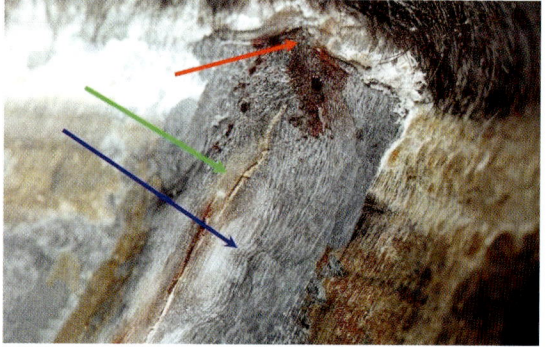

The coronary corium is filed away until a healthy attachment of horny tubules is found (red arrow). The horny tubules do not go straight down – as they are meant to – but in a defective wavy movement (blue arrow). Next to the wavy line of horny tubules is a glass-like hard horn; this indicates a keratoma (green arrow).

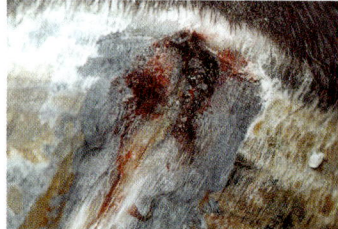

The coronary corium is cleaned carefully; if too much horn is removed, sometimes the hoof capsule can no longer develop.

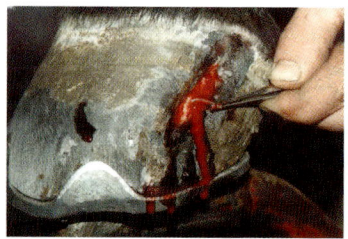

The keratoma is loosened and pulled away from the corium.

Part 2 – Disorders of the Limbs and Hooves

CASE HISTORY 2, PHOTOS BELOW

Cracks that develop higher up in the hoof capsule in the area of the coronary band always indicate a serious problem. It is not possible to say with certainty if it is a chronic crack or if it is a crack caused by a keratoma. Horses can become lame from a crack, as the area where the crack occurs is extremely flexible because of the hoof mechanism. The hoof capsule is divided in two by a sandcrack; each part then moves separately.

A horse was presented where the crack in the horny wall had opened up through drying out. The two parts of the horny wall could move separately, which caused lameness. The horny wall was filed out, all loose parts removed and on both sides of the crack a good attachment of healthy, strong horn was found. It was apparent that the cause of the crack was a traumatic sandcrack caused by inflamed laminae. The horny wall was broken at the germinating layer – the layer where horny wall is developed. The area where the break in the growth of the horny wall occurred was slightly stimulated with the file to be sure that a complete horny wall without cracks would be produced. This stimulation or light touching or filing of the germinating layer is applied at the germinating layer of the coronary band (coronary corium) and ensures that extra horn

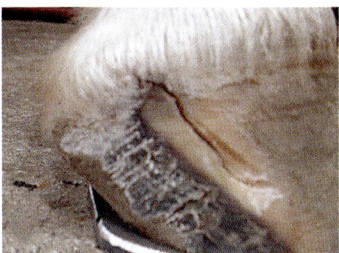

Sandcracks that occur at the top of the hoof capsule in the area of the coronary band always cause serious problems.

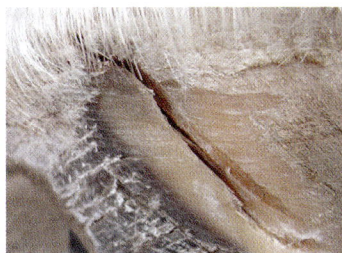

The horny wall has dried out somewhat, thus the parts become separated and can be moved separately.

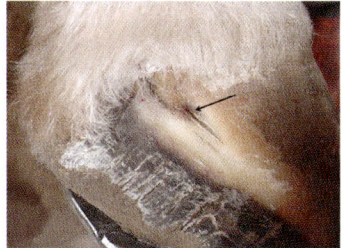

After filing out the horny wall, we reach the actual problem: the black line in the middle is inflamed laminae – the cause of the sandcrack.

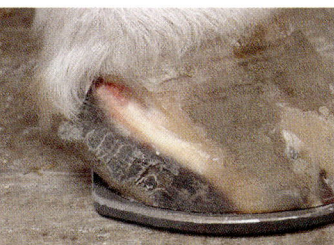

There is a break in the horny wall at the germinating layer. The area where the break in the germinating layer occurs is stimulated a little with the filing drill to ensure that a complete crack-free wall can be achieved.

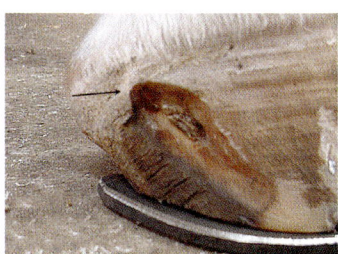

After eight weeks, a thick, healthy piece of horn is developed at the coronary band.

will be produced above the removed part. This extra horn production is necessary to give extra strength to the hoof capsule during the healing period.

CASE HISTORY 3, PHOTOS BELOW

Many farriers are of the opinion that you can fix all cracks in the horny wall by screwing them together with metal plates or glued-on plates, or even with clasps. Sandcracks are always caused by something and so the cause should be treated. Under the sandcrack on the horny wall, a metal plate is often screwed in the belief that the crack will then be immobilised. However, fixing this metal plate did not solve the problem; the opposite is true – the sandcrack will remain chronically defective.

The farrier had fixed a metal clasp low down on the sandcrack on a horse that was presented. After the horny wall had been filed away, it became clear that this horse's sandcrack was caused by chronically inflamed insensitive laminae. The whole area was cleaned out so that healthy wall corium was exposed. Thus the horny wall could once again grow healthily downwards.

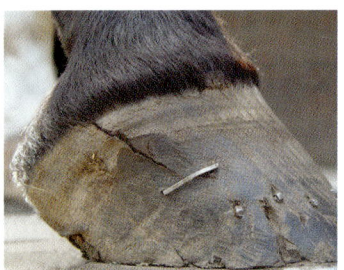

A sandcrack where a clasp has been placed below the crack.

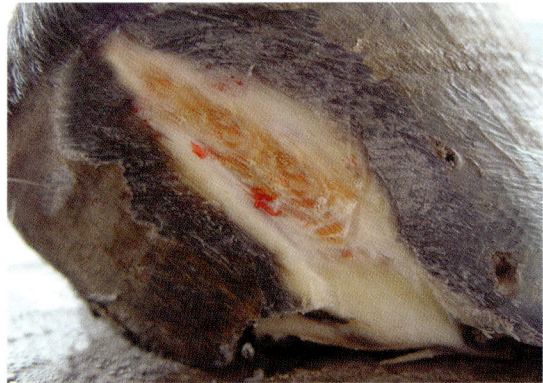

Inflammation of the wall corium appears to be the cause of the sandcrack.

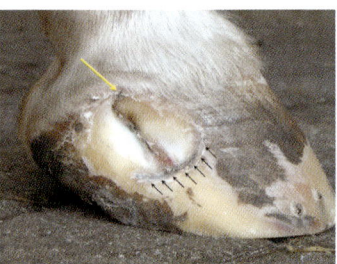

This sandcrack (yellow arrow) is a result of an eruption of an infection (black arrows). After the eruption, a permanent sandcrack developed.

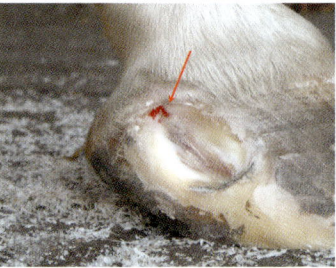

The horny wall is removed and the germinating layer of the coronary corium is slightly stimulated so that more horn will be produced.

4 THE HOOF: HORNY WALL

Poor Quality of Horn, and Chipped Hooves

Poor quality of horn is a hoof with a defective horn structure. The horny wall is composed of horny tubules that grow next to each other and downwards from the coronary corium; the horny tubules are interlocked by a semi-horny substance. From here to about 2 to 3 centimetres from the underside of the growing hoof capsule, the semi-horny substance comes away from the horny tubules. On the outside, it is clear to see that the horny tubules are loose.

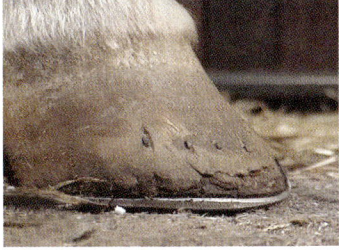

This is a side view of a hoof with poor quality horn. The semi-horny substance comes away from the tubules in the hoof capsule from the coronary band to about 2 centimetres from the bottom.

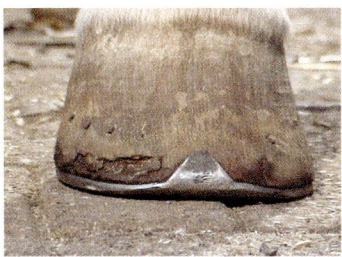

Front view of a hoof with poor quality of horn.

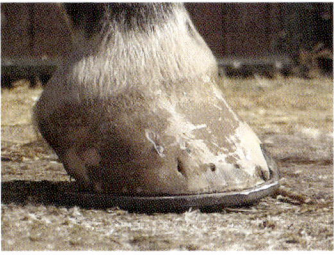

The same hoof after remedial shoeing. The farrier must fit the shoe extremely well and nail it on high.

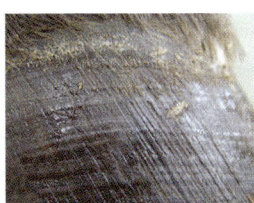

In a healthy hoof, the horny tubules lie close together and they grow downwards. This is the horny wall.

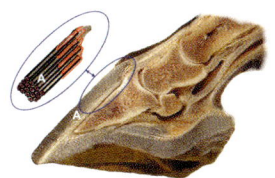

The horny tubules (A) are developed at the coronary band and lie in rows next to each other; the semi-horny substance keeps the tubules together.

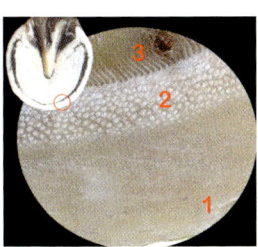

The picture shows the horny tubules; (1. thin tubule; 2. thick tubule; 3.white line) that are 'glued' together by the semi-horny substance. This substance disintegrates for no apparent reason: only after this, can one speak of a poor quality of horn.

The Hoof – Horny Wall

CAUSE

Poor quality of horn can, among other things, be caused by faulty shoeing. The stable bedding also plays a big role. Experience shows that horses that have a bedding of sawdust are more affected by poor quality of horn than horses with straw bedding. Sawdust draws moisture from the hoof and will also give off ammonia fumes from urine, which can cause a deterioration of the horn. Straw, on the other hand, has capillarity and easily absorbs urine. Straw can also be kept damp to keep the hooves more elastic.

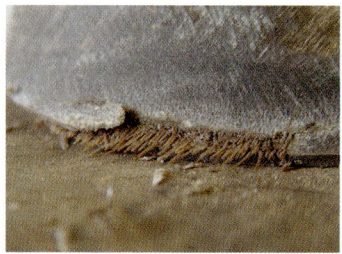 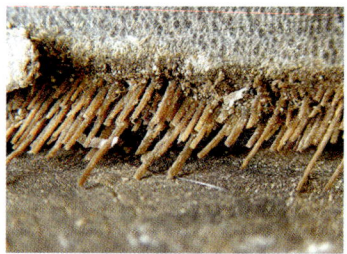 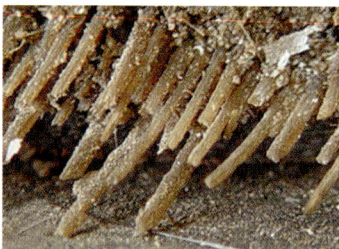

The beginnings of disintegration: a hoof with poor quality of horn.

In poor quality horn, the semi-horny substance releases the tubules. The loosened tubules make the weightbearing edge weak and thin.

The clearly loosened tubules are no longer held together by the semi-horny substance.

Many questions about the cause of poor quality of horn cannot yet be answered: poor quality suddenly arises under all kinds of conditions – dry or damp, variable temperatures, different seasons – and is found in various breeds.

TREATMENT AND HORSESHOES

For the treatment of a real case of poor quality of horn – which is quite rare – a really skilled farrier is needed. The farrier must apply a very good and very well-fitting shoe. The horseshoe should be large and preferably wide. The nails must fit exactly in the white line and be nailed high. Too large a shoe with a lot of extension – space that is needed to allow the hoof to move on the shoe – is disadvantageous for a poor quality of horn.

It is advised that a seriously poor quality of horn should be temporarily shod with clips to limit the movement of the hoof and to give the hoof capsule a chance to grow 'in peace'. A shoe with three clips will temporarily block the hoof mechanism, but without lasting side effects.

There is, up until the present, no remedy for poor quality of horn. It can sometimes be caused by a lack of elements in the feed. Experience shows that the use of more or less irritating salves, ointments and lotions to massage the coronary band to give better circulation to the coronary corium and the enhancement of strong horn production has little effect. As time goes by, these substances will irritate the coronary band and will sometimes lead to

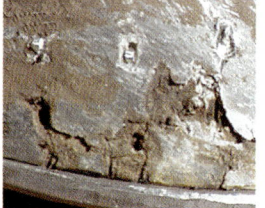 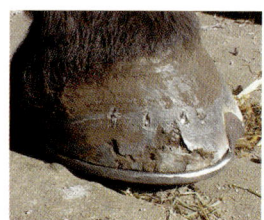

Poor quality horn needs a very well-fitted shoe with very high nailing. It is best to keep the hooves moist; oiling poor quality hooves dries out the wall and will make the problem worse.

inflammation of the skin above the coronet while the desired horn growth is lacking. Employing a skilled farrier will bring better results.

Chipped Hooves

Poor quality of horn should in no way be confused with chipped hooves. Chipped hooves can be caused in several ways: the weightbearing edge can chip due to a very dried-out horn, but chipping can also be caused by a softened horn and by neglect of the hooves. Thus we do not speak of poor horn but rather of neglect or incompetent treatment of the hooves. If hooves are badly looked after, pieces of horn can break off. It is understandable that if a hoof capsule is too long, pieces of horn can easily break off the weightbearing edge. A bad hoof capsule is not always a poor quality of horn.

A chipped hoof can become worse through the faulty work of a farrier, for example if the trimming does not conform to the foot axis, if the hooves are left too long, or if the horseshoe has not been fitted to the foot and thus the nails are driven outside the white line in the horny wall. If nailing is faulty, the horny tubules will be separated and the horny wall will crack. The horse will lose its shoes more frequently because the walls will be weaker. If action is not taken immediately, the quality of the hoof capsule will deteriorate. Special shoes must be fitted regularly to save the hooves but if the horse's hooves get worse and worse, this will no longer be possible.

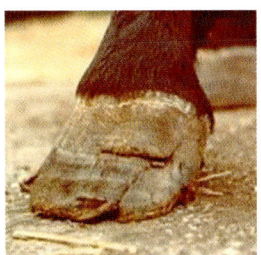

A chipped hoof – so not a poor quality of horn!

TREATMENT

Chipped hooves can be prevented by trimming the hooves in a proper manner. The wall thickness should be equal throughout. The hoof should be fitted with a normal and sufficient shoe so that the hoof mechanism can function well. As well as this, care should be taken that all nails are in the white line and preferably a little toward the inside, near the join with the sole. But be careful: don't fit a narrow shoe – that would mean too much of the wall being removed.

The nails must be driven well and nailed high so that the hoof can be left undisturbed for a very long time. If a horse's hooves have good hoof mechanism, the so-called 'blood pump' works optimally and the hoof receives adequate nutrients; in this way there will be healthy re-growth of horn.

CONCLUSION

A chipped or badly-maintained hoof can definitely be improved by a good farrier. A real poor quality of horn will be a little more problematical but this too can be treated successfully by expert shoeing from a skilled farrier.

Complete Horny Wall Cracks

A complete horny wall crack is a fissure in the horny wall between the coronary band and the weightbearing edge. A complete horny wall crack is usually superficial but can also be full-thickness.

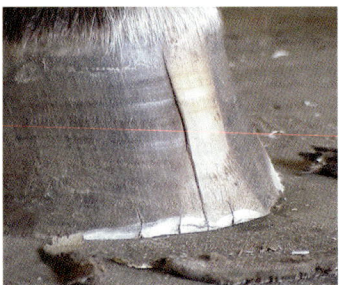

An example of a complete wall crack.

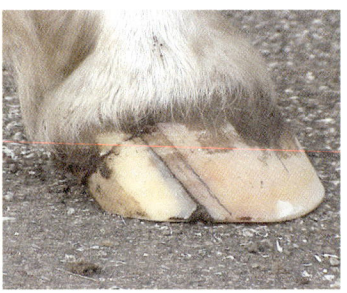

A complete side wall crack; the loose parts are removed until a good attachment is reached.

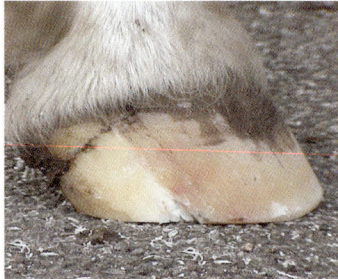

The crack is completely removed but the coronary band will not change. The horny wall will continue to grow down with an indentation in it.

A SUPERFICIAL COMPLETE HORNY WALL CRACK

CAUSE

Complete horny wall cracks are mostly a result of injury to the coronary band. When there is damage to the coronary band, the production of and the connection between the horny tubules is broken. This causes a crack. The consequences of such cracks are usually not serious because they affect the first layer of the horny tubules and are superficial. As the crack dries out a little, it seems as if the wall is splitting.

Older horses can develop many complete horny wall cracks. The cause of these cracks is the disappearance of the semi-horny substance – the substance that holds the horny tubules together. It is probably as a result of the effect of ultraviolet rays in combination with the age of the horse. These cracks are not serious; they do not cause lameness in the horse.

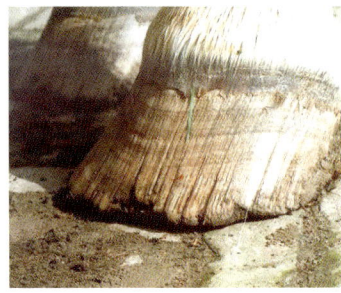

Old horses can develop many complete horny wall cracks. These cracks are not serious.

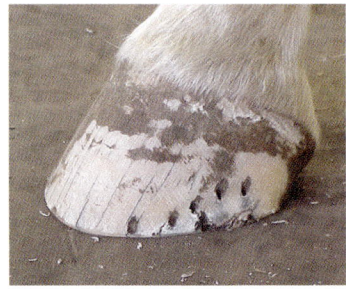

After the finishing of the hoof, many small superficial cracks can be seen.

Part 2 – Disorders of the Limbs and Hooves

TREATMENT

A complete horny wall crack can be treated by rasping or filing the wall thin where the crack is. The loose part is removed until the healthy attachments to the horny tubules are reached. This will weaken the wall a little. It is not necessary to treat a hoof with a superficial complete horn wall crack between toe clips as these cracks do not cause problems. What is important though, is that the horse has a roomy horseshoe.

A COMPLETE HORNY WALL CRACK

Complete wall cracks can also be full thickness so that they go through the whole thickness of the wall to the corium. They can cause lameness in the long-term and must be treated.

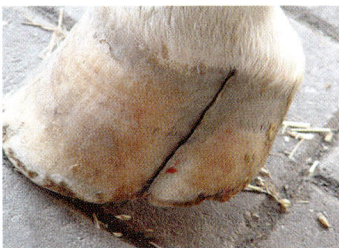

A complete full thickness horny wall crack. In the long-term it will cause lameness.

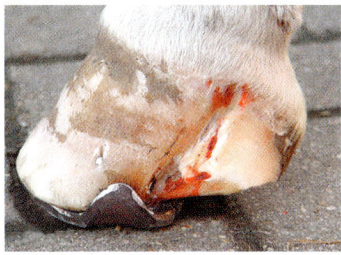

This crack is removed by filing out the horny wall. The germinating layer at the coronary band is also cleaned.

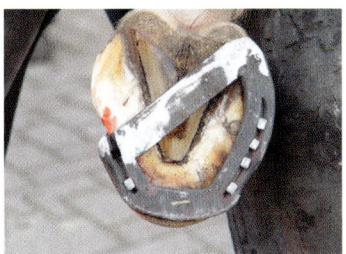

The hoof is shod with a three-quarter shoe. The heel part will be kept free to release it from weightbearing as long as possible.

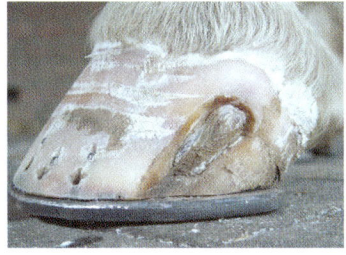

After ten weeks there is healthy horn development. The hoof is shod with a normal, roomy shoe.

TREATMENT

The crack is treated by filing away the horny wall until healthy attachments are reached. The germinating layer at the coronary corium is cleaned (see coronary band crack) so that the coronary corium can develop a healthy interlocking horn growth once more. This requires a thorough knowledge of the anatomy of the hoof capsule because if the farrier removes too much horny wall or if the coronary corium is damaged, no new horn can develop.

Grass Crack

Grass cracks are cracks that appear in the lower part of the hoof capsule by the breaking out of the wall. They can also be due to an irregularity in the white line. These cracks are usually of full thickness.

Grass cracks can be caused by:
- Stepping on stones
- Treading on uneven stones and a rough terrain
- Standing on edges
- Not trimming on time, so the toes become too long
- Neglect of the hooves
- Not picking out the hooves and not checking the white line for dirt and stones
- The disproportionate loading of the weightbearing edge. For example: a hoof is wrongly pared so that the toe is too long and thick and the heels too short. Thus the pressure on the heels is too great, which results in breaking out and cracking of the side walls
- Faulty shoeing. Weightbearing edge cracks can arise through badly fitting shoes and too much nailing outside the white line in the hoof capsule

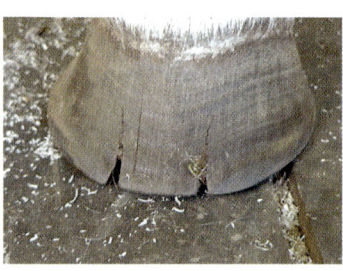

An example of a hoof with a grass crack.

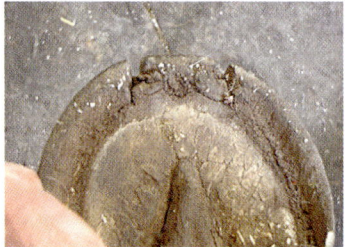

The same hoof as above but seen from underneath.

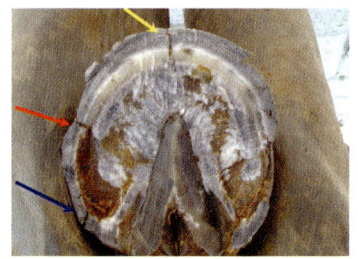

The hoof capsule grows straight down from the coronary band. If the wall is not properly treated and becomes concave (red arrow) problems can arise. As the wall is pushed outwards, grass cracks appear.

Under the hoof there are two grass cracks (red and blue arrows) and a toe wall crack (yellow arrow) caused by leaving the toe too long. There is a broadened white line in this hoof.

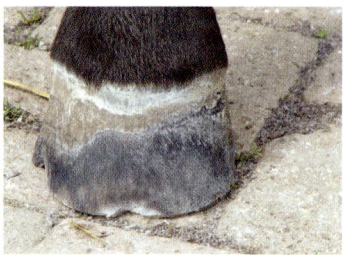

The hoof is made straight and the cracks are removed so that horn can develop that can bear weight without cracking.

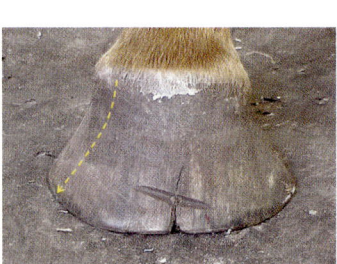

If the hoof is trimmed wrongly, it becomes concave (yellow line). A toe crack develops from too great pressure.

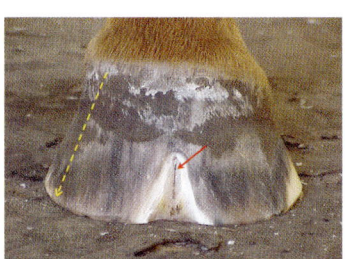

The horny wall is made straight (dotted yellow line) and the crack is removed. There is a black line (arrow) at the corium which indicates the place where bacteria have entered.

Part 2 – Disorders of the Limbs and Hooves

- Faulty trimming such as paring without taking the limb or foot conformation into account, or trimming the heels too much and leaving the toes too long
- Regularly striking a shoe off
- Shoeing too late

HORSESHOES

A hoof with grass cracks is mostly shod with a shoe without clips, as otherwise there would be too much pressure on the horny wall. The hoof should never be shod with double clips because it would hinder the hoof mechanism; the hoof mechanism can be so powerful that the walls can break at the places where the clips are. Treated toe wall cracks can be shod temporarily with a fore shoe with two toe clips. The aim of this shoe is to immobilise the treated area temporarily and to block the hoof mechanism. By intervening in this manner further cracking of the horny wall is prevented.

Grass cracks can easily develop in the toe through neglect because the walls spread and the toe cracks. As soon as the toe cracks, the wall of the wall corium is pulled off and a hoof inflammation can commence which makes the horse lame; this crack is parallel to the horny tubules. If

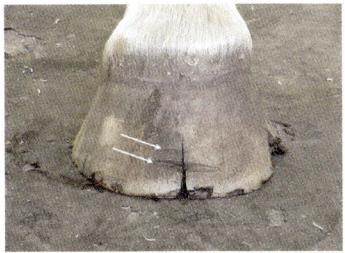

Unfortunately there are still grass cracks that are handled by scoring horizontally into the hoof or by burning a hole above the crack. This treatment leaves the horny wall weakened and the crack can easily split upwards.

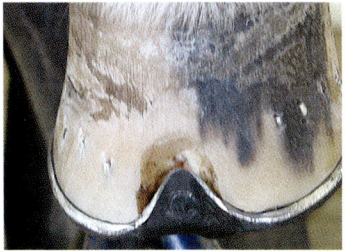

This crack has been removed and shod with a normal, well-fitted shoe.

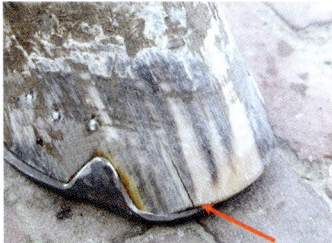

Even though this grass crack is between two clips it will continue splitting unless treated.

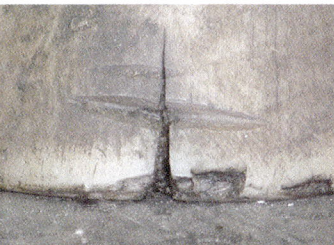

A toe wall crack as a result of inflammation. The crack runs parallel with the horny tubules.

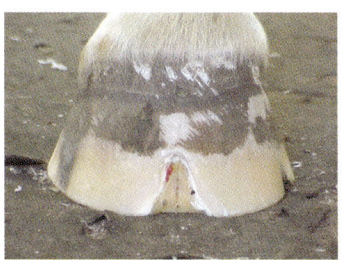

The same hoof as left after treatment. A yellowish tint is clearly seen after the cleaning of the corium. This indicates an inflammation.

an inflammation develops in this area, the chance is high that a fungus develops at the same time. This fungus – called white line disease – can loosen the whole toe wall. A crack where white line disease is involved is wavy. Grass cracks can also occur because a horse is shod too late or has its hooves wrongly treated. An example of this is a hoof which displays cracks in the side wall and the toe wall.

If we look under this hoof, we see that the weightbearing edge is of unequal thickness, causing a toe crack. The white line is broadened, and that is reflected in the horny wall – this runs from above to below in a curve outwards – but it should be straight and flat. A horny wall that is arched is weak as it has a tendency to collapse. A straight horny wall can carry the load. The horny wall is shortened and made flat, so that the hoof capsule can once again carry all the weight of the horse and the wall can no longer split.

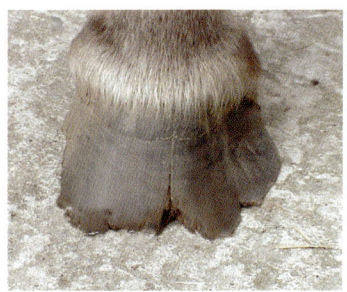

Most cracks appear at the toe and are always a result of faulty handling of the hooves.

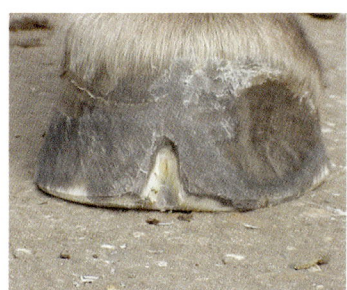

A treated toe edge crack; the hoof is trimmed correctly according to the foot axis. The crack has been cut open so that strong attachment of the horny wall is reached.

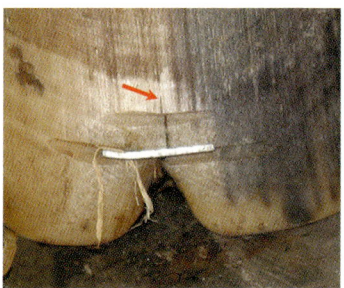

Many cracks are held together with clasps. This does not remove the cause of the crack so it continues to split (red arrow) and the horny wall becomes more and more weak.

A toe grass crack is a split in the horny wall of the toe area of the hoof. A toe wall crack can be superficial or deep, that is to say full thickness. The biggest cause of this sort of crack is faulty handling of the hooves. Grass cracks can develop because the horny wall in the toe area is too long and too thick, and when the toe rolls over it receives too much pressure, which also causes the wall to yield. Inflammation in this area can be the cause of cracks in the wall.

TREATMENT

Grass cracks in hooves need not occur: some cases can be very serious. Horses can have trouble with these cracks because the horny wall yields and splits further open.

Deep grass cracks are not helped by rasping the wall thin; the cause – be it a keratoma, an inflammation, dirt, etc. – is not removed, as is, of course, necessary.

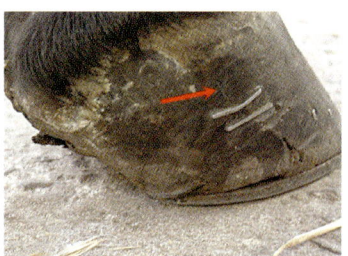

Grass cracks that have been wrongly treated can lead to serious lameness. This grass crack has been fixed twice with clasps without dealing with the cause. The horseshoe is not supporting the wall (it is too narrow) and does not solve the problem.

CASE HISTORY 1, PHOTOS BELOW

Grass cracks mostly occur because the horse has trodden on small stones which have become wedged into the white line. These stones work deeply into the white line so that bacteria can develop. In this way an inflammation of the corium can ensue; when this happens a fungus can also develop. The inflammation migrates upwards and subsequently breaks out at the coronary band. This brings with it all sorts of tiresome consequences (see False Quarter).

When treating, the cracks are removed as far as is possible. As much of the horny wall is removed as is needed to reach healthy attachment tissue; this can be seen by the corium that has become yellowish – normal corium should be white. The yellowish tint indicates that there has been inflammation; a black line is also visible – this is the dirt between the sensitive and insensitive laminae of the corium. After this line has been removed, the horny wall can grow normally without any further cracking. The most important thing is to protect the horse by fitting it with horseshoes.

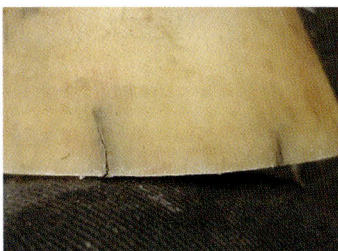

Grass cracks can be caused by dirt being trapped in the white line. They start small but can have disastrous results.

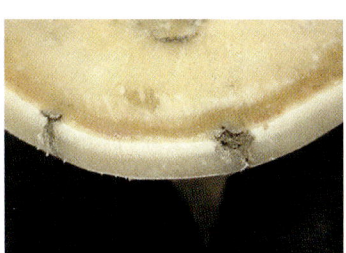

It is clear to see on the underside of the hoof that the problem began in the white line. Dirt has accumulated which has caused splitting in the hoof wall.

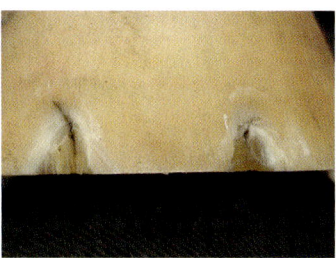

The horny wall is removed at the place where the cracks are; the crack is followed until it is no longer visible.

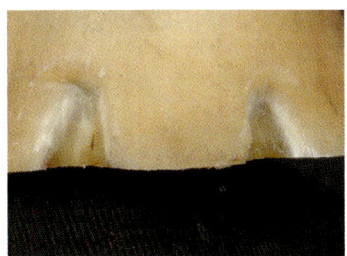

The crack is cut away and the yellow tint of inflamed wall corium is visible.

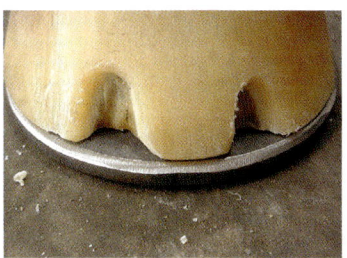

A hoof with grass cracks is usually shod with shoes without clips, otherwise there would be too much pressure on the horny wall.

CASE HISTORY 2, PHOTO RIGHT AND BELOW

A horse that was presented was troubled with a grass crack in the toe. After the horny wall had been filed away, the corium was cleaned. A yellowish tint was easily visible which indicated that there had been an inflammation in that spot. The horny wall was carefully cleaned out until there was healthy attachment around the wound. These types of cracks must be carefully removed to avoid worse problems.

CASE HISTORY 3

A horse that was presented had seriously neglected hooves. The whole wall had cracked and the horse was terribly lame. The side walls were broken and, because of the unequal weighting of the horny wall, these subsequently split. Not only had the horny wall cracked but also the solar surface. These cracks had to be completely removed to reduce the pain.

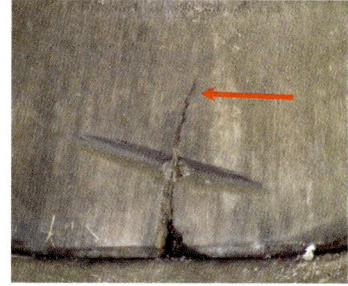

A toe wall crack as a result of inflammation in combination with a fungus: white line disease. The split is curved and does not run parallel with the horny tubules.

Rings of Horn

Rings of horn are rings that occur on the outside of the hoof following the shape of the coronary band.

Rings of horn can appear because of:
- Changes in feed
- Changes of season
- Overtaxing
- Lameness
- Hoof care
- Administering of medicine. When strong medicine is given, the coronary corium always reacts by producing extra horn
- Illness

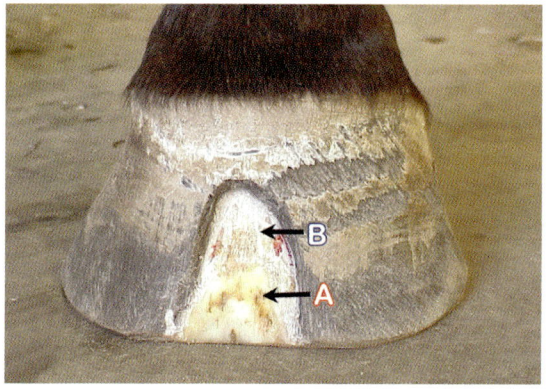

The affected part is thoroughly removed where this crack was. The yellow, inflamed area (A) is clearly visible with, above, the fungus (B). The hoof was shod temporarily with a shoe with two side clips.

The hoof reacts to the above-mentioned changes by increasing or decreasing horn growth; thereby rings of horn appear on the hoof. Rings of horn on the hoof indicate that the horse's normal pattern of living is changed; they do not indicate lameness.

Rings of horn are not always a negative sign; when a horse is laminitic, the rings of horn can be a positive sign – it can be concluded that the coronary corium is repairing the horn growth in the vicinity of the pedal bone. The moment a horse becomes laminitic, the coronary corium reacts by changing the direction of growth of the horny tubules. When the laminitis is properly treated, the coronary corium produces horny tubules growing in the right direction – the tubules follow the line of the pedal bone. The rings of horn that appear grow down with the horn growth; above the rings, the horny wall grows in a normal, healthy way. A reaction to thrush – an inflammation of the frog corium that has forced a way up to the coronary band – may produce rings of horn that are visible diagonally across the horny wall.

If the corium is viciously irritated by the treatment of the coronary band cracks, extra horny wall develops, which can also cause rings.

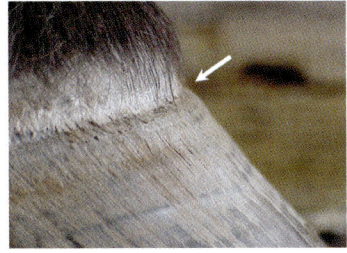

Rings of horn can have many causes. A ring of horn always indicates what a horse has gone through: in exercising, in feeding, in its stable or in sickness.

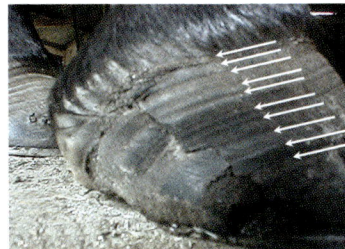

Defects in the horny wall continue to produce rings of horn if the problem isn't solved.

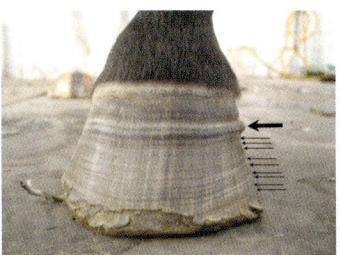

Hooves of horses that are neglected in the long-term display many rings of horn. The thickened edge of the horny wall (black arrow) is evidence that the horse has been lame for a long time.

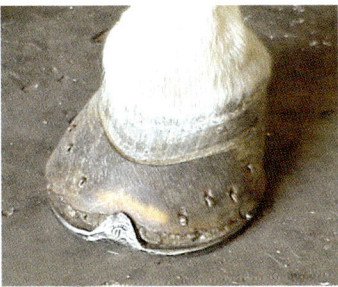

Laminitis is the only disease where extreme rings of horn are visible. The coronary band reacts by changing the direction of the horny tubules.

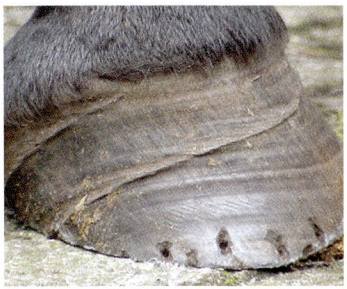

Rings of horn can develop as a result of thrush. They appear on the hoof in the shape of the coronary band. Rings on the horny wall are a typical characteristic of a coronary band inflammation.

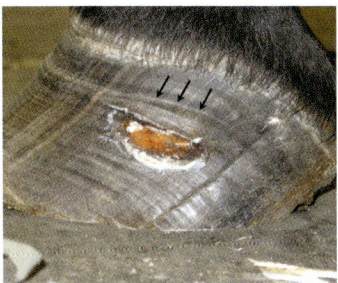

Inflammation that breaks out in the horny wall above causes a reaction in the whole coronary band – and an extra obstruction near the wound – which thus creates extra horn production in the form of very thick rings of horn.

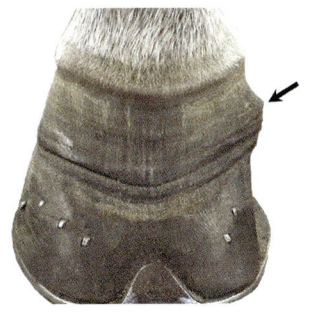

The horny wall crack is removed from the wall in an operation; the coronary corium is deliberately stimulated to activate extra horn production. The coronary band will develop a thicker wall; above this extra horn development the making of normal horny tubules is resumed.

Seedy Toe

The characteristic of seedy toe is the separating and deterioration of the horny tubules within the centre of the hoof wall. This results in a splitting off from the inner horny wall. The hoof capsule starts at the perioplic ring (the germinating layer) of the coronary band (coronary corium). The perioplic ring ensures that the horn grows longitudinally, in the form of tubes, along the sensitive laminae of the pedal bone to the ground surface. The hoof wall is made up of two different kinds of horny tubules: the outer layer of the thicker, insensitive laminae and the inner layer with the thinner, sensitive laminae (tubules of first and second kind).

CAUSE

Seedy toe is mostly found among horses that have to work frequently and for long periods on hard surfaces. The hooves of such horses are nearly always hard and dry. It is not yet clear why the horny tubules in the centre of the hoof wall begin to deteriorate. It has, however, been

The Hoof – Horny Wall

proved that seedy toe can be caused by horseshoes that do not fit and when the farrier does not place nails in the white line (or nail line) but in the hoof wall instead.

A horse is not necessarily made lame by seedy toe but it will be unwilling to put its hoof down heavily on a hard surface. When the hoof wall is tapped with a hard object, it sounds hollow. It is often the farrier who detects seedy toe, however it is also visible on X-rays.

TREATMENT

Seedy toe is easily treated. The loose, outside part of the wall is removed, after which the area is cleaned with Betadine (iodine). The hoof can be wrapped in a wet bandage at night in order to increase the hoof

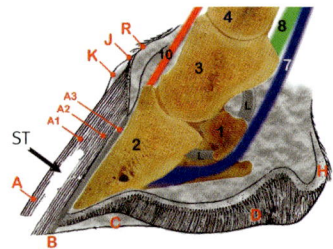

Seedy toe shows a separation in the horn wall (A) between A1 and A2.

1. Navicular bone; 2. Pedal bone; 3. Short pastern bone; 4. Long pastern bone; 7. Deep flexor tendon: 8. Superficial flexor tendon; 10. Extensor tendon

A. Horny wall; B. White line or nail line; C. Solar surface; D. Horn tubules; H. Digital cushion; R. Epidermis; J. Coronary band; K. Periople

A1. Outer layer horn tubules (thin)

A2. Inner layer horn tubules (thick)

A3. Laminal surface

ST. Seedy toe

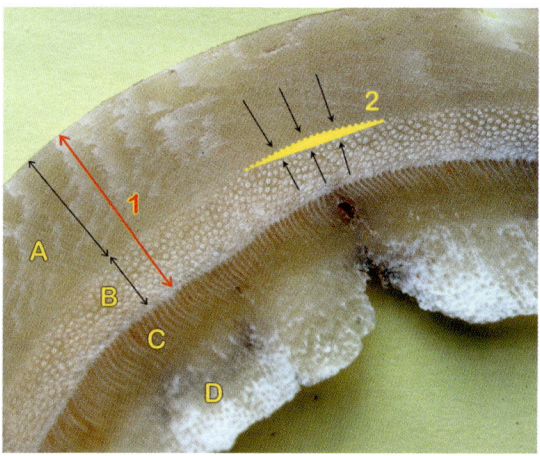

The horn wall (1) consists of two different types of horn tubules: on the outside they are thin (A) and further in they are thicker (B). Seedy toe develops between (2) these two types of horn tubules. The white line (C) and the sole (D) lie next to the horny wall.

humidity so that the elasticity of the hoof is encouraged. The horny wall can become loose from as far up as the coronary corium and can cause lameness. Since in this part of the horn there is a high risk that fungus develops, seedy toe demands a high level of care. (see White Line Disease.)

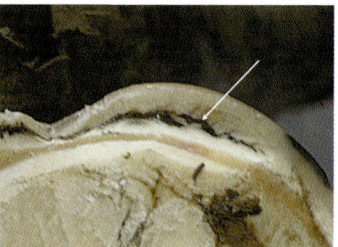

Dirt trapped in the seedy toe cavity can be the cause of pressure to the whole hoof wall. It is best to remove the outside part.

HORSESHOES

Horses with seedy toe should be shod with a bar shoe. In this type of horseshoe there is a light iron bar between both branches of the shoe to prevent movement. A skilled farrier is required for the treatment of a horse with seedy toe as the horse needs long-term supervision.

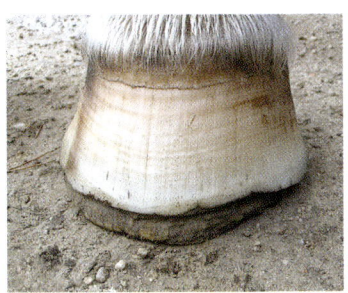

A case of seedy toe where the top layer of thick tubules has been removed; the horse need not become lame. The problem can only be solved with well-fitting shoes and by conscientious hoof care.

False Quarter

A false quarter is a horizontal crack in the horny wall caused by inflammation of the hoof corium.

CAUSE

False quarter develops on the underside of the hoof, mainly in the white line. As the horse treads dirt and little stones into the white line, an inflammation can develop in this area (pododermatitis). Due to the pressure of this bacterial inflammation, the horse moves alternately lamely and freely. As soon as the pressure in the hoof is reduced, when the inflammation has found an escape, the horse can move freely again. When nothing is done about the infection and it breaks out under the germinating layer of the coronary corium, a serious lameness results.

TREATMENT

Sometimes the horse is administered antibiotics (penicillin). The infection is calmed for a couple of days but it does not solve the real problem. After a while the inflammation moves upwards via the wall corium between the horny wall and the pedal bone. The infection breaks out again at the height of the coronary band under the germinating layer of the horny wall that produces horn. This breakout is explosive and can cause great havoc. Due to the pressure of the infection, the coronary corium bulges out. After the breakout, the coronary corium produces an abnormal amount of horn; the extra horn strengthens the wall and is not pared away until the horny wall has grown down half way. The horn growth temporarily stagnates at the spot where the infection breaks out. This appears on the hoof as a horizontal crack and is called a false quarter. As soon as the horse has an inflammation in the hoof, it must be sought out and treated before such outbreaks occur.

When a horse has an inflammation where the coronary corium bulges out violently, the horny wall under the breakout is removed a little. A Betadine (iodine) compress is applied to push the corium back in place.

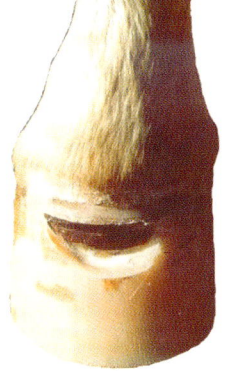

Here a false quarter can be seen. The horn growth is stopped temporarily.

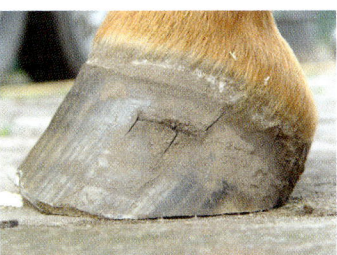

The false quarter: a permanent sign of breakout of inflammation.

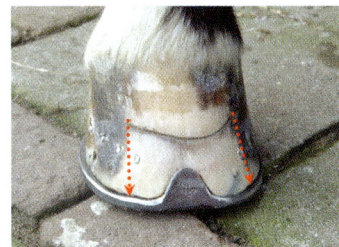

False quarter appears in all parts of the hoof capsule; if well-treated it need not cause problems.

The horny wall under the horizontal crack is separate from the corium; it is better to leave it be as it gives strength and protection to the hoof capsule. Further treatment is not required; the wall grows down by itself and the false quarter disappears after the hoof has grown down fully.

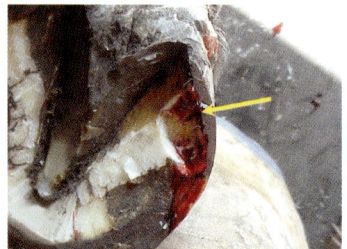 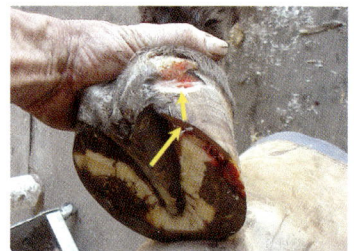 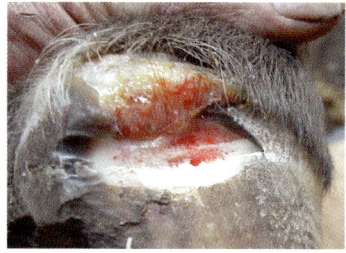

Left: there is inflammation in the buttress of the heel (yellow arrow). Middle: the inflammation has migrated upwards via the wall corium (yellow arrow). Right: the inflammation has broken out under the germinating layer. The colour of the wall is a glass-like yellow which indicates that penicillin has been administered.

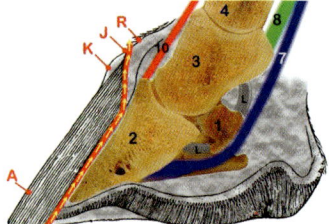

An inflammation begins in the sole; the inflammation migrates upwards via the wall corium (yellow/orange line) and breaks out in the coronary band area just under the germinating layer.

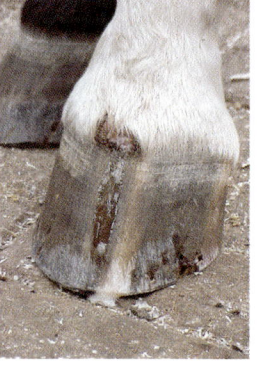 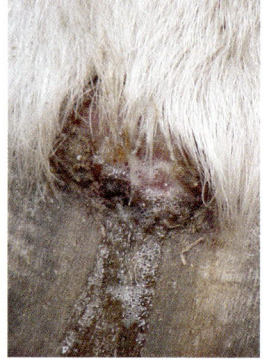

A breakout of an inflammation of the hoof that began underneath. This causes false quarter. The wound is dressed for a couple of days with a Betadine (iodine) compress.

HORSESHOES

Hooves with false quarters are shod normally. There will come a time when it is difficult to nail because the horny wall in the area of the false quarter will be loose.

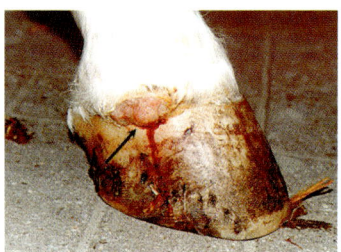 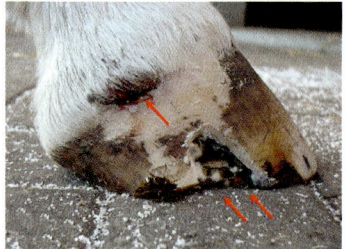 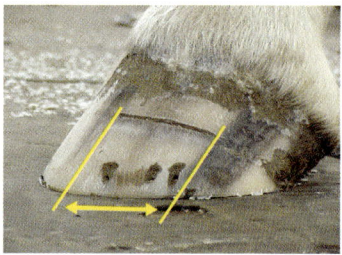

A breakout of a hoof inflammation that has not been treated properly. The coronary corium is bulging out terribly; this can cause the coronary corium to develop defective horn growth.

A serious inflammation has developed in the side wall that has broken out above in the coronary band. The hoof is dressed with a moist bandage with a fungicide solution, and a compress will be applied to the coronary band so that the corium stays in place. False quarter develops at the spot where the inflammation has broken out.

The wall under the false quarter is not removed as it keeps the hoof in shape.

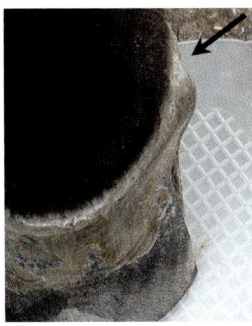

The coronary corium makes extra horn after the outbreak of an inflammation; the extra horn strengthens the wall. The extra horn is pared away only when it has grown down half way.

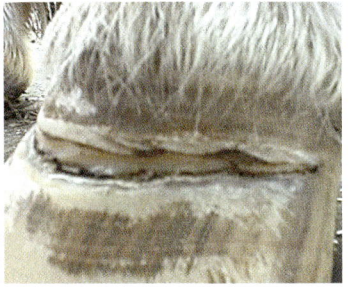

In some cases, three-quarters of the horny wall comes loose. It will definitely be a problem for the horse, but a farrier who knows his job can bring this to a satisfactory conclusion.

Separating Walls

Separating walls are when the connection between the horny wall and the wall corium is loosened. This is different from seedy toe where the wall corium remains covered with a layer of horny wall and the horn between the tubules (of the first and second sort) are loosened from the wall.

CAUSE

The origin of a separating wall has various causes:
- The horse or pony has had laminitis. The connections between the horny wall and the pedal bone have thus been broken, which allows for the possibility of a separating wall
- The breakout of an infection. The bacteria start to develop underneath at the white line with inflamed insensitive laminae and migrate above via the wall corium; a space is thus created between the horny wall and the wall corium
- White line disease. This fungus begins in the white line. The spores affect the sensitive and insensitive laminae that subsequently come loose
- Faulty trimming of the hoof, allowing the horny wall to be wrongly weighted
- Too narrow and too small horseshoes. Because the horseshoe is fitted too small and the horny wall filed down, the thin horny wall spreads beyond the shoe
- Neglect

A horse does not stand on its hooves but hangs by the pedal bone, from the hoof capsule. Thus the total weight of the horse is spread over the weightbearing edge of the hoof capsule. A separating wall can occur anywhere in the hoof and does not always lead to serious lameness, but the horse will tread carefully. Separating walls will cause many problems with normal growth of horn.

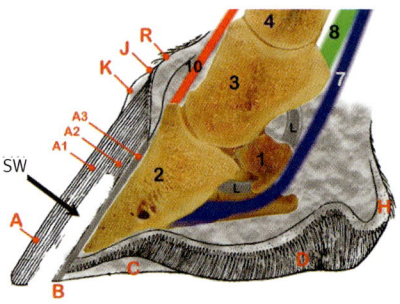

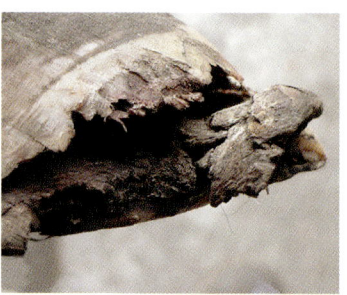

In a separating wall, there is a break between the horny wall (A) and the wall corium (A3). Because of this break, the hoof capsule is no longer connected to the pedal bone.
1. Navicular bone; 2. Pedal bone; 3. Short pastern bone; 4. Long pastern bone; 7. Deep flexor tendon; 8. Superficial flexor tendon; 10. Extensor tendon; A. Horny wall; B. White line or nailing line; C. Solar surface; D. Insensitive frog; H. Bulbs; R. Epidermis; J. Coronary band; K. Periople
A1. Outer layer of horny tubules (fine); A2. Inner layer of horny tubules (coarse); A3. Wall corium; SW. Separating wall

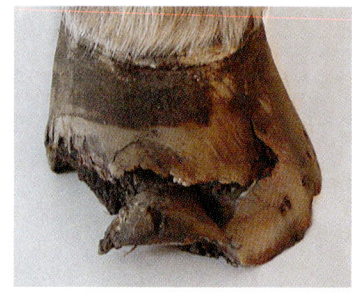

Separating walls can have disastrous consequences because the horse can tread only on the weightbearing edge and not on the sole.

TREATMENT
A separating wall does not heal easily, and there is no easy remedy. A separating wall must be professionally and adequately treated by a good farrier; it will not heal spontaneously.

HORSESHOES
Horseshoes can contribute substantially to the temporary relief of the horny wall. A good solution is a bar shoe where Equi-Thane Hoof Pak® (fast-drying silicone) has been injected in between to equalise the pressure on the lower foot.

CASE HISTORY 1, PHOTOS OPPOSITE AND PAGE 140 (TOP)
A cavity appeared in the white line – a separation between the horny wall and the wall corium – because of a neglected inflammation. Tweezers could easily be inserted into the cavity, indicating that the hoof had seedy toe and the wall had no more internal attachment. The wall could also be tapped to produce a hollow sound. When withdrawn, the tweezers had a greasy, granular substance on them which resembled the residue of woodworm; this indicated a fungus. The bacteria that caused the infection in the hoof are often accompanied by this fungus (see White Line Disease). It was extremely important that this separating wall was treated. First, the depth had to be established and marked off on the hoof capsule; it is important to follow the direction of the horny tubules. A cavity was then filed out in the horny wall, to the depth of the corium at the marked off area. The wall revealed pulverisation. When seeking in the filed out cavity for healthy attachment in the horny wall, the small opening that began underneath in the wall turned out to have a width of

20 centimetres above in the hoof capsule. The whole opening was laid bare by filing. Then the cavity was carefully examined to ensure that there was healthy horn attachment throughout. The remains of the horny wall were retained for strength and cohesion in the rest of the hoof capsule. A fungicidal agent was applied to the area where fungus was found. (The area can also be covered with honey which contains the fungicidal substance 'propolis'.) Afterwards the hoof was dressed.

After ten weeks, the horse was shod again. The opening was checked thoroughly for fungus spores, which appeared to be no longer present. The attachment of the hoof capsule was completely healed. The horny wall under the opening was still loose but would not be removed until the horny wall above the opening was strong enough and the hoof was able to heal completely. If necessary, extra nail holes can be put in the horseshoe so that the strongest parts can be nailed. After the hoof had again produced sufficient horn, the horse could return to equestrian sport.

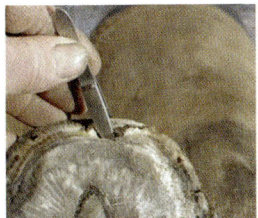

Tweezers can easily enter the cavity at the white line. It is apparent thus that internally the wall has no attachment: a clear example of a separating wall.

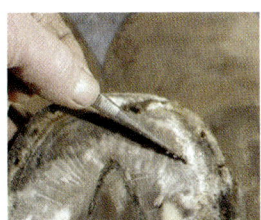

When investigating with the tweezers a greasy, granular substance appeared that resembled the residue of woodworm: this indicates a fungus.

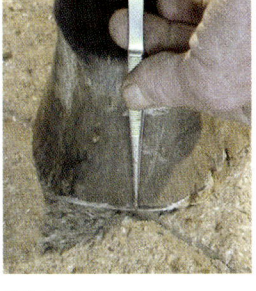

With the help of the tweezers, the depth of the separating wall was determined and marked off on the front of the hoof.

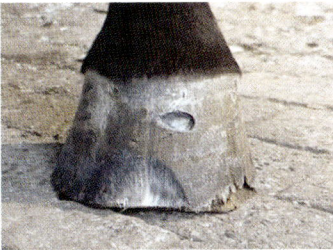

To save as much as possible of the wall, a cavity was filed out to the depth of the corium at the marked-off place on the wall; at this place the wall was loose and pulverised.

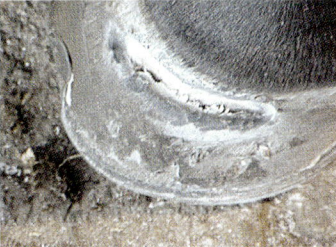

The attachment to the healthy wall is sought when filing out the cavity. Thus a tiny opening came to light, which began underneath and migrated upwards into the horny wall to a width of 20 centimetres. The whole area was filed out in the shape of a groove.

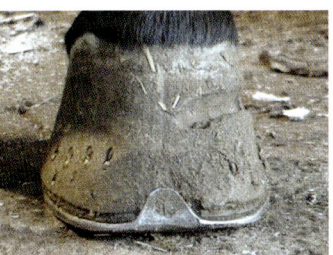

After eight weeks, the horse was re-shod. The fungus had completely gone and the hoof capsule had regained its original form.

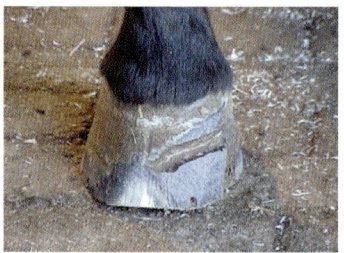 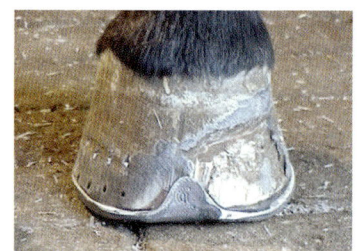 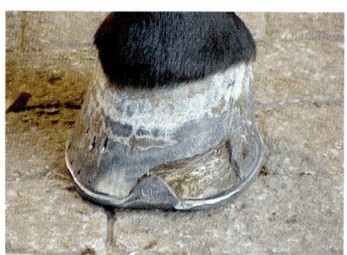

After another six weeks, enough horn had been produced and the loose wall was removed without it causing problems for the horse.

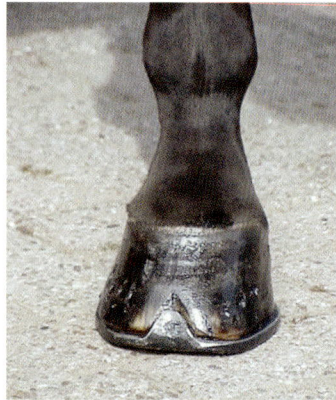

The end result: the horse can return to equestrian sports.

CASE HISTORY 2, PHOTOS BELOW AND PAGE 141 (TOP)

This horse's hoof grew with the utmost difficulty. The hoof had collapsed and needed to be supported. The horny wall was worked in such a manner that the farrier could replace the lost part of the weightbearing edge by a brace that took on the weight of the hoof capsule on the ground. Through this brace, the weight on the hoof capsule regained normality. After a number of weeks, a new hoof was formed.

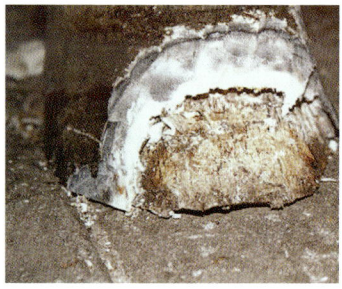 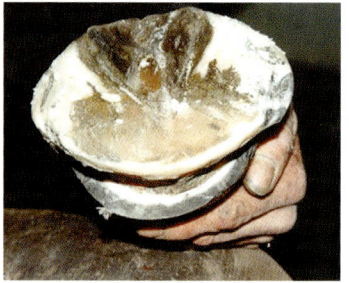 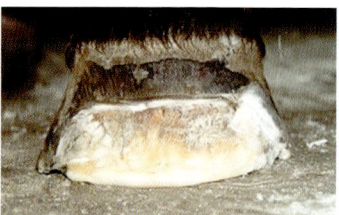

Due to laminitis, this horse has lost more than half the horny wall from separation. It will need shoes to support the hoof capsule and prevent the collapse of the coronary band.

The loose parts are entirely removed. A section is formed in the top of the hoof capsule to support it.

A normal horseshoe is made in the form of the coronary band as the hoof was originally. A bridge is made which fits exactly into the straight cut-away part.

Part 2 – Disorders of the Limbs and Hooves

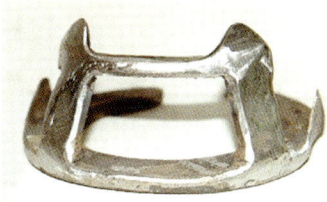

The hoof capsule must be supported on all sides to prevent serious lameness.

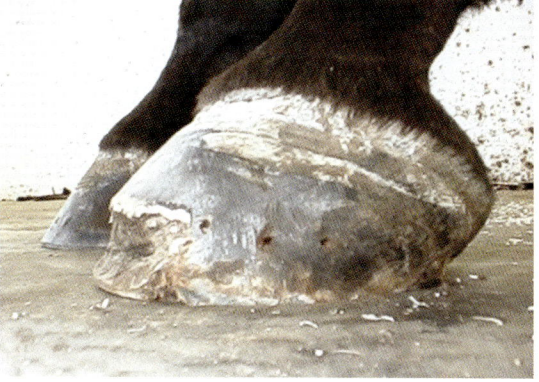

After ten weeks, the hoof capsule has grown a bit and the pedal bone – that is attached to the horny wall – has more support. The hoof no longer needs extra support and can be shod normally.

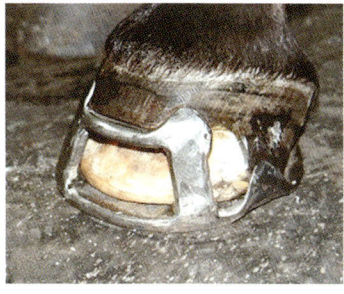

The horseshoe also has two clips so that the hoof capsule cannot spread sideways. Two clips are drawn into the bridge so that the corium is not under pressure.

CASE HISTORY 3, PHOTOS BELOW AND PAGE 142 (TOP)

Separating walls are frequently seen in donkeys because a temperate climate does not suit them and they are usually much too fat and thus have hoof problems. A donkey was presented where all horny wall had vanished because a fungus had attacked the whole hoof capsule. The fungus had caused a separating wall. The horny wall of the donkey's hoof was loose all round the sole and had no more attachment with the insensitive laminae. The pedal bone could thus rock in the hoof capsule as is seen in laminitis. The solar surface had to take on all the pressure of the horny wall, which is easier for donkeys than other solidungulates.

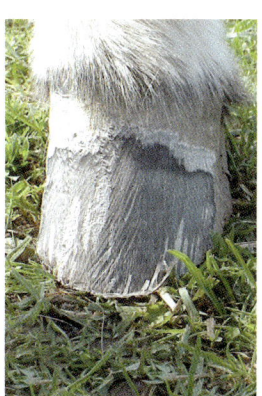

Separating walls can also develop when the hoof is affected by a fungus; this can be seen by the white stripes on the horny wall.

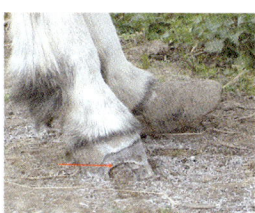

Laminitis with separating walls is often seen in donkeys. People still think that donkeys should be fat but this causes hoof problems. The form of the hoof and the structure of the horn are different from that of horses.

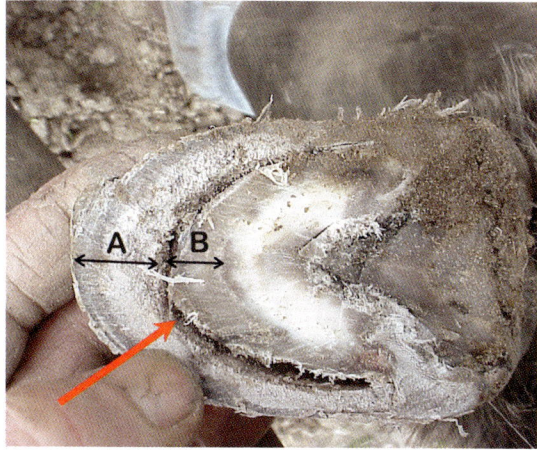

This donkey's hoof displays a separating wall: the break between the horny wall (A) and the broadened white line (B).

The Hoof – Horny Wall

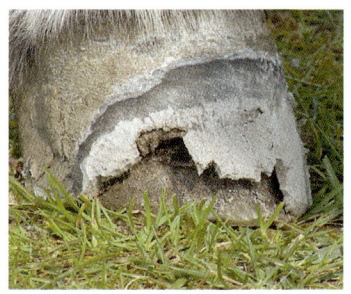
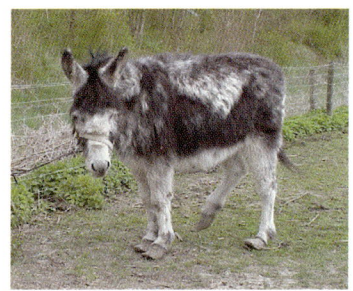
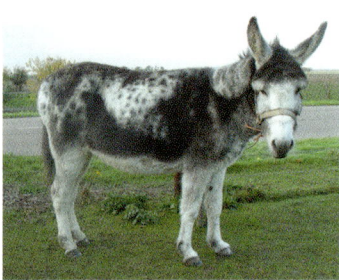

A total loosening of the horny wall.

The life of a donkey can be much improved by good farriery and a suitable diet.

Superficial Horny Wall Cracks

Superficial horny wall cracks are cracks in the horny tubules of the wall. There are two sorts: the first runs parallel to the horny tubules. This crack is mostly caused by damage to the coronary band. Through this, there is a break between the downward growing tubules which leads to a crack. In this sort of crack, the coronary corium can heal spontaneously and continue to develop normal horny wall.

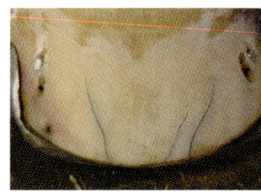

Cross-grained superficial horny wall cracks are not removed – if the horse is not lame – as this weakens the wall.

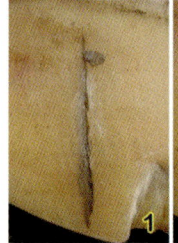 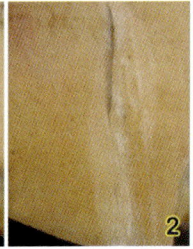 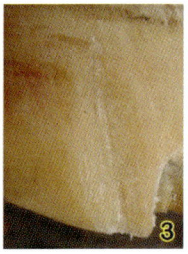

An example of a superficial wall crack.
1. *The crack is about half a centimetre wide.*
2. *The lower part of the crack is filed away.*
3. *All loose horny tubules are filed away and the crack is removed.*

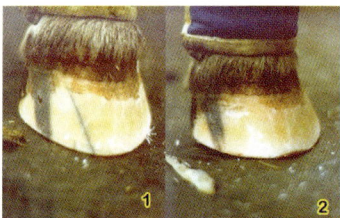

An example of a superficial wall crack that runs across the grain of the horny tubules and which covers more than half the hoof (1). This crack was removed to prevent possible future problems.

The second type of superficial horny wall crack, on the contrary, does not split parallel to the tubules. Horses that 'brush' – strike the fore hoof with the hind hoof – often display cracks that are at right-angles to the horny tubules. This crack on the fore hoof is also seen with horses that constantly kick against a hard stone wall.

CAUSE

Horses with superficial horny wall cracks in their hooves do not become lame. Superficial cracks have many causes. They are never spontaneous but always have a reason; type can be determined by where it occurs. The treatment also depends on the place where the crack appears.

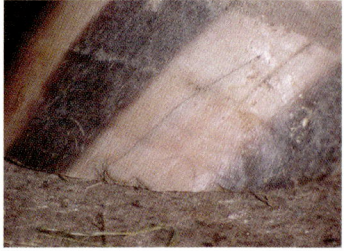

A superficial side wall crack that runs diagonally across the horny tubules at the end; the cause is usually kicking against a wall and it rarely causes problems.

Part 2 – Disorders of the Limbs and Hooves

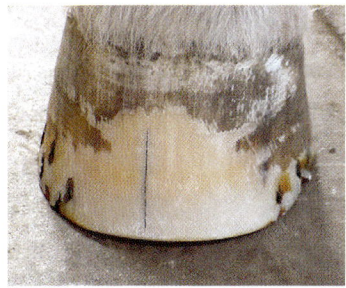

Neither the filing of horizontal grooves nor the burning of a hole is used on superficial grass cracks; this weakens the horny wall and does not prevent further splitting.

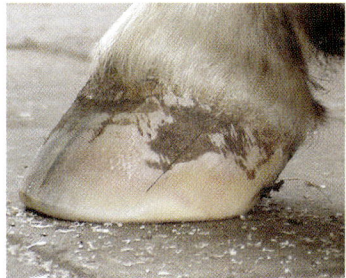

A superficial side wall crack caused by damage to the coronary band does not cause problems.

TREATMENT

A superficial horny wall crack that is parallel with the horny tubules is mostly filed out. This is not harmful to the hoof. The hoof grows down normally from the coronary band. The farrier often files a groove or burns holes to prevent the crack from splitting further. The biggest disadvantage of filing out, making a groove or burning holes is that the horny wall is weakened too much. Therefore, it is better not to file out the crack but to ensure that the horse can no longer kick against the hard surface by, for example, fixing rubber to the doors and walls.

A superficial crack that runs at right-angles across the horny tubules must be checked and then filed out; here, the horny wall is somewhat weakened.

HORSESHOES

Firstly, the farrier must determine what sort of crack it is before deciding whether to remove it or not. With superficial cracks, it is important to shoe the horse with roomy and well-fitting shoes to help protect the hoof from damage caused by kicking against walls. If the horse becomes lame, removing cracks is necessary.

CASE HISTORY 1, PHOTOS LEFT AND BELOW

A horse that was presented had a superficial horny wall crack at the toe. This crack was caused by injury to the coronary band or the coronary corium. The horny tubules were no longer attached at the site of injury, so the coronary corium was completely filed out which allowed for healthy horn growth again.

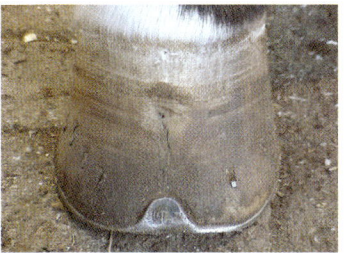

The superficial crack has healed completely after treatment. Perfect horny wall grows down again from the coronary band; this picture shows 2.5 centimetres of healthy horn.

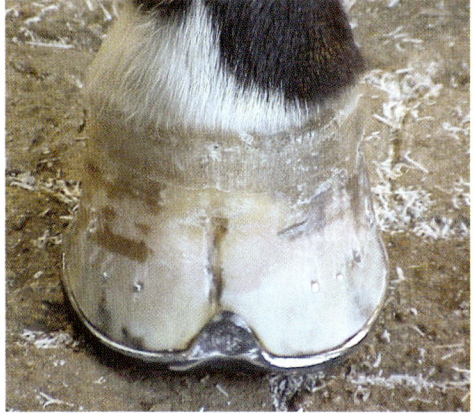

This hoof has been re-shod. The horny wall crack has been cleaned without weakening the wall unnecessarily.

Full Thickness Horny Wall Cracks

Full thickness horny wall cracks are the depth of the horny wall to the corium. Horses are nearly always seriously lame from this type. If the cracks are not treated, the chances of healing are minimal.

Full thickness horny wall cracks can be caused by:
- Kicking against a door or wall
- Too short or too narrow horseshoes
- Horseshoes with double clips
- Damage to the coronary corium
- The outbreak of infection
- Inflamed keratoma

Full thickness horny wall cracks can occur at any place on the horny wall, but mostly at the side walls and particularly in the heel area. As the movement in these parts of the wall is greatest – due to the hoof mechanism – they are very difficult to get under control. If the horse is not lame, the walls can be reasonably kept under control with the help of horseshoes. Cracks do not close up of their own accord and not even with the help of shoes. It is important that the veterinary surgeon or the farrier also tackle the root cause.

A suppurating hoof corium inflammation can easily develop with full thickness horny wall cracks because dirt enters readily and causes infection. The horny wall will be divided into two by the crack and will move separately from the rest of the hoof capsule. This usually causes bleeding at the coronary band. Full thickness cracks are always serious and in most cases lead to serious lameness.

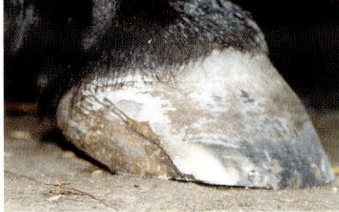

A full thickness hoof crack in the heel area causes more acute lameness because it is constantly being forced open by the hoof mechanism.

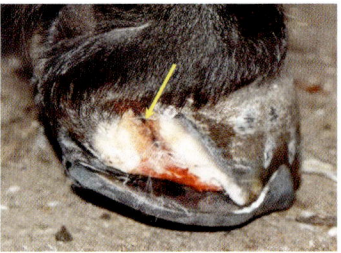

The part behind the crack is removed; the cause is now visible (arrow) – chronically inflamed insensitive and sensitive laminae.

TREATMENT
There are many treatments possible for holding a full thickness horny wall crack together. Clasps, screws and metal or synthetic plates are often used – without results. A full thickness horny wall crack is always as a result of a deeper problem such as injury to the coronary band,

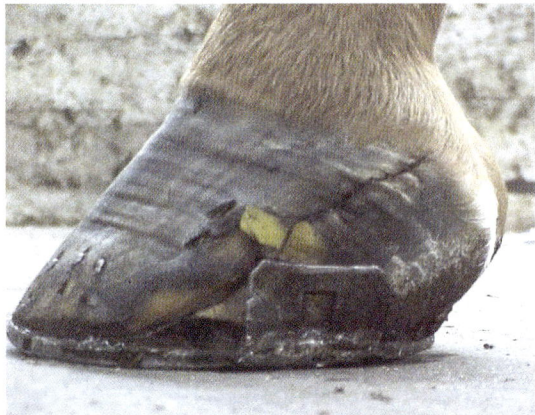

Full thickness cracks are treated in all kinds of ways but mostly the remedy is worse than the disease.

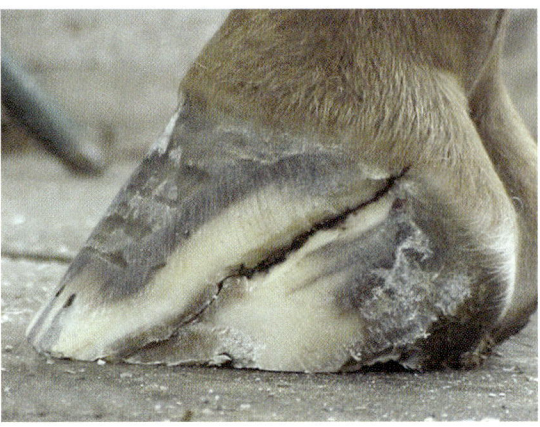

This picture clearly shows that the wall corium is completely inflamed.

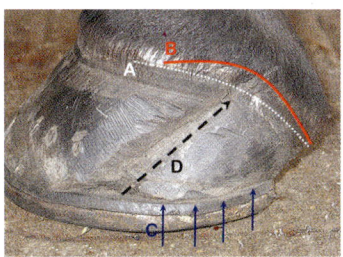
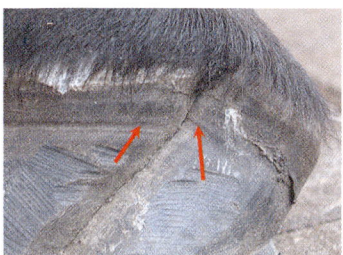
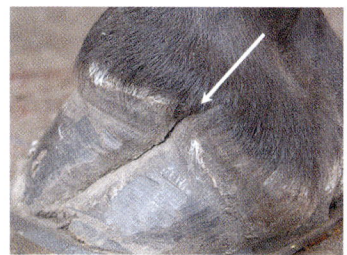

Pressure from the ground (C) causes the part behind the crack to be forced upwards, which pushes up the coronary band (B); (A) shows the normal coronary band profile.

The enormous pressure rubs the two parts of the wall together.

The full thickness makes the horny wall split in two; both parts move separately, which causes lameness.

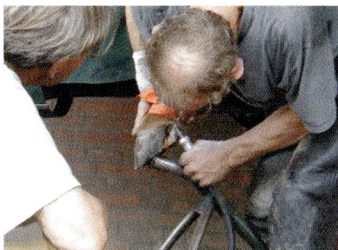
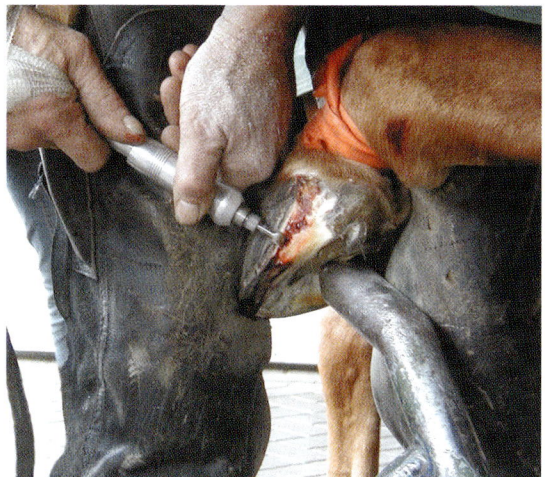

The hoof is temporarily tied with a ligature to block blood circulation. Here, I am filing out the coronary corium; a veterinary surgeon is always present.

The horny wall is filed out until healthy horn is reached.

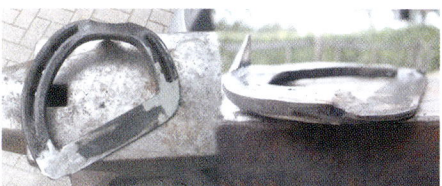

The horseshoe – which was prepared before we began the resection – is applied after the operation. Thus we can prevent the hoof being too long without blood.

inflammation of the wall corium or a keratoma. The coronary band cannot normally heal the crack by itself. Therefore, the germinating layer of the coronary band is stimulated by the filing drill to encourage new growth. This is extremely specialised treatment. When a full thickness horny wall crack is not treated the horse can stay lame.

When full thickness heel wall cracks cause lameness, the loose part at the back must be removed because it is in this part behind the crack that there is the most movement. The horseshoe must be fitted with a light

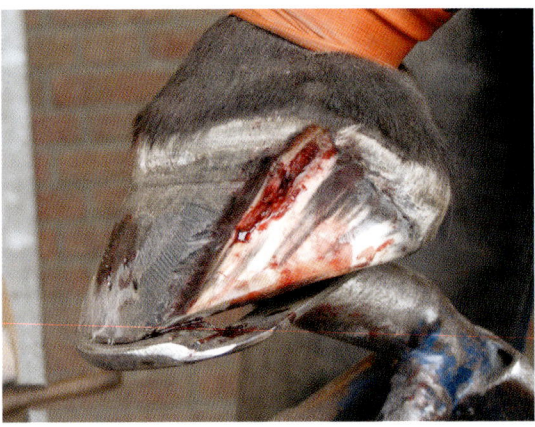

The wound will be dressed with a Betadine (iodine) compress so that the corium does not bulge out, and to prevent infection.

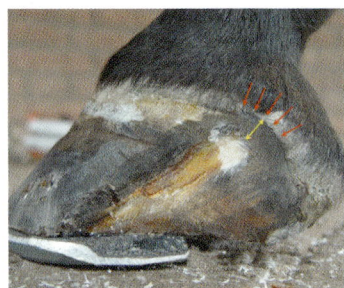

After eight weeks, the wound is dry and hardened. There is already 3 centimetres of new horn (yellow arrow) and the coronary band (red arrows) will return to normal without any cracks.

bar so that there is no movement in the shoe. It is important that the cut-away part of the hoof is not supported by the horseshoe and is free of weightbearing.

HORSESHOES

The shoes for full thickness heel wall cracks are different for each horse. Before the heel wall crack is treated, it must first be determined whether the horse bears weight on the hoof, by making it walk a bit. Then, at shoeing, the manner of weightbearing can be taken into consideration. The horse must always be able to place the hoof flat on the ground. The shoeing nearly always consists of a bar shoe to take any movement out of the shoe.

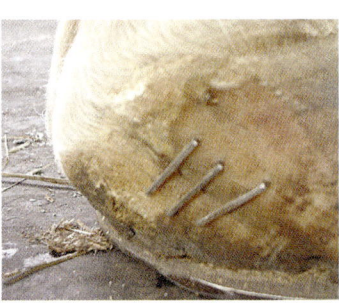

Clasps are not the answer to full thickness hoof cracks.

CASE HISTORY 1, PHOTOS BELOW

A horse that was presented had the commencement of a full thickness horny wall crack which had had little attention, thus the crack had run right to the coronary band. The crack had to be removed as did all irregularities in the wall, to prevent serious problems. Under the crack on the wall corium there appeared to be bruising, which seemed to be the cause of the full thickness horny wall crack. The horny wall had to be removed until a good attachment was reached in all parts of the horny wall and the wall corium. After this the horny wall could heal again.

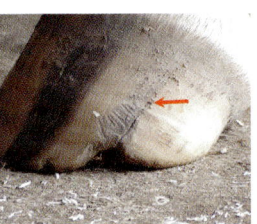

The development of a new full thickness hoof crack which has received too little attention.

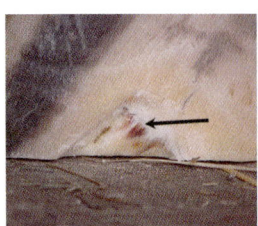

Under the full thickness crack, the bruising that caused the crack is visible in the wall corium.

CASE HISTORY 2, PHOTOS BELOW

A horse was presented where someone had tried to contain the full thickness wall crack with the help of metal plates. The metal plate had caused the horse to become lame due to too great a counter pressure. When the crack was being filed out it appeared that the wall corium was completely inflamed. The crack never could have healed because of the metal plate. The whole heel part of the hoof had to be removed because the corium was completely infected. The hoof was shod in a way that protected the treated part but did not bring weight to bear (upward pressure from the ground on the hoof). In this way, the hoof could grow again properly.

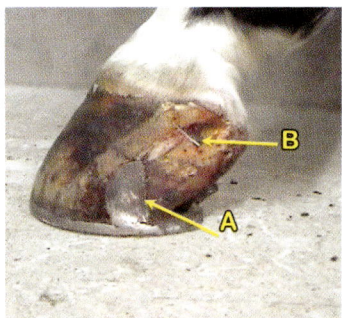 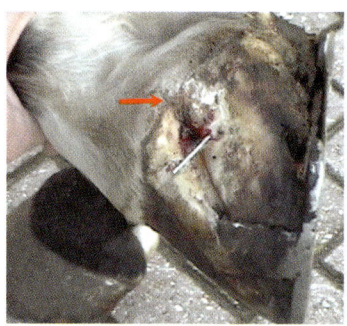 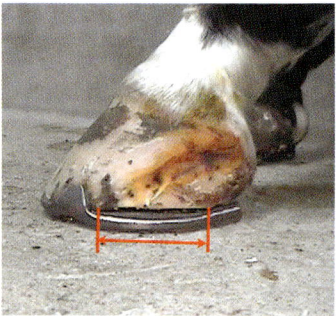

The farrier tried to repair the full thickness crack by welding a metal plate on to the horseshoe (A) so that the wall would not shift. He also put in a clasp – without success – over the crack (B). Because the hoof was too upright, the pressure on the heels was too great so the wall was pushed inwards, which caused serious lameness.

The full thickness crack goes through the coronary band or coronary corium. The part around the clasp is completely infected – it is a big mistake to put in a clasp here.

The hoof is first trimmed in accordance with the foot axis (lower heels) and then the crack is completely filed out. The hoof is not fixed but shod with a large horseshoe whereby part of the side wall is kept completely unburdened (arrow).

CASE HISTORY 3, PHOTOS LEFT AND PAGE 148 (TOP)

A horse that was presented appeared to have a crack in the side wall that had given no problem for years but now was the cause of serious lameness. At examination there appeared to be a dent – a break – in the coronary band. The heel area pressure had forced the heel wall up, which resulted in a full thickness wall crack which continued to bleed a little at the coronary band. The only option was to remove the part of the heel wall that was causing the problem.

    Such treatment always takes place in cooperation with the carer, veterinary surgeon and farrier. The lower foot is anaesthetised and a tight rubber band (ligature) is put on the pastern cavity to temporarily close down the blood circulation in the lower foot. The full thickness crack is filed out until good horn attachment is reached, and the germinating layer of the coronary corium is stimulated. Because of this, the coronary corium gives an extra impulse to the horn to make the horny wall thicker. This treatment requires extremely exact work: if too much is filed away, good horn growth will not take place. The horse was dressed with a Betadine (iodine) compress to prevent the bulging out of the corium. After eight weeks, the horny wall had grown about 2 centimetres and the coronary band had a beautiful profile without a dent. After six months, the horse had a new, healthy hoof capsule.

If a hoof crack is not treated at an early stage, tough measures are needed for the hoof to heal. The wall parts (1 and 2) can move separately and create lameness in the long term.

The Hoof – Horny Wall

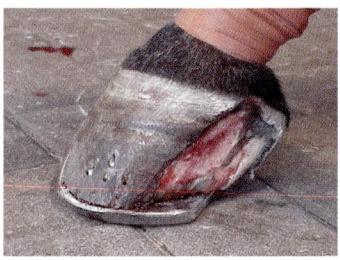 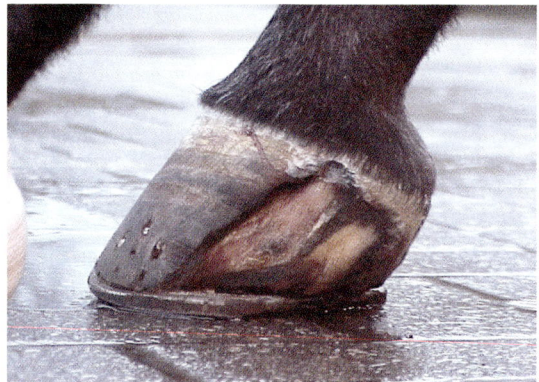

The hoof is anaesthetised and the blood circulation is temporarily blocked by a ligature (tight rubber band). The part behind the crack is filed out until healthy horn attachment is reached. The hoof is shod with a three-quarter shoe – the part with the wound is left unburdened – and afterwards dressed with a compress.

After two weeks, the wound is dry and the horse may be exercised.

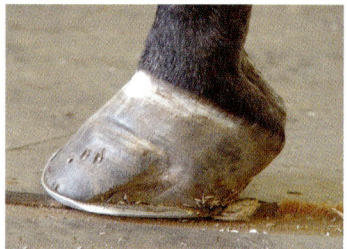

After three months, the hoof has re-grown by more than half. The horse is fitted with a normal horseshoe with a light bar added between the branches, and may be exercised normally.

CASE HISTORY 4, PHOTOS BELOW AND OPPOSITE

Horses can damage their hooves seriously in every imaginable way. This horse had got its hoof wedged, and had torn off the side of the hoof capsule. The owner had taken good measures by dressing the injury immediately and calling the veterinary surgeon and the farrier. This meant the horse was helped rapidly.

There was nothing else for it but to completely remove the loose heel part. In so doing, not only the side wall but half the solar surface was pulled off. The horse had to be shod with a special remedial shoe to protect the wound and control it properly. The horse was fitted with a shoe with a diagonal bar for the necessary stability. The healthy part of

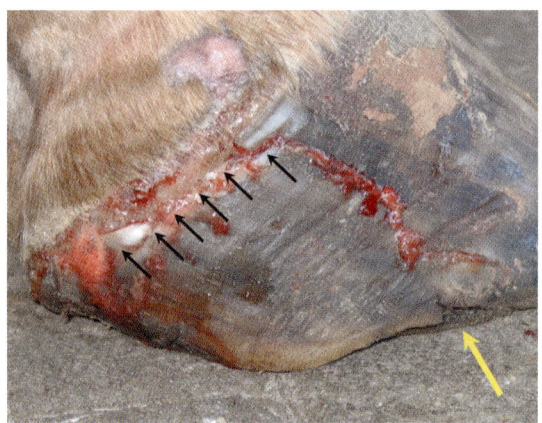 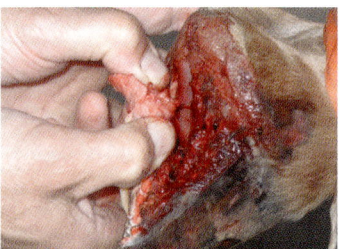

A serious case: the horse pulled off part of its hoof. A grass crack – a weakness in the wall – can be seen clearly.

The whole quarter part can be pulled off from the top; this part can never be stitched back and must be removed.

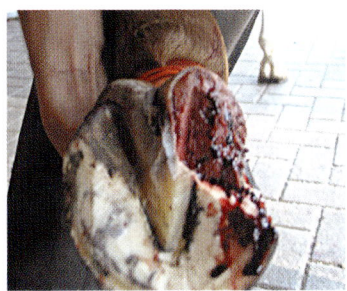
A good view showing the underneath of the hoof. A quarter of the sole and a piece of the frog are missing.

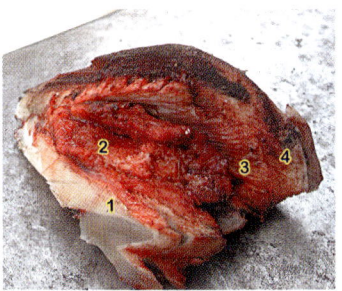
The torn off part.
1. Frog; 2. Sole; 3. Horny wall laminae 4. Coronary band

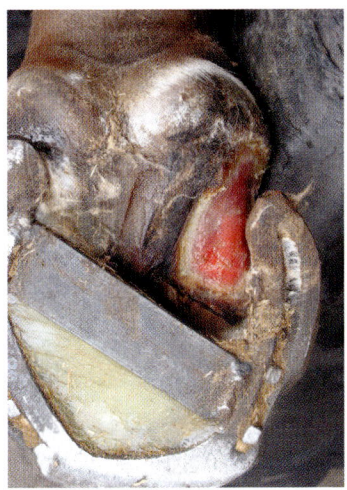
After eight weeks, the wound is properly healed. The white line next to the wound indicates that the closure is going well. Part of the hoof is supported with a metal bar where Equi-Thane Hoof Pak® has been squirted in underneath.

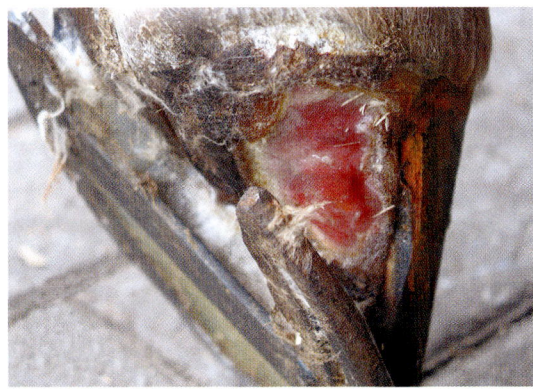
The side of the hoof is also healing very well. The horse can return to full equestrian sport in due course.

the sole was also brought into service by using Equi-Thane Hoof Pak® to provide equal pressure so that the hoof could not collapse.

The hoof was dressed with a Betadine (iodine) compress to prevent the bulging out of the sole and wall corium. After two months, the wound was looking better and the 'white edges' appeared that indicate good healing. The wound had to be protected for a while so that the sole and wall could heal.

4 THE HOOF: TOE

Long Toes and Low Heels

When the length of the toe results in faulty weightbearing of the whole hoof, it is too long. The heels receive too much pressure through this faulty weightbearing, which means that they wear down more than normal – causing low heels – and sometimes even roll under.

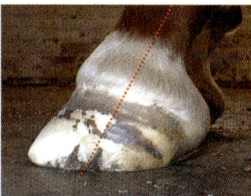

The farrier has trimmed in accordance with the foot axis. The horse can thus place its foot normally.

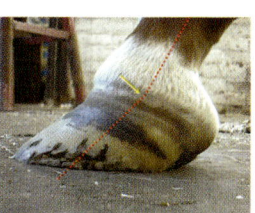

This horse's toe is too long. It is clear to see that the foot axis is broken backwards (yellow arrow). The short and long pastern bones and the pedal bone are no longer an extension of each other. The pressure on the heels becomes greater, with greater wear as a result.

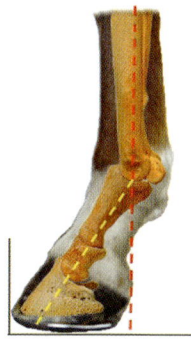

The foot axis is an imaginary line that starts in the middle of the pastern and runs down parallel with the toe of the horny wall. Thus the long and short pastern bones and the pedal bone – that lie along the imaginary line – are an extension of each other.

CAUSE

The greatest cause of hooves with long toes and low heels is faulty treatment of the hoof capsule. This causes changes in the foot axis – the position of the lower foot from below the pastern to the ground. The foot axis is an imaginary line starting at the middle of the pastern and running downwards parallel to the toe wall. The long pastern bone, the short pastern bone and the pedal bone are all in a row on this imaginary line. If the foot axis is broken backwards, then the long and short pastern bones and the pedal bone are no longer an extension of each other. A foot axis broken backwards is caused by the toe of the hoof being left too long so that the total pressure of the hoof capsule moves to the heels. The upshot is more wear and low heels.

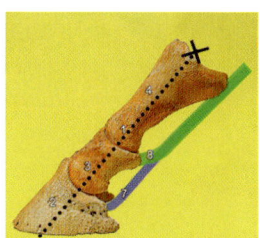

The foot axis of a horse's hoof as it should be. The bones and joints fit together and form a line.

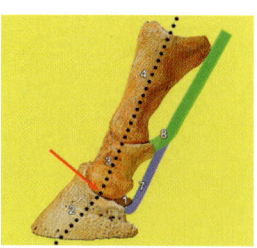

Long toes and low heels give a foot axis where the hoof joint is broken backwards (red arrow). The pedal bone (2) is not an extension of the short pastern bone (3) and long pastern bone (4). This causes more tension on the deep digital flexor tendon.

Part 2 – Disorders of the Limbs and Hooves

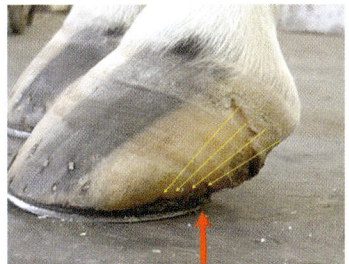

This picture shows clearly that the heel area has become flatter (red arrow) because of the horseshoe. The yellow arrows show the direction of the horny tubules that have become nearly horizontal at the back. What is more, this hoof has been shod with wedges to heighten the heel part; this actually has the opposite effect – the heels have become lower from the extra pressure.

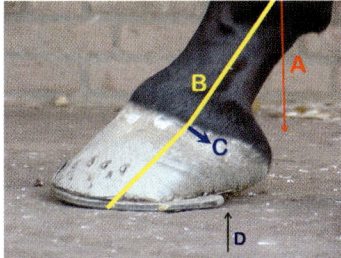

The hoof before treatment. The yellow line (B) shows the foot axis broken backwards at the hoof joint because the toe has been left too long. The pressure that is caused by this broken axis (arrow C) influences the heel area; this causes the line of force (A) to fall behind the bulbs. Thus the horseshoes fall short so that there is insufficient support (D).

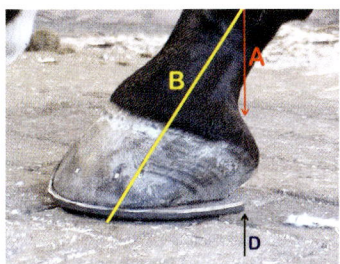

The hoof after treatment. The foot axis (B) has been brought back to the normal conformation and the toe has been shortened. Thus the line of force has clearly been brought forward with a reduction of pressure on the heel area. The branches of the shoe are longer and give good support (D). A Belgian bar shoe has been fitted temporarily to give extra support.

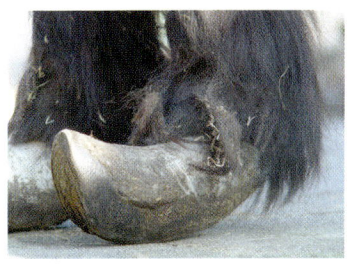

This hoof is badly neglected.

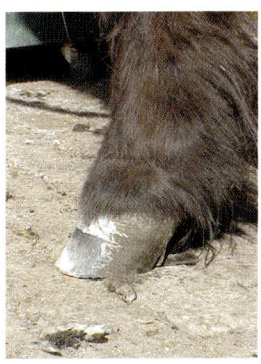

At treatment, the whole toe wall is removed, which returns the hoof to its normal shape.

Horse hooves with long toes and low heels are also caused by faulty trimming or shoeing or lameness where one of the hooves is overburdened. Hooves with long toes and low heels can also be inherited. In a hoof with a long toe and low heel, the solar surface becomes flatter and flatter and can no longer tolerate pressure from the ground, so that sensitive soles ensue.

Horses with long toes and low heels are forced to have the hoof in a deviant foot axis conformation. This can cause trouble in the ligaments and tendons. Above all, a horse with long toes can no longer 'roll' the hoof over well, and steps off with its hoof tardily. The result of this is that, with every step, it catches its shoes – the horse strikes the ends of the branches of the fore shoe or the bulbs of the fore hoof – with its hind hoof (see Over-reaching). The horse can seriously injure itself in this way. As the position of the hoof is defective, the quality of the gait is affected. Back problems can also be caused by long toes and low heels.

DIAGNOSIS

A hoof with long toes and low heels is recognised by the following characteristics:

- A flat solar surface
- A horny wall that is thick in the toe and becomes thinner toward the heels
- Collapsed or rolled-under heels
- The vaulting of the sole surface disappears and the sole becomes flatter
- A wide hoof
- Low, under-run heels and bulbs
- Wide and flat frog

The Hoof – Toe

Hooves with long toes and low heels fall into two categories:
1. **Hooves with long toes, low heels and a straight foot axis.** These hooves should be trimmed normally with no extreme changes in the foot axis. With a generous and long horseshoe the horse can do its work well. Such horseshoes ensure that the hoof receives more support in the heel area. This is not to say that the problem is solved, but nice hooves can be kept intact. These hooves are sometimes unjustly called 'flat feet'; people often try to change these types of hooves by fitting them with shoes with synthetic or metal wedges – a heightening under both branches. This does more bad than good, because this presses the heels down and makes them even lower.
2. **Hooves with long toes, low heels and a foot axis broken backwards.** This category often has problems that are difficult to solve. For example, when trimming the hoof, care has not been taken with the foot axis or the thickness of the wall. As well as this, sometimes the hoof capsule is not filed correctly, the toe wall is left too wide or the side walls are filed too much. Sometimes, too, the horseshoe does not follow the shape of the coronary band.

CASE HISTORY 1, PHOTOS UNDER AND PAGE 153

Not trimming, or insufficient trimming, can lead to the hoof having long toes. At first sight, there was nothing wrong with this horse's hoof except that it had very long toes. After the hoof was thoroughly examined and trimmed, it was apparent that the thickness of the hoof was variable. The left wall was thicker than the right wall. A thinner wall wears down more quickly than a thick wall. If the walls had been of even thickness, the hoof would have worn down evenly. The hoof had a thick wall in the toe part and a thin wall in the heel part. The hoof mechanism ensured that the heel part could move so that the wall – already thin at this point – would wear out more quickly. Because the toe wall was thick and hardly moved, this part wore out less quickly and became stronger, resulting in a long toe.

A hoof with too thick and long toes creates the following problems for the farrier:

1. Each nail hole is at the same distance from the outside edge of the shoe and must correspond exactly to the hoof's white line. When the hoof is thicker than normal, the farrier can never drive the nails into the white line.
2. The nails will be driven outside the white line into the horny wall, which leads to the horny tubules splitting. The wall is made of horny tubules that are not flexible; thus the horny wall will tear and the nails will quickly become loose. In treating these hooves, the toe part is shortened as much as possible, the horny wall is evened up and the heels are touched as little as possible. The horse should be temporarily shod with a Belgian bar shoe – a shoe with a broad, light, metal bar forged between the two branches. Equi-Thane Hoof Pak® is

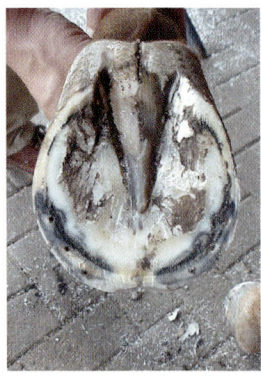

As soon as the hoof was trimmed it was apparent that the horny wall which the horse stood on was of uneven thickness.

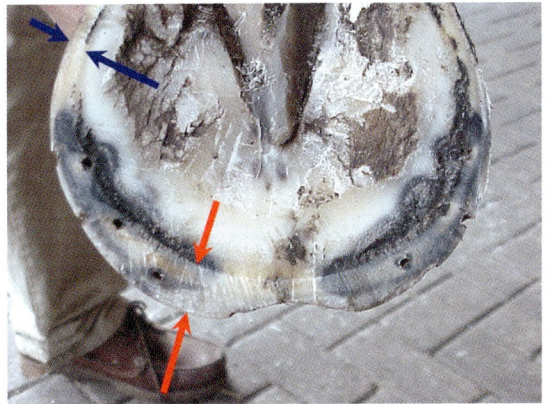

The wall is thicker at the toe (red arrow) than on the sides (blue arrows). Because the toe wall is thicker and hardly moves, it becomes stronger. The horny wall is thinner at the heel area which results in more wear – this develops a long toe.

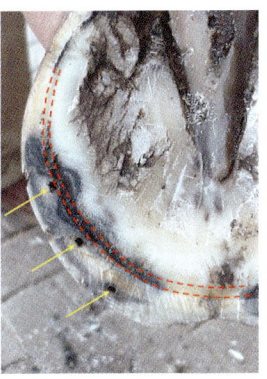

A horseshoe has nail holes that are of equal distance from the outer edge. If the horny wall is thick, the farrier cannot drive the nails into the white line (between the red lines). This picture shows that the last shoes were nailed on, in the toe area, outside the white line.

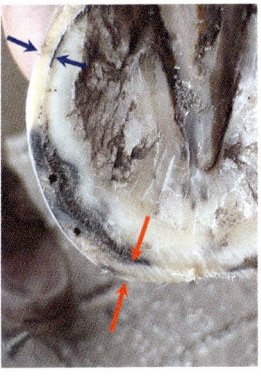

When trimming, the thicker wall at the toe is made as thin as the side of the hoof. This ensures even weightbearing and wearing down of the hoof capsule.

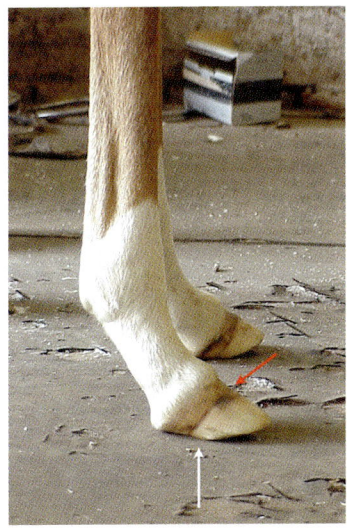

Some foals stand flat on the heels or bulbs, causing the toe point upwards. This problem rights itself after a few weeks.

brought in under the bar to spread the pressure over a greater area. The pressure that the heel walls must bear is, by the effect of the Hoof Pak, shared by the sole and the frog, which creates a greater surface; the pressure on the heels is reduced and heels can be restored.

CASE HISTORY 2, PHOTO LEFT
Sometimes foals stand on the bulbs or the heels of the hoof, which makes the toe point upwards. This position is caused by the fact that the young limbs of foals are still weak. Given time, the problem rights itself. A ring can be clearly seen (red arrow) on the hoof of this foal; the strong yearling hoof is already developing above the ring while under the ring there is still the weak foal hoof.

CASE HISTORY 3, PHOTOS PAGE 154
The owner of a horse that was presented said that the horse took short steps, would not turn, stumbled a lot and had a sensitive hoof. On examination of the hoof, it was apparent that there had been an attempt to heighten the heels by using synthetic wedges. This had caused the destruction of part of the hoof capsule. Because of faulty pressure on the

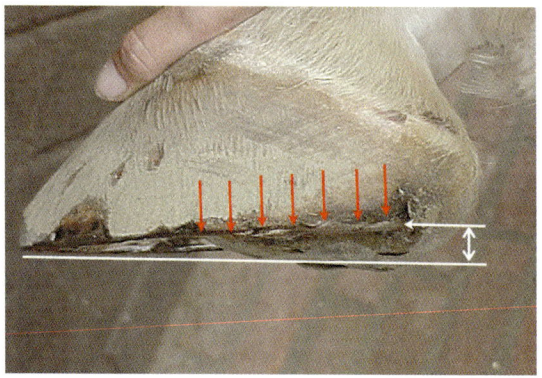

An attempt was made to raise the heels with synthetic wedges, which resulted in the heels being completely pushed down (white arrow).

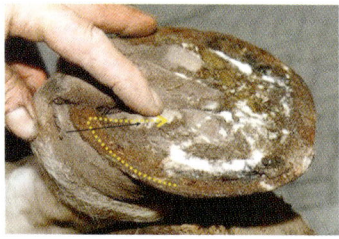

The buttresses of the heel display extra horn growth. This area can be supported with the help of Equi-Thane Hoof Pak® so that the horny wall can repair.

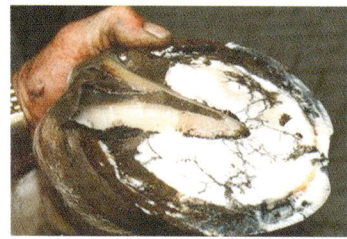

When trimming the hoof, almost nothing should be removed; only the white horn can be pared. Only the toe area is removed. It is important that as much horn as possible is saved and that the solar surface is left as thick as possible.

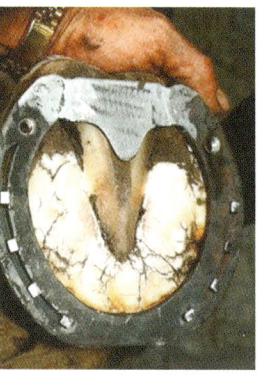

The hoof is fitted with a Dutch bar shoe; only the frog is under pressure when the horse moves.

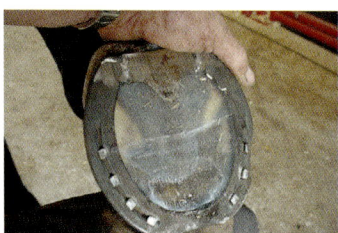

In order to unburden the horny wall, the sole can be put under pressure with the help of Equi-Thane Hoof Pak® inserted in the shoe.

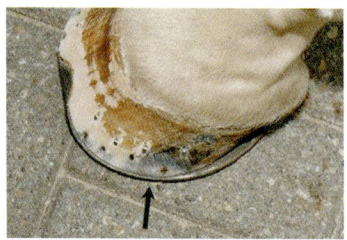

After the third nail hole, the shoe must be wider to allow the hoof mechanism to function well.

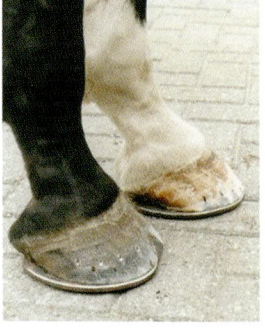

The position of the hooves has been restored as much as possible and, after being shod several more times, the horse will again have healthy hooves. The shoe must be broad and long so that the horny wall can move properly and so that the hoof has not extended over the shoe after two weeks.

heels they had been pushed away and the horse had to put too much weight on the frog. This caused the horse to be lame. On picking up the feet, it was seen that the buttresses of the heel displayed extra horn growth. If necessary, this area can be made to bear weight by applying Equi-Thane Hoof Pak® to unburden the horny wall.

When trimming this hoof it was important to remove as little of the horn as possible. After trimming, a Dutch bar shoe was fitted – a shoe with a bar, whereby the frog receives pressure when weight is borne by the hoof. From the third nail hole, the shoe offers sufficient space (extension) to the hoof. The branches were long enough and gave the hoof enough support. The horseshoe had to be wide and long enough so that the hoof capsule could move well on the shoe and so that the hoof, after two weeks, would not extend beyond the shoe.

CASE HISTORY 4, PHOTOS BELOW

A horse that was presented had collapsed walls because the buttress of the heels was interrupted and turned under – this adversely affected the position of the hoof. When horses have under-run heels and thereby a foot axis broken backwards, immediate action must be taken. The under-run heels must be removed completely so that the heel wall regains its former shape. A horseshoe with a broad bar is fitted. The heels are also supported by Equi-Thane Hoof Pak®. The fit of the shoe is generous.

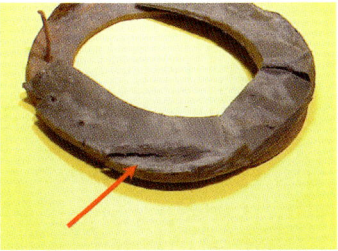

In order to heighten heels, synthetic wedges are often used. The heels will press into the wedges and thus not be able to move or roll under; the use of synthetic wedges is usually a case of the remedy being worse than the disease.

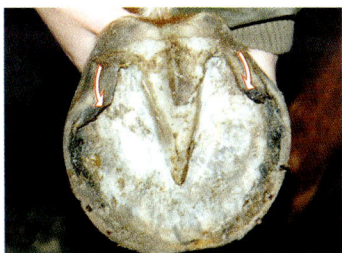

The heel area is rolled under, which has a bad effect on limb conformation. This rolled-under horny wall at the heel can also cause bruising and inflammation in the solar surface.

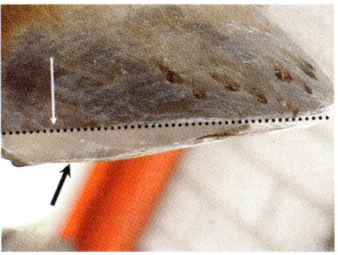

The heel wall is vigorously removed so that the frog even bulges out from under the bearing edge.

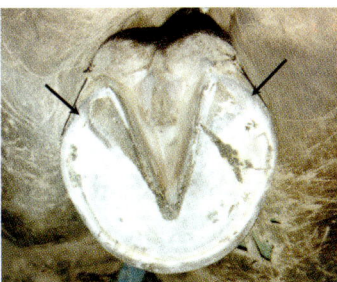

By removing the rolled-under parts, a healthy heel wall can grow down again normally. A shoe with a broad bar can be fitted. The hoof is shod with a wide shoe.

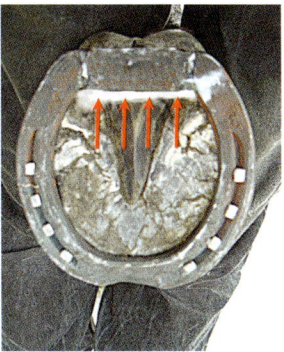

This is a Belgian bar shoe where Equi-Thane Hoof Pak® has been packed between the bar and the hoof so that the heels can no longer roll under and can be properly supported. This allows them to grow back normally.

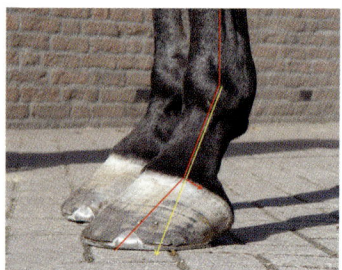
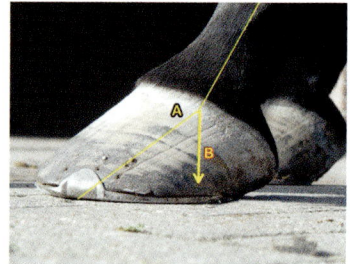
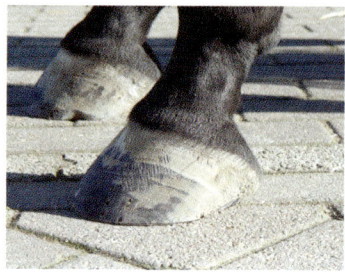

Fore shoes with double clips cause big problems: the hoof mechanism is blocked and the hooves become narrower.

The foot axis (A) is broken backwards in the hoof joint, which causes greater pressure on the heel area. As a result of the side clips, the hoof becomes even longer. Moreover, the horny wall extends beyond the shoe.

This neatly trimmed hoof will be shod normally with a shoe with a toe clip, so that the hoof mechanism can operate again.

CASE HISTORY 5, PHOTOS ABOVE

A very serious problem here was shoes with double clips; a fashion fad which hinders the hoof's mechanism and which changes the shape of the hoof: the hoof becomes narrower. With these shoes, the toes will become longer and the heels will receive more pressure, which means more wear and the heels becoming lower. The foot axis is automatically broken backwards. Because the toe becomes longer, the horseshoe is also 'pulled' forward so that the heel walls are no longer supported. The horny wall behind the clips will break because of this restraint. Anybody with a bit of understanding of horse anatomy can only come to the conclusion that a horseshoe with double clips on the fore hooves is undesirable.

CASE HISTORY 6, PHOTOS RIGHT AND OPPOSITE

The paring of hooves and the measuring up of a well modelled horseshoe seems to be a great problem for some farriers. Many hoof problems can be traced back to bad, sloppy or tardy (not always the fault of the farrier) shoeing.

Before treatment: a horseshoe on a fore hoof that unfortunately is seen too often; an oval shoe that does not fit. This horse will roll its hoof over more at the outer side because the pointed front of the shoe is in the way. The heels have grown over the shoe and are blocking the hoof mechanism. This shoe will cause the heel part to break off and become lower.

After treatment: the same fore hoof but with a horseshoe that fits. A fore hoof should be round, because the shape of the coronary band and the coffin bone in the hoof capsule are equally rounded. The hoof is shod with a shoe two sizes bigger that is sufficient in length to support the heels.

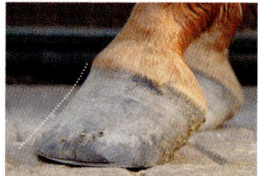

A hoof where the toe runs forward in a curved line (white line). The toe wall should be straight.

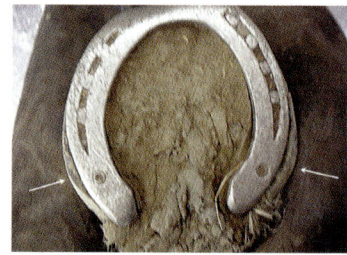

There are still quite a few horses shod with an oval shoe that does not fit. This horse will break over with its hoof more to the outside, because the pointed front is in the way. The heels have grown over the shoe and block the mechanism of the hoof. This horseshoe will cause the heel area to break off and become lower.

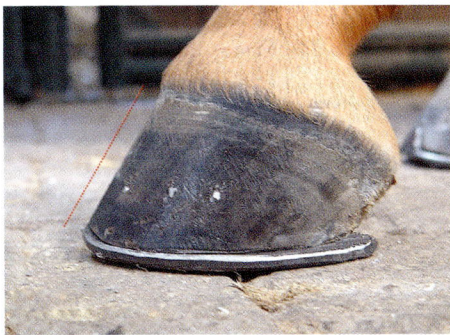

Correct shoeing. The horny wall runs straight (red line) which allows the hoof capsule to bear the weight of the horse easily.

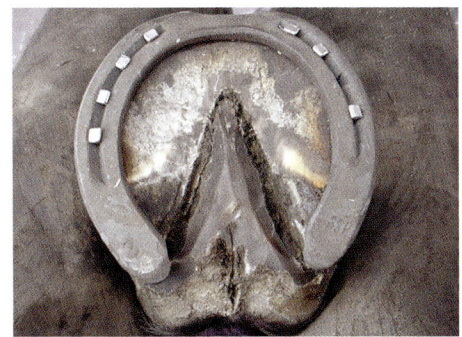

A fore hoof should be round just as its horseshoe should be. The farrier has now fitted a shoe that fits correctly. The shoe is two sizes bigger than the former horseshoe and it has enough length to support the heels.

Inflammation of the Toe

An inflammation in the toe is usually a simple, infected hoof corium inflammation accompanied by pus formation. This inflammation is also called *Pododermatitis purulenta*.

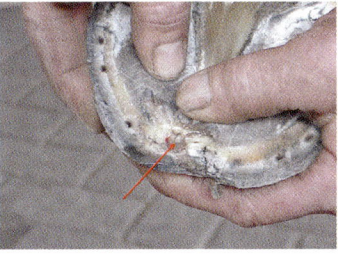

An inflammation in the toe of the hoof (arrow). This inflammation does not migrate upwards via the horny tubules but creeps further along the white line and under the solar surface.

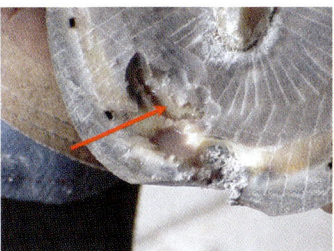

The inflammation can loosen the whole sole from the sole corium. Here, a piece has been opened up so that the pus can drain out (red arrow shows the edge of the pedal bone).

CAUSE

Inflammation mostly starts because dirt from outside works its way into the white line where bacteria get the chance to develop. An inflammation in the toe causes pressure in the hoof capsule which is painful for the horse. An infected inflammation will always seek a route between the insensitive and the sensitive laminae, up to the coronary band. The lameness can vary from slow and slight to sudden and very serious, interspersed with days of no lameness. An inflammation of the corium can also be a result of a sharp object puncturing the solar surface and wounding the corium directly underneath. (See Puncture Wounds.)

SYMPTOMS

A horse that has an inflammation in the hoof suddenly becomes acutely lame. The horse has a high pulse rate – the pulse can be felt at both hoof arteries found on the inner and outer sides of the pastern cavity – and puts its foot down in a certain way; it mostly puts its hoof forward and keeps it stretched to rest the inflamed part as much as possible. The horse may also sweat and paw the ground restlessly. The limb displays a build-up of fluid. The farrier can determine where the inflammation is by observing how the horse sets its feet down.

DIAGNOSIS

An inflammation of the toe can usually be confirmed by observing the way the horse stands and moves. In some cases, other problems can display the same lameness – such as a crack in the pedal bone, separating walls, a keratoma, thrush and ligament problems.

TREATMENT

An inflammation must always be treated. The veterinary surgeon and/or the farrier examine the sole with probing pincers; by squeezing the hoof with the pincers the place with pain can be determined. The horse reacts to pressure on the painful spot, indicating where the inflammation is. With a hoof knife, the horn is removed layer by layer at the inflamed spot until it is exposed. The inflammation is opened up so that pus and dirt can be removed. By taking the pressure off the inflammation the horse has less pain and moves better.

After treatment, it is extremely important to keep the wound clean. Usually, the farrier will fit a shoe immediately so that the inflamed area is protected from ground pressure and the wound is kept properly visible so that it can be kept clean and be checked every day. After shoeing, the hoof is dressed for two days with a wet bandage with a bactericidal solution.

HORSESHOES

A horse with an inflammation in the hoof is best shod with a normal horseshoe. If necessary, the toe part is forged in a way that relieves pressure on the inflamed area. Also, if necessary a cotton pad can be put between the shoe and the inflammation so that no dirt can get into the wound. If the inflammation is very serious, a horseshoe with a surgical plate can be fitted: this is a normal shoe with four screw holes where a metal plate can be fixed. Padding can be inserted between the plate and the hoof so that the solar surface is under pressure and/or so that the wound is kept clean.

CASE HISTORY 1

A horse had an inflamed sole. The cause of the inflammation was unevenness – probably from sand or pebbles – between the horseshoe and the solar surface. The inflammation was cut open and cleaned. A shoe was fitted with a forged-out toe area so that the sole could not burden the shoe and the area was protected from dirt and ground pressure.

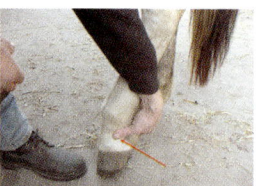

The pulse rate of a horse can be easily felt on the hoof arteries which are to be found on the inner and outer sides of the pastern cavity. The pulse is more evident than in the other limbs.

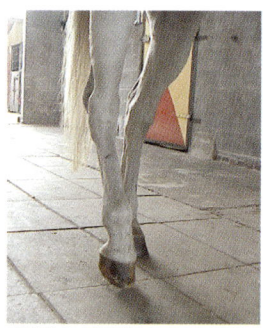

The farrier or the veterinary surgeon can determine where the inflammation is according to the way the horse places its hoof.

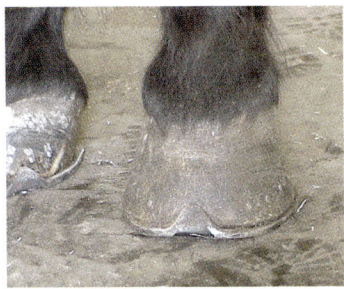
This apparently healthy hoof made the horse seriously lame.

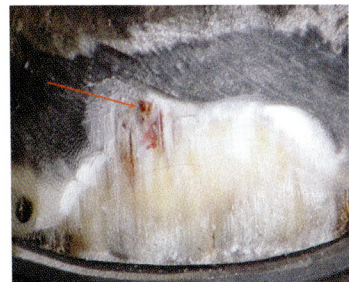
In the middle of the hoof, an aseptic (without bacteria) inflammation had developed. A horse with an aseptic inflammation will be seriously lame.

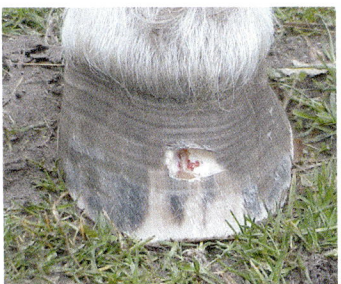
In order to save as much of the horn as possible, the hoof is filed out in the middle. This kind of treatment demands much experience and skill.

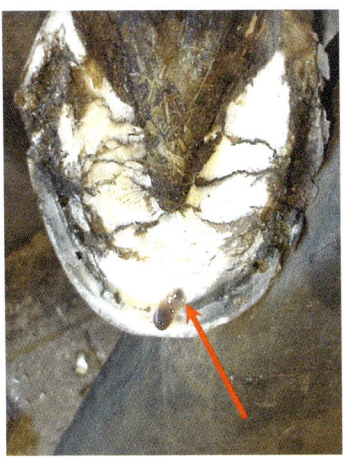
The toe inflammation in the sole is caused by the friction of sand or unevenness between the solar surface and the horseshoe.

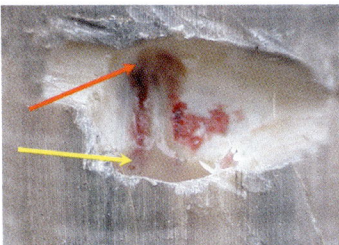
A tiny channel is visible between the horny tubules (red arrow) that led the inflammation to the coronary band. When the horny tubules were pulled open, the pus came out (yellow arrow) which will prevent further damage.

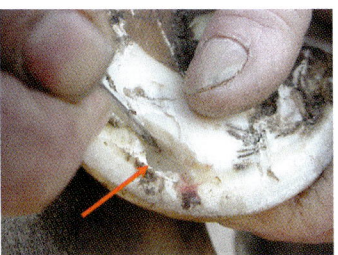
A lot of experience is needed to find an inflammation and afterwards to treat it in such a way that the horn or the weightbearing edge receives as little damage as possible.

CASE HISTORY 2, PHOTOS ABOVE

A horse that was presented was seriously lame. The hoof artery pulse rate on the inner and outer side of the pastern cavity was extremely high. The hoof was placed down only at the toe and the horse could barely walk. Under the hoof a channel was visible between two insensitive laminae in the white line. The channel was opened up but without success: the pressure remained and the pulse rate remained extremely high. The hoof capsule was warm in the toe area. After consultation, the hoof capsule was opened in the middle; this way of working prevents the hoof from being made too weak. A tiny channel was visible, between the insensitive laminae; on opening the laminae, the pus came out and thus the pressure was relieved and the horse could weight its foot normally again. The corium was cleaned so that this could not close up and the inflammation continue to develop. Afterwards, the whole hoof was dressed with a wet bandage with bactericidal solution. After a couple of days, the horse was free from inflammation.

CASE HISTORY 3, PHOTOS THIS PAGE AND OPPOSITE

A horse that was presented had suddenly become lame. The owner had immediately called the farrier but nothing could be found so the horse had been sent on to us. The horse placed its foot more and more to the side. When moving, the horse turned its hoof out exaggeratedly and placed it down on the inner side. The owner said the horse had not been right for a few of weeks but that had passed. When probing the hoof, the outer side of the hoof appeared to have a lot of pain and the white line had changed in shape at the painful spot. The horse had a rapid pulse rate which possibly indicated an inflammation. It was decided to file out a small hole at the place where it was thought the problem was, to save the wall as much as possible. When the corium was reached, a black discharge flowed out; the horny wall had to be removed after all in order to reach the corium. The corium appeared to be inflamed and had to be removed. The wall was removed until healthy horn attachment was reached. A horseshoe was immediately fitted, with a clip behind the wound so that the hoof would not break out. The hoof was dressed with a Betadine (iodine) compress. After a week, the wound had dried well;

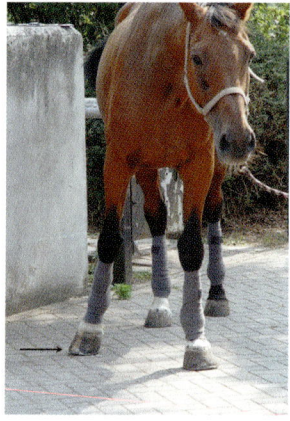

This very lame horse puts its right fore hoof to the outside.

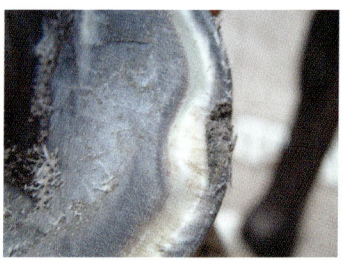

Examination showed that the white line had undergone a change of form; this could be from an inflammation or a keratoma.

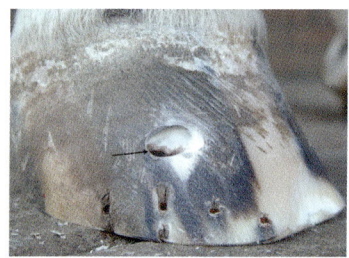

A hole is filed so that the horny wall is saved as much as possible.

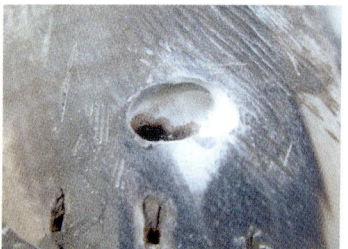

When the wall corium is reached, the black discharge flows out. This indicates that an area of horny wall must also be removed.

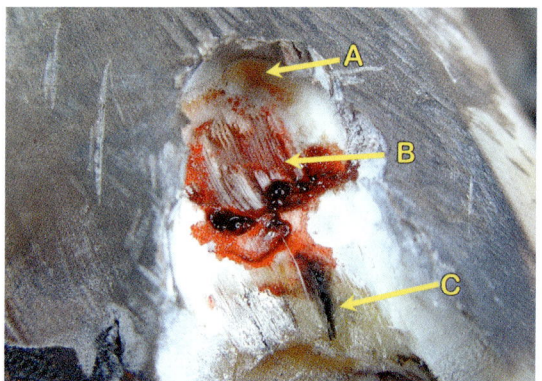

After the wall is removed, the root cause is visible (C): inflamed laminae in the white line (B). The inflamed insensitive and sensitive laminae at the pedal bone (A). The yellow insensitive laminae – which should have been ivory white – are removed.

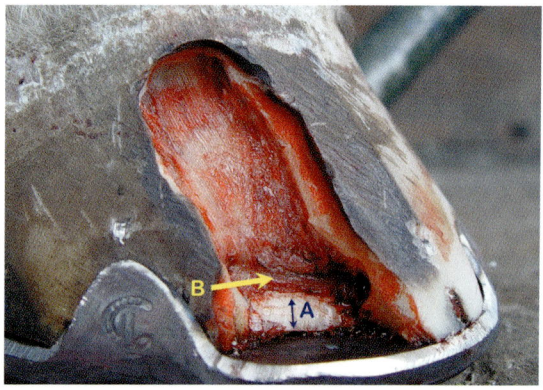

A clean wound with all parts visible. The thickness of the sole corium (A). The underside of the pedal bone (B).

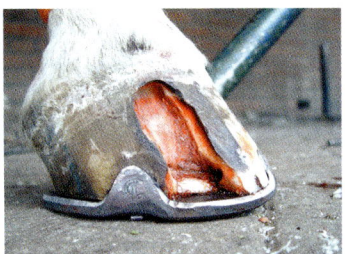

The hoof is dressed with a Betadine (iodine) compress to prevent the corium from bulging out. The horseshoe with the side clip ensures that the hoof cannot break out.

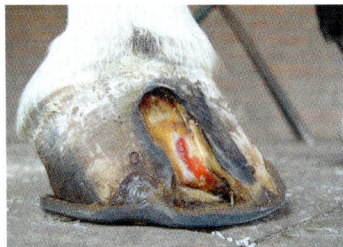

After one week, the hoof is healing well and is dry; the corium has stayed in place.

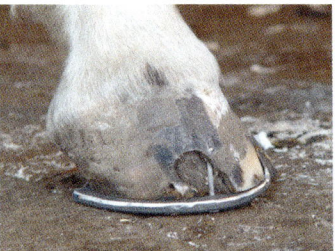

After two months the wound has closed. The wall must never be packed with filling material to try to prevent inflammation.

because of the compress the corium had not bulged out, and the lameness had also disappeared. After two weeks, the wound closed well and an ordinary bandage was put on: the horse was allowed daily exercise.

CASE HISTORY 4, PHOTOS BELOW

This is an example of a serious and rare breakout at the area of the coronary band. A septic (staphylococcus bacteria) inflammation infected the bone membrane and bone and had migrated to the coronary band. Such cases deteriorate very quickly and treatment is practically impossible.

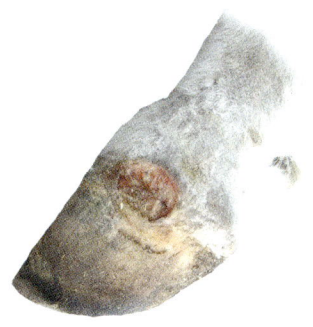

An extremely serious and rare breakout in the coronary band area. A septic (staphylococcus) inflammation in this area affects the bone membrane and bone and forces a way to the coronary band.

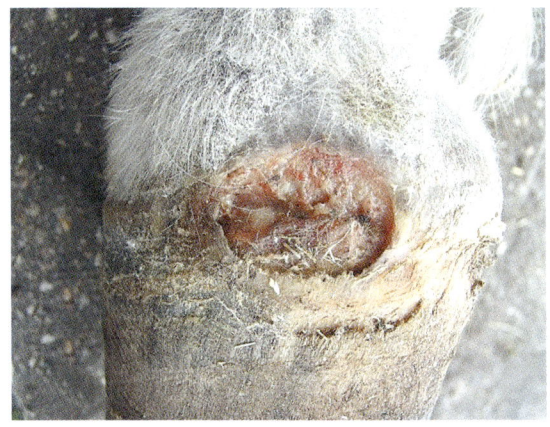

These staphylococci destroy the area and they affect all the bones and tissues. In the end, there is nothing for it but to have the horse put down.

4 THE HOOF: HEELS

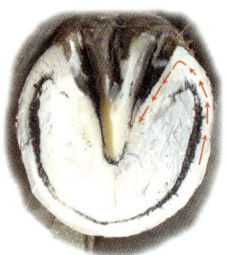 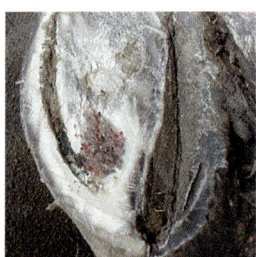 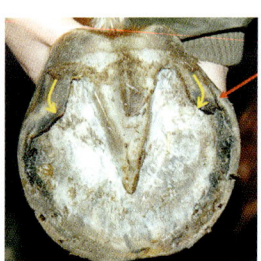 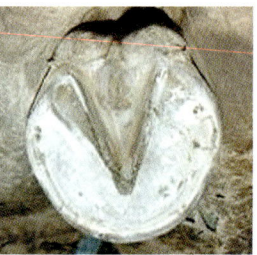

Normally the horny wall at the buttresses of the heels runs parallel with the lateral clefts (red arrows). This angle – called the 'bar' – must not have a break in it. By removing too much at trimming the bars can become too weak, enabling the horny wall to break in or out.

Rolled-under heels can press into the solar surface and cause bruising. The horse becomes even lamer; the pressure and movement in the solar surface can cause inflammation in the hoof.

Rolled-under heels must be treated properly because the horny wall, which rolls under, can break off (red arrow). The yellow arrow shows how the wall rolls under.

The hoof has been trimmed and the rolled-under heels removed. Thus the heels are made stronger ('blocked') and they can produce a straight and healthy horny wall.

Rolled-Under Heels

Rolled-under heels are recognised when the walls of the lateral clefts curl inwards, due either to faulty trimming or to incorrect limb conformation of the horse.

CAUSE

Rolled-under heels can be caused by, among other things, the horse's hoof being shod without paying attention to the foot axis. A foot axis is an imaginary line that begins in the middle of the pastern joint and is drawn through the long and short pastern bones and the pedal bone. This line runs parallel to the front of the hoof capsule. When the foot axis is broken, the line is straight from the long pastern bone to the short pastern bone; at the short pastern bone the line is 'broken' backwards and then is drawn, at an angle, parallel to the front of the hoof capsule to the ground. In trimming, a broken foot axis is caused by allowing the toe to be too long. The pressure on the heels becomes greater and causes curling under.

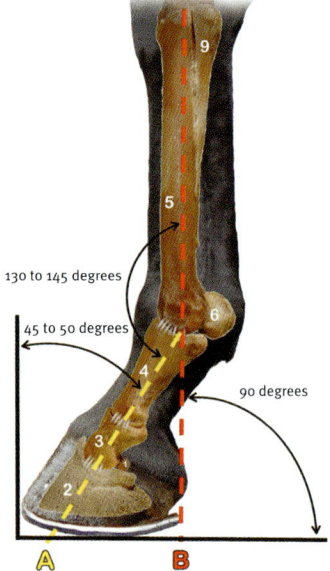

Angles of 130 to 145 degrees; angle of toe wall 45 to 50 degrees; 90 degrees angle with ground surface.

A foot axis is an imaginary line (A) that begins in the pastern and runs through the long pastern and short pastern bones and the pedal bone. This line runs parallel to the front of the hoof capsule.

Part 2 – Disorders of the Limbs and Hooves

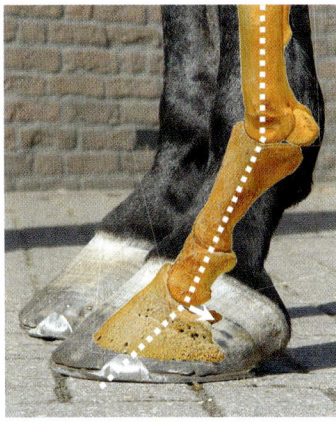

A foot axis broken backwards, caused by too long a toe. This causes great pressure on the rear part of the hoof or the heels.

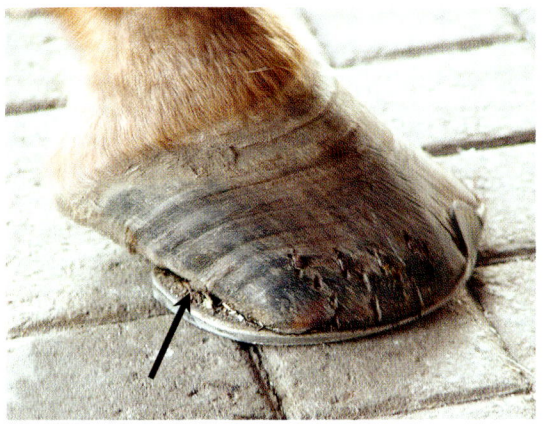

This horse's problem was caused by a toe that was too long and too small a horseshoe; the branches of the shoe are too short. The hoof walls have extended over the inner side of the shoe. The heels will flatten due to the enormous pressure and the horny wall will roll under. If an imaginary vertical line is drawn down from the bulbs, one finds the place where the branches of the shoe should end.

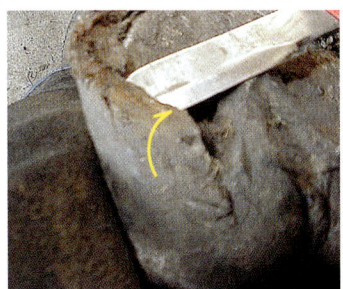

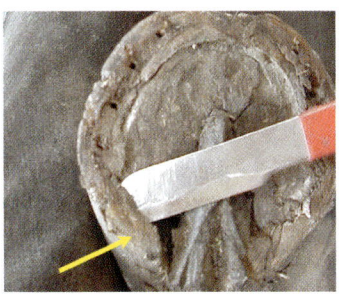

By shoeing this horse with synthetic wedges, the problem has merely worsened. The heels are pushed into the wedge and can no longer function. The hoof will grow down normally, causing the horn capsule to become a little wider; the heels cannot grow outwards and thus will roll under.

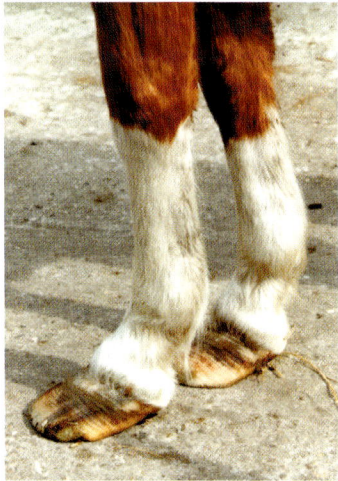

Due to neglect, these heels will roll under extremely and the horse will use the horny wall as heels.

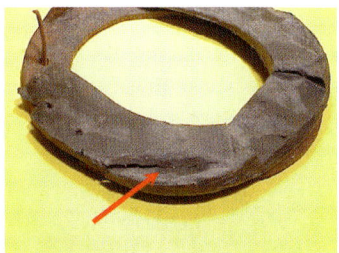

There was an attempt to raise the heels with the help of synthetic wedges. However, the horse will stand according to its normal foot axis and thus will press the heels into the wedges, putting more pressure on the heels. The wall becomes fixed and rolls under; because the heels can no longer move there is a chance they may break.

Rolled-under heels can also be caused by placing synthetic wedges between the horseshoe and the hoof. The placing of wedges is an attempt at raising the heels; by so doing, the foot axis is changed. The horse will try to set down its hoof according to its normal foot axis and will, thus, intensify the pressure on the heels, whereby they will be pressed into the synthetic wedges. The consequence of this is that the walls get fixed into the wedge and can no longer 'slide' (hoof mechanism) and they therefore curl under and can tear.

Rolled-under heels can also press against or into the solar surface, resulting in bruising and/or inflammation. This can be compared to an ingrowing toenail in humans. When the rolled-under heels put pressure on the sole the horse can suffer serious lameness.

The Hoof – Heels

TREATMENT

There is only one way to treat rolled-under heels. When trimming, all rolled-under parts must be removed. The hoof must be trimmed in such a way that a continuous weightbearing edge and heel area are created. The heel area must be enlarged; this is also called 'blocking'. For the present, one cannot take the position of the hoof into account; the hoof will have, temporarily, low heels. Fortunately, the heels are quickly restored.

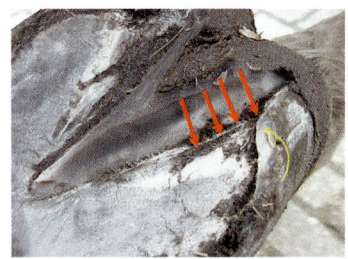

By removing too much of the bar, or by the use of wedges, loose heel walls arise (red arrows). The bar, by the movement of the heel wall (yellow arrow), will gradually attach itself. A skilled farrier can find a solution here.

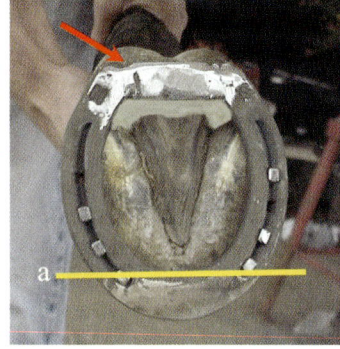

An example of a shoe for horses with rolled-under heel walls. A light bar is welded between the branch ends. Equi-Thane Hoof Pak® is inserted (red arrow) under the bar so that the heels can no longer roll inwards. The hoof is shod with a Hoofcare® Breakover horseshoe so that the point that the horseshoe rolls its toe over is further back than with a normal shoe.

Under-Run Heels

If the wall at the buttress of the heel – the farthest back part of the heel – turns under and the horny wall becomes flatter and serves as the weightbearing surface, this is called under-run heels.

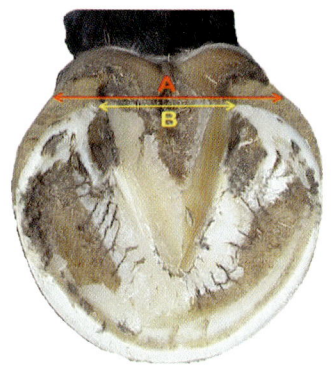

Under-run heels are hoof defects. The heel buttresses no longer have a sharp angle but turn gradually. The horn doesn't grow outwards but inwards. Thus the horny wall lies flatter and acts as the weightbearing surface of the hoof, which forces the heels inwards. Normal width of the heels (A). The heel buttresses lie far under the hoof (B).

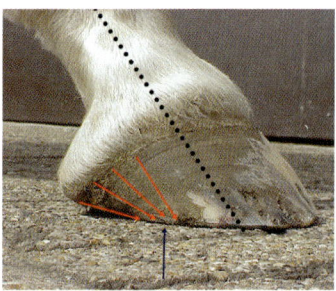

Horses with under-run heels can have a normal foot axis. That does not mean that the pressure on the heels is correct. In this example, the heel walls are actually lying flat.

CAUSE

There are a number of causes of under-run heels:
- Narrow hooves and hooves with a less-developed frog
- The foot axis is normal but the back half of the hoof is narrow, which causes the horny wall, in the back half, to turn in
- Too-short horseshoes, which give the heels too little support
- Too-narrow horseshoes, which cause the walls to drop down over the shoes and become seriously damaged. The walls become too thin and weak
- Removing too much of the turn at the buttresses of the heel, which undermines the strength of the heels

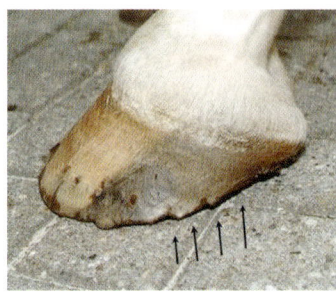

The heels are lying under the vertical line and have become extremely thin and broken.

Part 2 – Disorders of the Limbs and Hooves

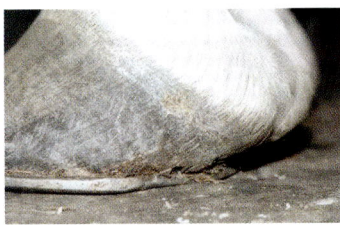

A horseshoe that is too short and too narrow causes the heels to hang over the shoe.

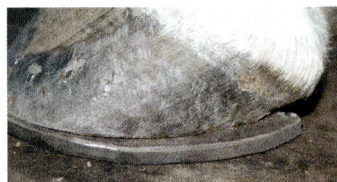

This well-fitted horseshoe – broad and long – supports the heels sufficiently.

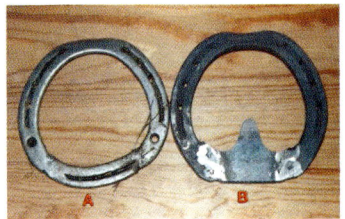

A horse that was presented had been fitted with the horseshoe on the left. The shoe is two sizes too small, and a round piece of old horseshoe has been welded between the branches. Moreover, the horseshoe is lopsided. The horseshoe on the right is the shoe that was subsequently fitted; it is a beautifully forged Belgian bar shoe.

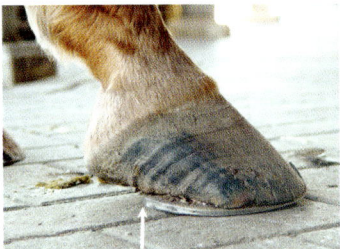

A hoof capsule that is hanging over the horseshoe. The heels are lying completely flat; they should be at 45 degrees.

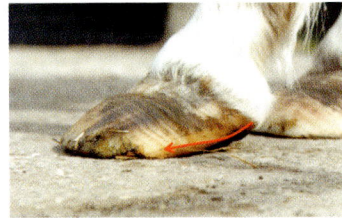

A neglected hoof caused by laminitis. This can cause under-run heels (red line; heels).

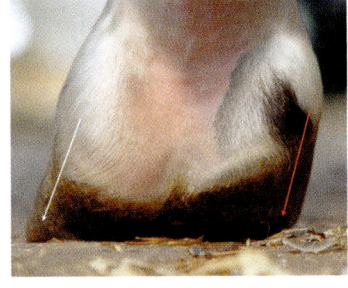

A base-wide conformation can produce under-run heels. Horses with this defect can be helped by a skilled farrier. This conformation should not be changed in any way.

- Defective horseshoes; for example, the use of synthetic wedges that break the horny wall. The heels receive too much pressure from such defective shoes and break down
- The neglect of the hoof; for example, by neglecting laminitis
- A defective conformation, such as a base-narrow or base-wide conformation. These conformations can usually be rectified by good shoeing

The pressure of the hoof on the ground is usually equal. When the horse has a foot axis broken to the back, the line of the foot axis lies more toward the back half of the hoof: the two halves of the hoof are loaded unequally. The result of this is that the pressure is greater at the back of the hoof than at the front. Thus, uneven wear ensues.

Horses with low heels or flat feet can, with the loading at the back half of the foot, have heels that do not stand at an angle of 45 degrees but lie extremely horizontally. Under-run heels are more common in fore hooves than in hind hooves.

TREATMENT

A horse with under-run heels must be shod temporarily with a broad and long horseshoe. A bar is welded into the shoe, preventing pressure on the frog when the hoof bears weight. The whole under-foot is packed with Equi-Thane Hoof Pak®; this is a stiff, fluid substance which can be worked and which dries in 20 seconds. When the solar surface bears weight, the heels are unburdened.

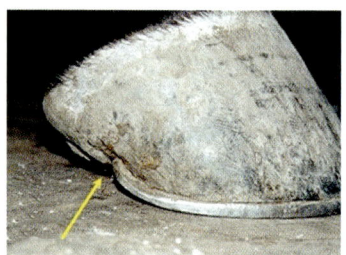

There are numerous horseshoes that merely make problems worse. The horse on the left was constantly pulling shoes off, so the branch ends were fitted to curve into the heels, causing malfunction; the heels were forced inwards.

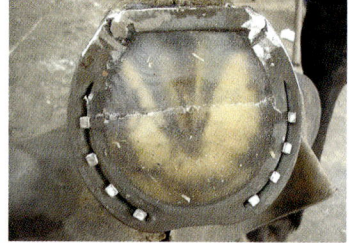

The whole under foot is packed with Equi-Thane Hoof Pak®; this distributes the pressure over the hoof, thus unburdening the heels.

CASE HISTORY 1, PHOTO BELOW RIGHT
A horse was standing on the bulbs of the hoof, which had put so much pressure on the heels that it was using the horny wall as a weightbearing surface. When being treated, a very wide and long horseshoe was fitted to support the hoof capsule. The horse must be trimmed and shod every six weeks. By shortening the toe each time, the farrier could gradually bring the pressure forward.

Inflammation of the Heels

An inflammation in the heels of the hoof is an infected hoof corium inflammation with pus formation. This type of inflammation is also called *Pododermatitis purulenta*.

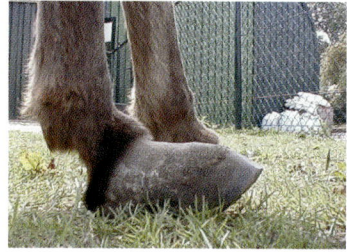

This horse is standing on the heel bulbs. Thus there is too much pressure on the heels and the horse uses the horny wall to bear bodyweight. The hoof no longer grows downwards but forwards.

CAUSE
Heel inflammations are caused mostly by dirt, such as small stones or wood chips, working up into the white line (the white line is composed of insensitive laminae) so that bacteria entering have a chance of multiplying. The heels, due to the hoof mechanism of the hoof being weighted and unweighted, change form and slide over the ground; it is therefore easy for tiny stones and dirt to be forced in and cause an inflammation. There is also the chance – through this movement – that the buttresses of the heels tear, so that bacteria can be forced in. An inflammation in the heels causes pressure in the hoof capsule, and thus pain. The inflammation will always force its way up between the insensitive and sensitive laminae to the coronary band. Lameness can be sporadic.

SYMPTOMS
A horse that has inflammation in one of its hooves suddenly becomes seriously lame. The horse has a high pulse rate – the pulse can be felt at both hoof arteries, on the inner and outer sides of the pastern cavity – and places its foot in a certain way; it mostly places its hoof forward and keeps the hoof stretched out to unburden the spot with the inflammation as much as possible. The horse may also sweat and paw the ground restlessly. The limb has an accumulation of fluid. The farrier and the veterinary surgeon can determine where the inflammation is by observing the way the horse places its foot.

DIAGNOSIS

An inflammation of the heel can usually be confirmed by observing the way the horse stands and moves. In some cases, other problems can display the same lameness – such as a crack in the pedal bone, separating walls, a keratoma, thrush and ligament problems.

CASE HISTORY 1, PHOTOS THIS PAGE

A horse that was presented was seriously lame. It had a large swelling on the inside of the hoof. The cannon had swollen and the contours of the pastern cavity and the heels could barely be seen. The horse had already been lame for three weeks, had laid down a lot and had had a temperature. The hoof was warm and there was a fast pulse rate. The horse had been given penicillin. The penicillin temporarily suppressed the inflammation but could not cure it. Thus, the inflammation appeared cured but it was actually just in a non-active phase. Thus treatment had been too slow. The swelling was so large that the whole bulb area bulged out above the coronary band. Under this area there was a huge inflammation that had to be removed. Because treatment had been too slow it was clear that there would be ruination in the internal hoof. Filing out was the only answer.

With this horse, the inflammation began in the buttresses of the heels and had migrated upwards via the horny wall; it had forced a way in between the solar surface and the pedal bone. The affected part of the solar surface and the heels had to be cleaned out

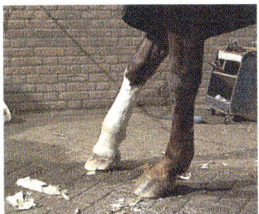

An extremely lame horse. It does not want to put weight on the hoof and, at rest, places the hoof far forward.

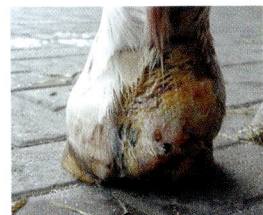

The horse has an enormous swelling on the inside on the heel bulb. The cannon is swollen. The contours of the pastern cavity and the heels are barely visible.

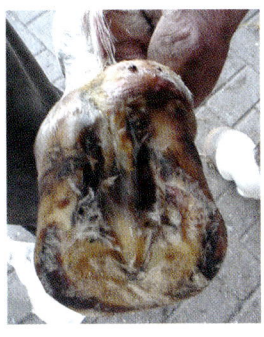

The swelling is so great that the bulb area is bulging over the coronary band. Under this area is a huge inflammation that must be removed.

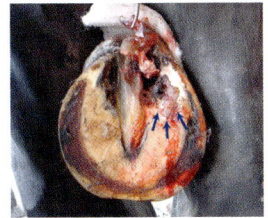

The whole heel area had to be removed, because the sole and the wall corium displayed signs or rotting. The inflammation had already worked its way under the sole (blue arrows).

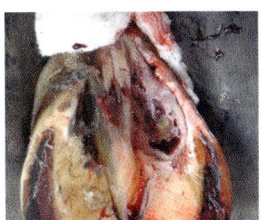

The heel area (horny wall, bar and sole) is partly removed and the sole corium is cleaned.

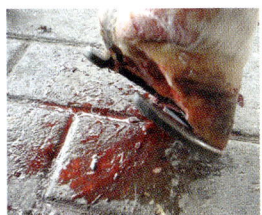

The side heel wall is also partly removed because it has been weakened by the removal of the sole and the bar.

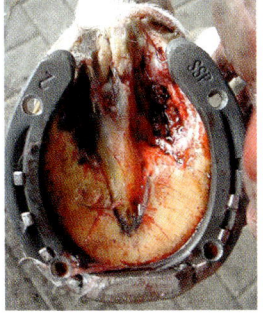

The horse is shod with a surgical plate shoe to give counter-pressure to the wound. The counter-pressure prevents the bulging out or collapsing of the corium.

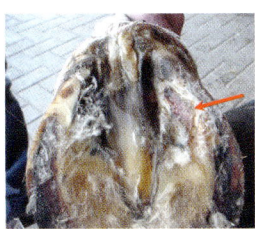

After five weeks, the wound is dry and nearly closed up, bar a tiny area (red arrow). The horse may start with light exercise but needs to have special horseshoes for a while to protect the affected parts of the hoof.

because the solar surface – which already displayed a rotten appearance – had been affected by the inflammation. The buttresses of the heel were removed for three reasons. Firstly, the wall had been weakened and had become thin by the removal of the buttress of the heel and had lost its strength. Secondly, the wound could be better looked after and thirdly, the pressure would be removed from the coronary band and the bulbs.

The horse was shod with a surgical plate shoe so that there could be counter-pressure placed on the wound. If the inflammation is very serious, surgical plate horseshoes may be fitted: this is a normal shoe with four screw holes where a metal plate can be fixed. Padding can be inserted between the plate and the hoof so that the solar surface is under pressure. No side clips may be added to the shoe, because this would put too much pressure on the horny wall, which would hinder the hoof mechanism. The applied counter-pressure prevents the corium from collapsing or bulging out. After a couple of weeks, the wound was suitably dried out and the hoof could function again. The horse could begin light exercise but still had to be shod with special shoes to protect the affected parts.

CASE HISTORY 2, PHOTOS BELOW

A horse was presented that was lame. Because the horse had been used on hard and uneven ground without shoes, cracks had developed in the

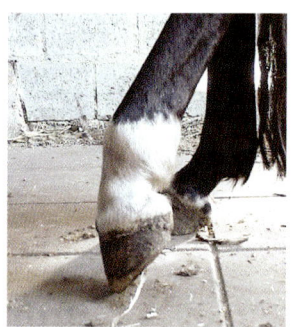

A typical conformation of a hind hoof that is inflamed in the heel area. When moving, the horse will barely place its heel on the ground and the steps will be short.

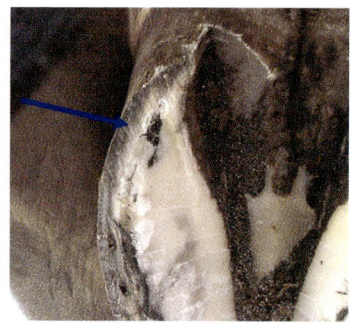

The farrier must first trim the hoof to check that the horny wall and the white line do not have any irregularities.

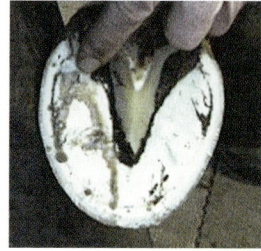

The buttresses of the heels were pared out with a hoof knife – with a curved blade – which caused the pus to be spontaneously released.

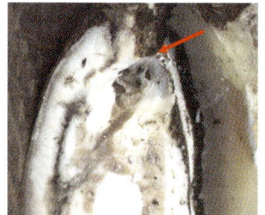

As soon as the place was cut out, the cavity where the inflammation was became visible. The heel angle was also broken in the corner.

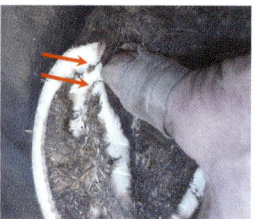

The bars – the turned-in angle of the horny wall – are interrupted and there are two cracks (red arrows) visible that will cause trouble. As soon as pressure is applied, the pus is released.

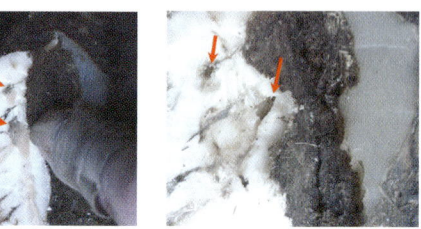

This example shows two cavities where bacteria can multiply.

Part 2 – Disorders of the Limbs and Hooves

buttresses of the heel wall. Due to the movement in the hoof capsule, the heels and buttresses, dirt and stones had worked their way in and an inflammation had developed.

First of all, the hoof was trimmed to check whether the horny wall showed any irregularities and if the buttresses of the heels were without breaks in them. The horny wall goes round at the heel buttresses, turns sharply inwards and then runs parallel to the frog – these are the so-called bars. They are actually a continuation of the horny wall. When the point of inflammation has been determined, the horn is cut away, layer by layer. In the angle of the hoof capsule – the heel area – the inflammation was even visible in two places. By making an opening, the pus could be released; this allowed pain caused by the pressure to diminish and the horse moved more freely. The inflamed area was cleaned thoroughly and the horse was shod with normal shoes. Afterwards, the hoof was treated with a bactericidal solution and bandaged. No further treatment with medicine was necessary because the inflammation had been properly dealt with and after a few days had disappeared.

CASE HISTORY 3, PHOTOS THIS PAGE

It is not always easy to reach an inflammation; if one is not sure whether the inflammation as been completely removed, then the side wall of the hoof must be opened up; in so doing one tries to leave as much of the horny wall intact as possible in order that it stays as strong as possible. A hole is made in the place where the inflammation is. A drain drenched in a bactericidal solution may be inserted in the horny wall, reaching down to the solar surface. The drain ensures that no more inflammation will develop between the horny wall and the wall corium. After the treatment, the whole wound is dressed with a moist bandage to keep it temporarily free from dirt and dung.

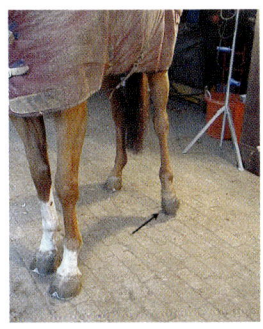

This horse is very seriously lame. It places its hind hoof to the side and bears its body weight on the toe area. The horse has a rapid pulse rate and there is extreme warmth in the area above the heels.

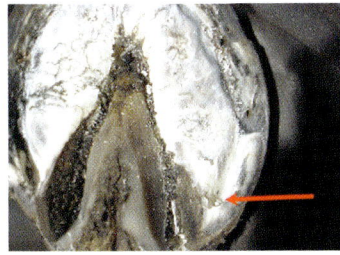

At first sight, there is little to see, but indeed there is a minuscule hole that indicates inflammation. The horse is extremely sensitive at the top side of the buttresses of the heel. To keep the hoof capsule as strong as possible, an opening is made in the side wall at the place of inflammation. This type of treatment requires great skill.

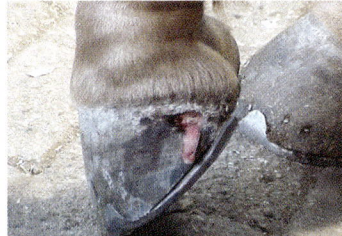

A drain can be inserted in the hoof because the opening has been made in the side wall. The drain, or piece of gauze, is led from the hole in the wall via the wall corium to the sole; the sole is treated with a bactericidal solution so that the internal area stays clean and there is no chance of a return of the inflammation.

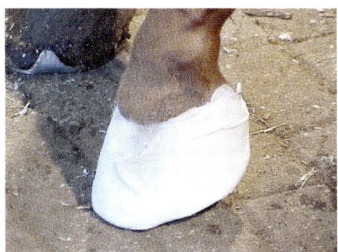

After treatment, the hoof is dressed with a bactericidal bandage so that the whole hoof is temporarily protected from dirt and dung and can be 'left to soak'.

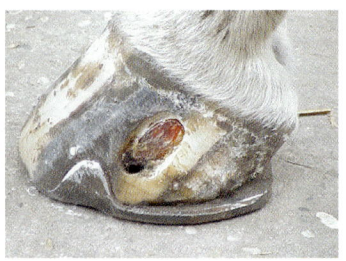

This is a splendid example of a horse that was treated for serious lameness but nevertheless could return quickly to equestrian sport. With this treatment technique the hoof capsule properly retains its shape and the foot position is not changed. The cavity in the wall is not filled, because otherwise the chance of inflammation can be repeated.

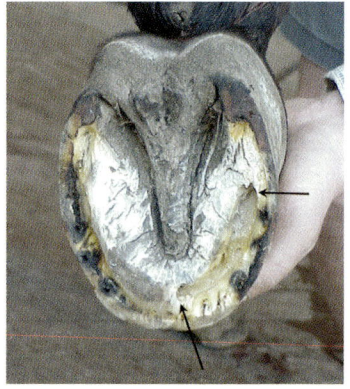

A long-term lameness. The inflammation has worked its way from the buttresses of the heel via the solar surface to the toe. The area is cleaned and the horse is shod with a quarter bar shoe to prevent ground pressure and to keep dirt out.

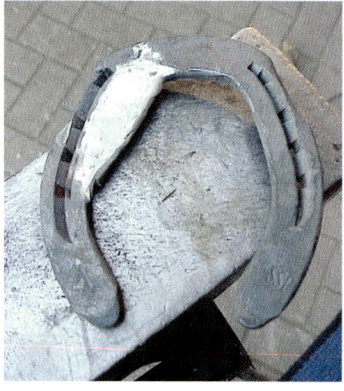

A light side bar is welded onto the shoe which allows the affected area to be examined. A piece of gauze with Betadine (iodine) can be inserted between the horseshoe and the hoof.

CASE HISTORY 4, PHOTOS ABOVE

Usually the inflammation rises up via the wall corium. The inflammation of the heel of this horse had, however, worked its way to the toe via the solar surface at the buttresses of the heels. This place had to be protected from ground pressure and dirt that could accumulate in the cavity.

On such hooves, two sorts of horseshoe can be fitted:
1. A shoe with a thin, open bar. The wound can be dressed by putting a gauze bandage with Betadine (iodine) between the bar and the solar surface. This can easily be changed daily so that the wound remains clean.
2. A horseshoe with a forged-out heel, so that the wound remains visible. The advantage of this shoe is that there is no extra weight on the shoe.

At the subsequent shoeing, the solar surface had grown sufficiently and the hoof could be shod normally.

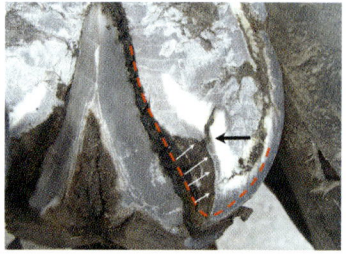

From the buttresses of the heel, the bar angle (red dotted line) does not run parallel with the lateral cleft but curves inwards (white arrows). Thus there is an interruption in the bar (black arrow).

CASE HISTORY 5, PHOTOS RIGHT

If the horse is getting good hoof care and if the owner arranges for the farrier to come in good time, inflammation can often be prevented.

The angle of the bar of this horse was defective. From the angle of the heel, the bar angle did not run parallel with the collateral groove but had turned inwards. Because this bar displayed a defective line, a break had ensued that had filled with dirt, which could easily lead to an inflammation. The angle of the heel with the bar was cut away so that there was a flat surface. The insensitive laminae had a yellow tint and were clearly inflamed. Speedy treatment prevented this horse from becoming lame.

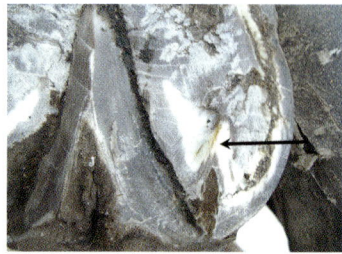

The buttress of the heel is cut out with the bar until there is a flat surface. Inflamed insensitive laminae are present (arrow).

4 THE HOOF: FROG

Thrush

Thrush is an inflammation in the frog, caused by bacterial decay which leads to deterioration.

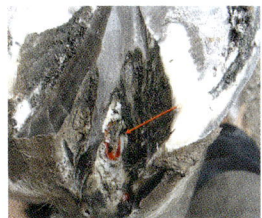

Thrush is damage to the horny digital cushion, but the frog corium can also be affected; In that case, one speaks of an inflammation of the frog corium.

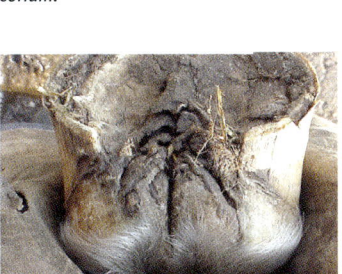

The openings in the bulbs at the back of the hoof indicate a breakout of the inflamed frog.

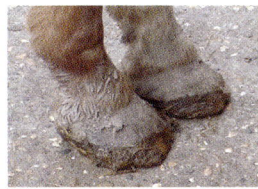

Thrush develops more quickly in hooves standing frequently in dirt and dung.

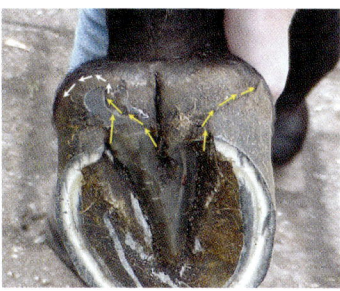

A typical form of thrush is an inflammation under and between the frog tissues. This thrush has broken out in the back part of hoof on both sides of the heels. This is the only escape for the inflammation because this is where the hoof is most mobile. The yellow line indicates the path where the inflammation breaks out. In the coronary band above, this inflammation (white arrows) can further undermine the perioplic ring.

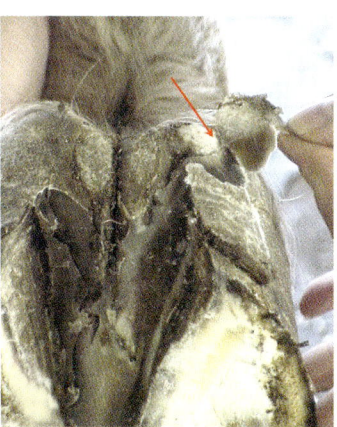

The inflammation breaks out at the bulb and will travel further along the coronary band under the horn (red arrow).

CAUSE

Thrush can be caused in various ways:
- Too little movement. Horses that are stabled have more trouble from thrush than horses out at grass. Horses should move a lot so that the hoof mechanism can function well
- Lack of care and cleanliness in the hooves. This allows dirt to remain in the hooves, which can lead to bacterial inflammation and, possibly, to maggots
- Dirty stables. This causes the frog to have more contact with urine and to deteriorate because of the ammonia in the urine
- Faulty shoeing. When horseshoes are too small, the hoof capsule sags over the shoe and the hoof mechanism cannot function well
- Certain hoof shapes. A narrow hoof has less hoof mechanism than a

broad hoof. Narrow hooves spread out less and therefore dirt is more likely to build up. This makes the chance of inflammation of the frog more likely
- The ground. Bark and wood chips on an arena surface covering can easily get wedged into the frog, which causes inflammation
- By penetrating into the frog groove too deeply with a sharp instrument; this can unintentionally push bacteria into the hoof. Bacteria multiply best in a dark, oxygen-free and moist environment; the hoof is uncommonly suited to this

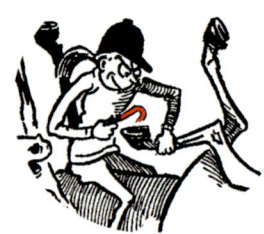

A lot of scraping with a sharp implement can make thrush worse. Because some horn is scraped away each time, there is a chance that the sole can be pierced; this gives bacteria a chance to enter.

Thrush is more common in hind hooves than in fore hooves. Usually, the horn is undermined from within the central groove of the frog. Thus the rest of the frog and frog corium can easily be affected.

A horse that is troubled by thrush need not necessarily be lame. If the thrush has advanced to such an extent that the horse is indeed lame, then it will display more lameness on soft going than on a hard ground. This is because there is more pressure on the frog from soft ground than there is on hard ground.

TREATMENT

Thrush is easy to cure but it does mean daily care. The farrier cuts away the affected frog with a hoof knife until healthy attachment horn is reached all round and not one bit of inflamed horn remains. The stable must be cleaned so that the horse does not stand in its own dung or urine; the frog cannot tolerate urine. It is important not to dig too deeply into the groove of the frog with a sharp instrument, and the grooves should be cleaned out each time with water so that oxygen can penetrate into even the deepest parts. After this treatment, if the hoof is dry, Egyptian salve can be applied to the frog. This is an acidic tar. Above all, do not apply a thick layer on the frog as this will seal it off from oxygen, which will only enhance the thrush. In place of Egyptian salve, Socatyl salve can also be used. Socatyl is a drying, bactericidal salve. These remedies should not be used for too long because they harden the frog which would then lose its function; the digital cushion must be soft and

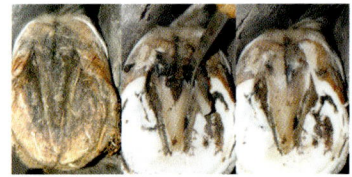

If thrush appears, the farrier must cut away all infected parts so that only healthy horn is left and no trace of infection remains.

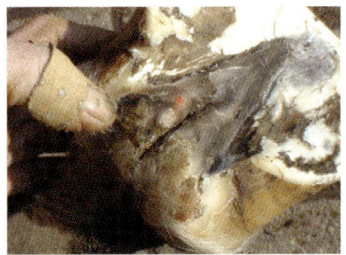

A hoof with thrush after it has been carefully cut away.

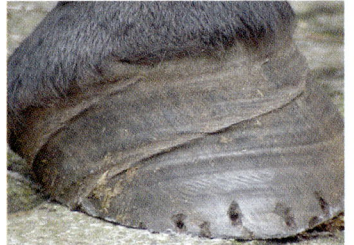

Thrush does not harm the hoof. If the inflammation disappears under the perioplic corium, a reaction takes place; an extra layer of horn will be produced that has the shape of the coronary band and grows down normally.

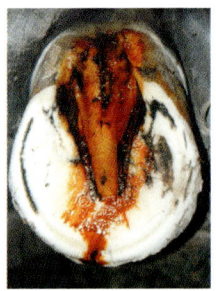

Betadine (iodine) is the most common remedy for tackling thrush. Betadine (iodine) is drying and is bactericidal. The digital cushion must remain elastic otherwise it loses its function.

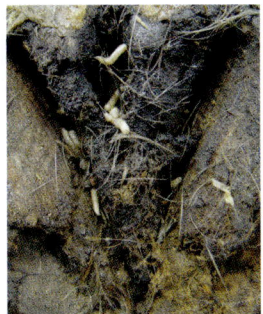

Frogs can be so neglected and inflamed that they are full of maggots.

elastic. However, it is Betadine (iodine) that is most used. The frog is sprayed clean and then dried. After that, it is sprayed with Betadine (iodine). Betadine is a drying, bactericidal solution and can easily be pushed into spots hard to reach.

HORSESHOES

A horse with thrush is fitted with a broad shoe so that the hoof mechanism can optimally function. Efficient care and a good farrier can cure a horse of thrush.

Canker of the Frog

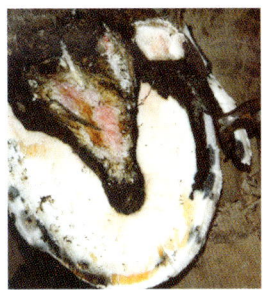

An example of canker; there is proliferation of growth in the whole digital cushion, which bleeds at the slightest touch.

Canker is a hoof corium inflammation that is accompanied by a lot of morbid growth of tissue of the inflamed corium. This form of carcinoma is found mainly in the sensitive frog – thus the name frog canker – but it can also spread to the bulb, bar and sole corium and, in extremely serious cases, also to the wall corium. As canker does not appear only in the frog, it is better to use the term 'hoof canker'.

CAUSE

The cause of canker is unknown. Although there is an essential difference between thrush (primarily a process of deterioration) and canker (primarily a process of tumour growth) in some cases it is difficult to distinguish one from the other. Thus, among the horses that are presented at the clinic, this disease is always in a far advanced state, which makes the illness infinitely more difficult to treat. Canker is an inflammation process in the sensitive frog – and in some cases, also in the surrounding area of the bulb bars and sole corium – with proliferating growth in the germinating layer. Normally, the germinating layer produces solid, robust horn, but in canker this is an abnormal amount and of a soft and cheesy quality where deterioration occurs easily and where bacteria later (secondarily) develop an inflammation process: it seems as if the tissue is decomposing. Canker is always characterised by proliferating growth and swelling. The canker bleeds easily and profusely when it is handled. It is clearly a persistent process that sometimes develops explosively and which is difficult to stop. Some horses with

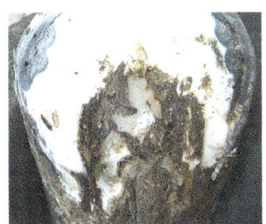

In very bad cases, canker can affect the wall corium. These areas are nearly impossible to treat.

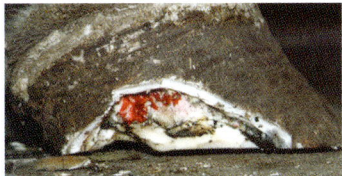

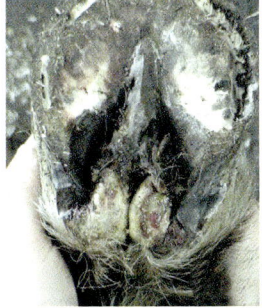

The difference between thrush (left) and canker (right) is very difficult to distinguish.

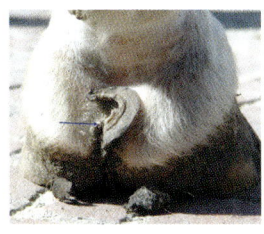

Some horses with canker are recognised by an extremely fast-growing curly, horny stalk projecting out from the central groove of the frog.

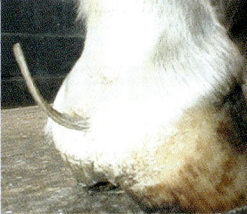

The horny stalk can take on a different appearance with each horse; this horse has an explosive growth of a straight horny stalk.

canker can be recognised by an extremely fast-growing horny stalk growing out of the central groove of the frog.

If canker is not recognised in time, it can take on disastrous forms and affect the whole coronary band and perioplic corium. In the worst cases, the only solution is to have the horse put down.

Horses with canker – or hoof canker – are not, or are seldom, lame. Thrush does, though, cause lameness in horses. Canker can occur in one or more hooves, in both the fore and hind hooves. There is absolutely no proof that canker is contagious for the unaffected hooves or for other horses.

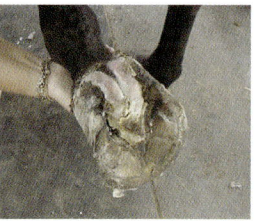

This is a form of canker that has affected not only the frog but also the bulbs.

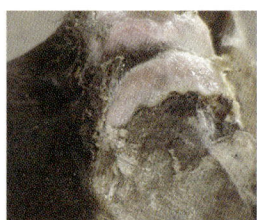 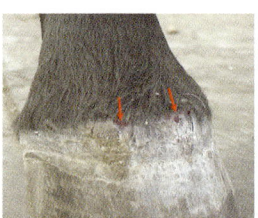 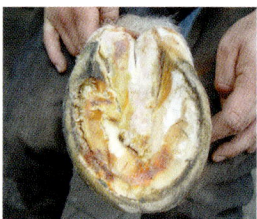

The horny bulbs proliferate in the form of a glass-like inflamed line to the coronary corium.

After a while, this canker will affect the whole coronary corium (red arrows). The horse will no longer be able to develop a good hoof capsule, which is its death knell.

This is a disastrous form of hoof canker. The frog and the sole are entirely affected; it is clear to see that the wall corium is affected. This is the result of bad treatment for a year: one can say without question that this is animal torture.

TREATMENT

Canker is difficult to cure. although we have had positive results with our method of treatment. Over the years, my twin brother and I have developed a method of treatment with which we have been able to help many horses. The operation is always done with a team consisting of a veterinary surgeon and a hoof specialist. The treatment consists of the rigorous removal of the whole frog, the removal of the sole including the germinating layer of the sensitive frog and/or the sole with the sole corium and, in the worst cases, the bulb with the bulb corium and wall with the wall corium. This specialist treatment is highly intensive and difficult; it requires extremely careful work. The way of operating must represent a guarantee for a quick cure.

CONCLUSION

Canker is a disease which farriers and veterinary surgeons often do not respond to sufficiently rapidly, adopting a 'wait and see' attitude or starting with the wrong treatment. Unfortunately, this leads to many horses falling into the hands of alternative practitioners which finally results in their death while they could have been saved.

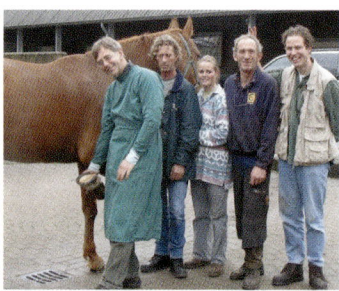

Canker is always treated by a professional team. From left to right: Drs B. Boschker, equine veterinary surgeon; P. van Dijke, assistant veterinary head of stable management; M. Verbocht, assistant veterinary stable management; A. van Nassau, State qualified teaching instructor and specialist farrier; Drs T. van Loon, veterinary surgeon.

CASE HISTORY 1, PHOTOS BELOW

A horse that was presented had a serious form of frog and bulb canker and had to be operated upon. The whole operation took place under absence of blood – that is to say, the hoof was temporarily tied off so that the bloodstream came to a standstill and the blood remained limited. The frogs, both bulbs and the heels of the hoof were affected and had to be removed and were cut out in such a way that every part of the diseased organism was completely removed. Examination during treatment was of great importance: if an affected part had been overlooked, then cutting away had to be resumed. The original form of the frog had to be maintained, thus during the operation the future digital cushion was shaped in the hoof by cutting the form of the frog in the remaining cushion

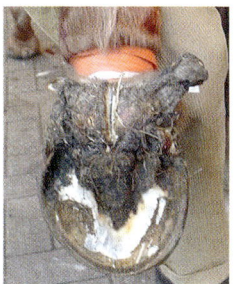

Horse with prolific growth of hoof canker.

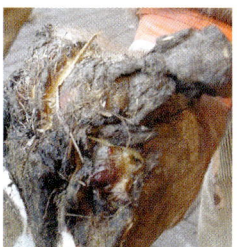

The whole heel area is in a state of tissue destruction. Canker is always characterised by proliferation of growth and swelling.

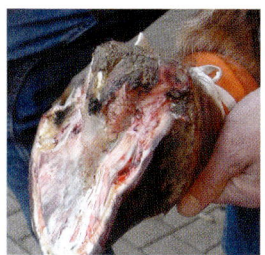

The hoof is cut away so that all pathogenic organisms have been removed. The heels must also be removed. The wall corium has been partly affected.

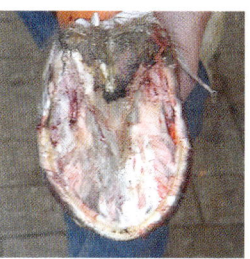

A general view of a cut-away hoof; a healthy part of the bulb has been retained and will cover the future frog.

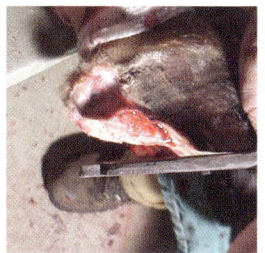

The horseshoe is fitted; it is now clear how much of the heels had to be removed.

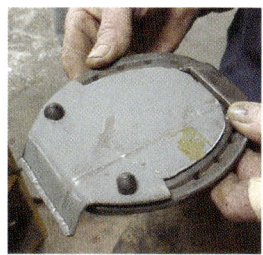

The horseshoe is a surgical plate shoe.

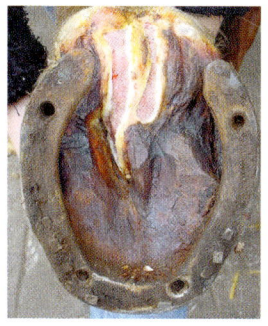

After ten weeks, the sole and the bulb corium have nearly covered the wound with horn.

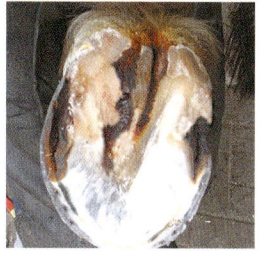

This is an excellent and healthy outcome.

of fat. After the operation, the hoof was shod with a surgical plate horseshoe; this is a normal shoe with four screw holes where a metal plate can be fixed. Thus no dirt or dung can enter the hoof and the wound can be easily treated. After the horseshoe was fixed, the wound was covered with iodine crystals (iodum). These have an aggressive and etching-like effect which ensures that all remaining diseased cells are killed. After a while, the remaining sole corium slowly covers the cut-away digital cushion – the geminating layer of the frog was no longer present but was replaced by the germinating layer of the sole so that the preshaped digital cushion had a horny construction. After the digital cushion had healed closed, it regained its sensitive frog structure and could fulfil its original function.

The treatment of canker is extremely labour-intensive and takes many months. With the surgical plate horseshoe, the horse can nevertheless go out to grass as long as the hoof stays dry and clean.

CASE HISTORY 2, PHOTOS PAGES 176, 177 AND 178

A horse was presented at the clinic that had canker and had to be operated upon. Under the hoof a fungus-shaped area was visible that had spread to both bulbs and under the buttresses. The tissue was thread-like and while being treated began to bleed profusely. It also exuded a penetrating smell which is characteristic of canker. Another characteristic of canker is the presence of a protuberance from the central groove of the frog that grows explosively and is extremely hard. The horse that was being treated also had such a protuberance.

The lower foot was anaesthetised and tied off so that work could

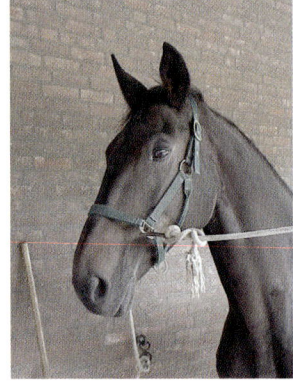

This is the horse with canker in case history 2.

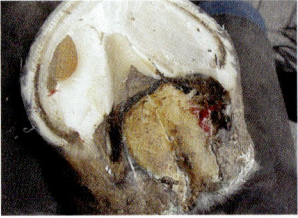 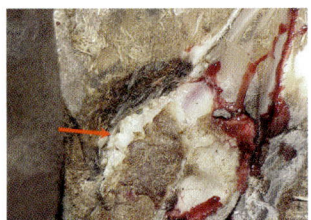 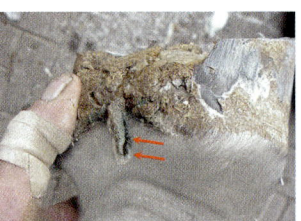

Left: a fungus-shaped part that had proliferated to both bulbs and under both buttresses. Centre: the heel angle (red arrow) has changed position because of the canker. The tissue is thread-like and bleeds when touched. Right: the protuberance from the central cleft of the frog is characteristic of canker.

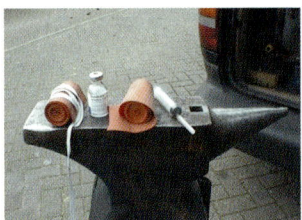 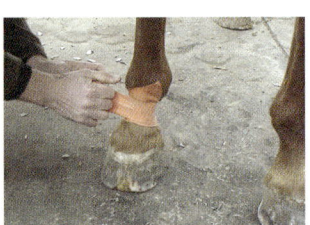 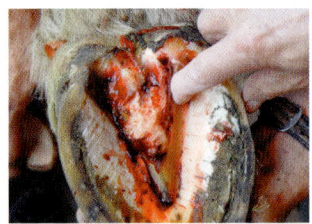

Left: the lower foot is anaesthetised. Centre: the hooves are tied off with a ligature (an elastic band) so that work can proceed with a complete absence of blood. Right: all the diseased germinating layer of the frog and bulb is removed; even the sole is removed.

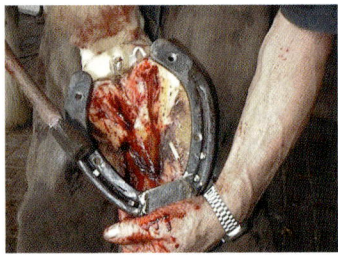 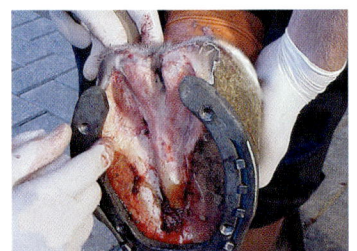 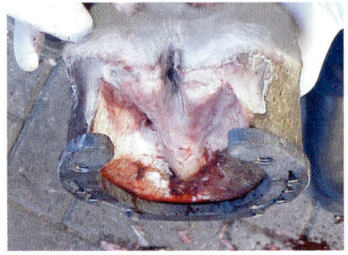

Left: The surgical plate horseshoe is prepared in advance and is nailed to the hoof. Centre: the hoof is entirely free of diseased tissue and is checked one last time. Right: the form of the digital cushion is cut into the hoof. The germinating layer of the bulb, the frog and part of the sole corium have been completely removed.

proceed in the absence of blood. The whole diseased germinating layer of the frog, the bulb and the sole were removed. After this, the hoof could be shod. A made-to-measure surgical plate horseshoe had been prepared earlier so that it could be nailed on immediately after the operation. The treated area was covered with iodine crystals. To prevent excessive blood loss, the hoof was taped up. After a week, the wound was thoroughly etched, the blood vessels had been cauterised and the healing process had begun. White edges formed around the wound; this indicates new horn development of the sole and the bulb that closed in the frog with sole horn. The wound was covered with a gel – that is also used for people with burns – so that the frog stayed healthy. The white edges must not grow too rapidly and were thus regularly cut back. The white edges must grow together unbroken; too-rapid growth can lead to interruptions that are not desirable for a good closure.

After a time, the whole digital cushion was covered with sole tissue and the digital cushion was able to heal and provide a healthy hoof mechanism.

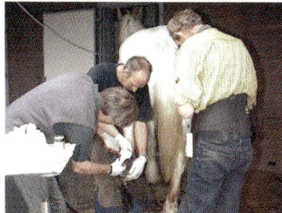
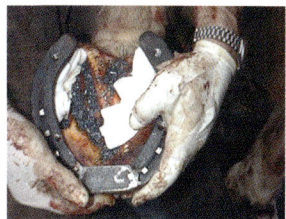
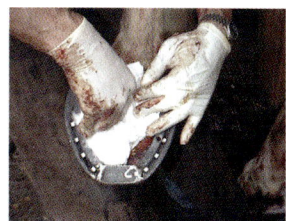

Left: a team of farriers and veterinary surgeons treated this horse for many months. Centre: the wound is treated with iodine crystals. Right: the hoof is packed with gauze bandages.

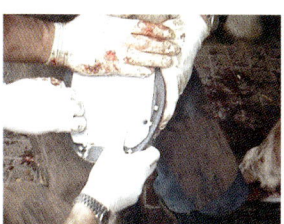
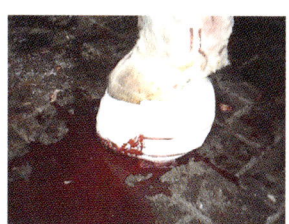
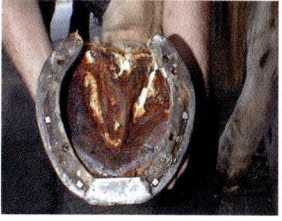

Left: the steel plate is screwed to the horseshoe under pressure. Centre: the hoof is taped up to prevent too much blood loss. Right: the hoof after a week; the hoof is well etched, which allows the healing process to begin.

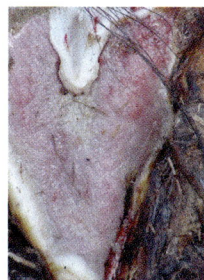
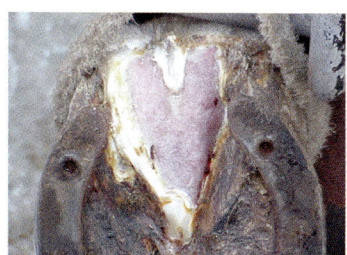
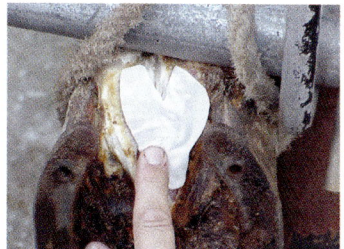

Left: a white border develops rapidly around the wound; a sign that the healing has started. Centre: the white borders form the new horn growth from the sole and the bulb. These close the frog in. Right: the wound is covered with a gel that is also used for people with burns.

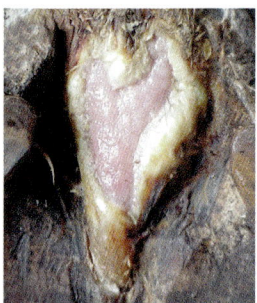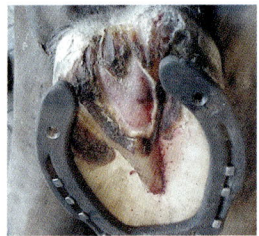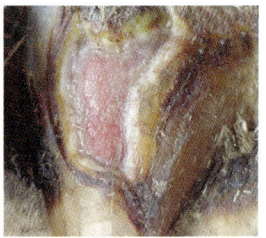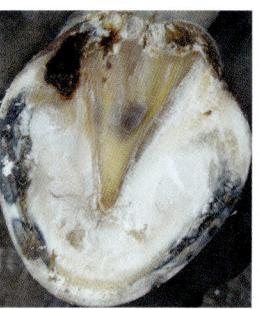

Left: horn originating in the germinating layer of the sole and bulb closes over quickly and is checked daily. Centre: the healing process going well. At this stage, the wound has a dry bandage. Right: the wound is closing. The whole digital cushion is covered with a sole tissue and will be restored to a normal digital cushion within a short period of time.

The end result of a successful treatment.

CASE HISTORY 3, PHOTOS BELOW

A horse was presented that had an extremely serious form of canker. The whole frog and a part of the outer quarter part of the sole were completely affected and were completely removed. During the operation, the whole germinating layer of the frog was removed. As well as this, a part of the sole was removed right up to the pedal bone. The subsequent treatment was the same as in case history 2. This horse was administered painkillers for a long period to prevent it overburdening the other healthy hooves unnecessarily, which could have led to problems. After six months intensive treatment, the whole lower foot had closed up with an extremely strong horn construction. The shape that the frog had been given at the operation was still present. After a couple of months, the digital cushion had regained its original elastic surface which ensured an optimum hoof mechanism.

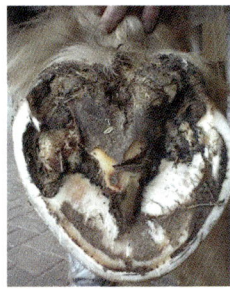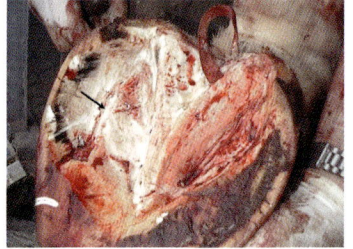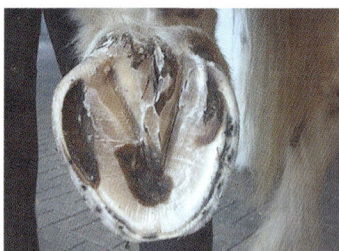

This is an extremely serious form of canker where the frog and sole must be removed.

A rigorous intervention; the contours of the pedal bone (arrow) can be clearly seen. This treatment requires thorough knowledge.

This is the hoof after six months of treatment.

CONCLUSION

The method of treatment that has been developed by my twin brother and I has been a breakthrough for the treatment of frog canker that has enabled us to help many horses.

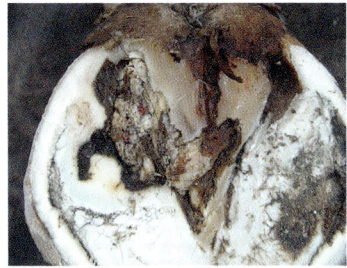
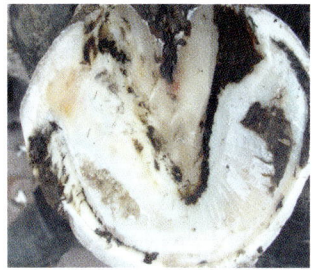

This is a case of canker where a part of the frog and a small part of the sole are affected. Do not delay and do not go to alternative practitioners, but take serious measures; the horse will be saved from a long road of suffering.

Inflammation of the Frog

In inflammation of the frog, the digital cushion of the hoof is inflamed.

CAUSE

Inflammation of the frog can come about because the horse steps on a sharp object or stone. Usually, the horse is not lame from inflammation of the frog, as the sensitive frog is not inflamed. The horse's digital cushion consists of an extremely soft and elastic but strong connective tissue and has little blood. It also has a lot of fatty tissue with countless little islands of cartilage. If, at the time of trimming, there is a sudden escape of pus, then this indicates an inflammation of the frog; a cavity must be looked for in the digital cushion. An inflammation of the frog usually does not cause lameness: in general, the inflammation is in the digital cushion and produces little or no pressure – seeing that the digital cushion is very mobile – unlike the wall corium.

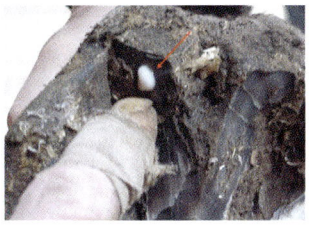

This is an example of an inflammation of the frog.

As soon as pressure is put on the frog, there is an escape of pus.

The function of the digital cushion is enhancement of the hoof mechanism. The moment the horse sets its hoof on the ground, the digital cushion is pressed upwards by the ground, and both heels expand outwards; this action causes blood to be sucked into the hoof. The moment the horse lifts its hoof, the digital cushion and the heels return to their original position – which presses the blood back again. The continuous back and forth flow of blood in the hoof supplies the hoof with nutrients. This movement of the hoof is called the hoof mechanism.

An inflammation of the frog or digital cushion can not harm the hoof. On the other hand, an inflammation in the sensitive frog does cause hoof problems.

A horse with inflammation of the sensitive frog does not want to bear weight fully on the hoof, but rests it on the point of the hoof. It will be very lame on soft going but will move better on hard ground.

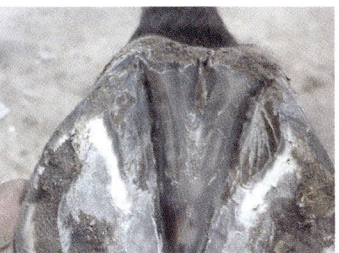
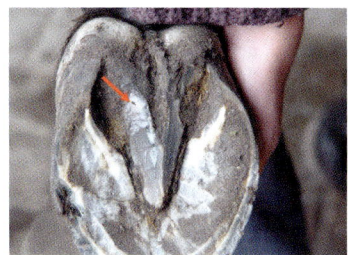

The digital cushion has been neatly trimmed; a beautiful frog without irregularities.

An enormous amount of pus, that had been under pressure, escaped spontaneously when the hoof was pared. This does not cause lameness in the horse. The entrance to the cavity in the digital cushion can be seen clearly.

TREATMENT

It is important that the farrier treats an inflammation of the frog carefully, because it can easily lead to thrush. The treatment of an inflammation of the frog corium consists of cleaning the frog corium and dressing the wound with a Betadine (iodine) bandage.

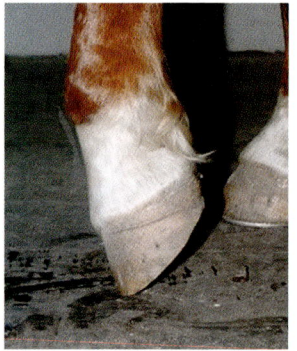

A horse with an inflammation of the sensitive frog is extremely lame and rests its hoof on the point of the toe.

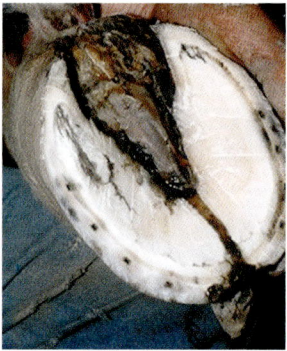

The frog corium is completely inflamed; the black discharge flows spontaneously from the hoof.

CASE HISTORY 1, PHOTOS RIGHT AND BELOW

A lame horse was presented that had an inflammation of the frog corium which had already worked its way to the bulbs of the hoof. The inflammation had caused the frog to come loose. The inflamed part was completely removed. The hoof was dressed with a Betadine (iodine) compress to kill the bacteria and to ensure that the frog corium could once again develop a healthy frog. The hoof was shod with a shoe with two light bars. The bars in the shoe protected the frog from ground pressure. A piece of gauze soaked in Betadine (iodine) could be inserted between the bars to keep the wound clean.

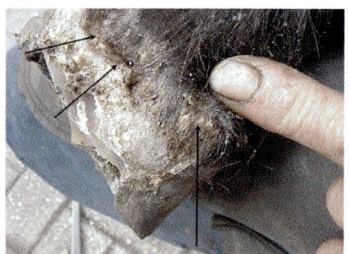

The inflammation of the frog corium in the hoof of this horse has worked its way to, and broken out at, the horny bulbs (black arrows).

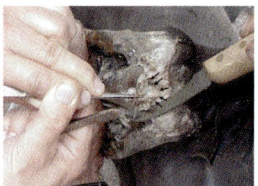

The inflamed body of the frog is carefully cut away from the bulb corium. Both sides are also cut away.

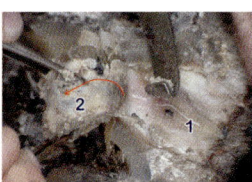

The whole frog pad (2) is cut away from the frog corium (1). The hoof is fitted with a horseshoe that has two bars to prevent ground pressure.

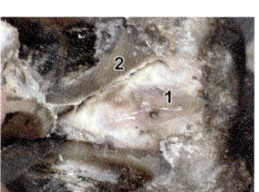

Clear image of the frog corium (1) that will reform the frog pad.

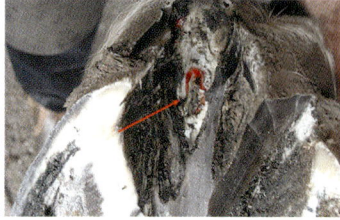

Inflammation of the frog corium caused by a piece of wedged-in wood. If this inflammation is not treated, thrush can develop.

Part 2 – Disorders of the Limbs and Hooves

4 THE HOOF: SOLE

Dropped Sole

If the sole is lower than the weightbearing edge, then this is called a dropped sole. This problem is seen all too often in horses. It is simply called dropped sole, but is in fact a collapse of the solar surface caused by too much pressure from the pedal bone on to the sole.

CAUSE

A dropped sole occurs in horses that have, or have had, chronic (gradual) or acute (sudden) laminitis. In laminitic horses, the pedal bone tips over and the point of the pedal bone puts more pressure on the sole, which causes it to drop. The cause of this tipping over that the pedal bone, due to inflammation of the wall corium that occurs in laminitis, can no longer be held in place.

In a worse phase of laminitis, the pedal bone tips over in its whole circumference to a vertical position in the hoof capsule – this is called 'sinker'. This causes too much pressure in the sole and it drops. Laminitis can have the effect of the walls no longer growing along the pedal bone and downwards. This then results in the internal connection between the hoof capsule and the pedal bone no longer being renewed, which brings

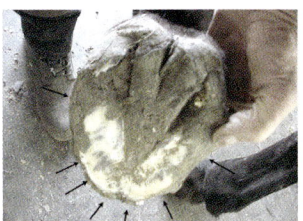

In normal hooves, the sole is concave. When the hoof is weighted, the sole becomes flat and the heels move outwards. This is part of the hoof mechanism.

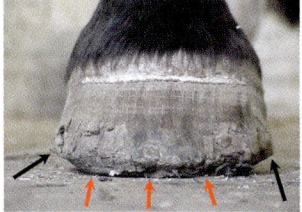

When a hoof is convex and no longer concave, the hoof mechanism can no longer fulfil its function well. This is the root of many hoof problems.

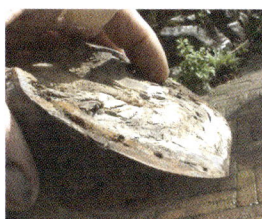

A horse with a dropped sole; the sole is proud of the weightbearing edge.

too much pressure to bear on the sole which then drops. In the long run, the horse will have weightbearing problems because it can only tread on the weightbearing edge of the hoof capsule and not on the sole, which leads to enormous bruising in the hoof.

A dropped sole is not only due to laminitis; horn wall problems can also be the cause.

HORSESHOES

Horses with dropped soles are a big problem for all farriers. The farrier has to fit shoes with sometimes only a tiny piece of wall for nailing and he has to reduce pressure on the sole. The hoof must, nevertheless, be shod otherwise the horse cannot function. In so doing, the sole must be left as thick and as strong as possible so that it can be carried in part by the shoe. The weightbearing edge must be trimmed extremely carefully. The farrier checks to see if one or more parts of the weightbearing edge can be carried by the shoe. This requires a farrier who really knows what he is doing.

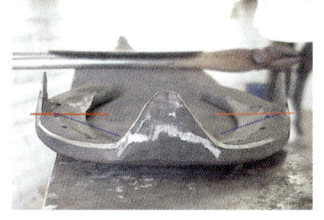

An example of a 'seated out' shoe. The red lines indicate the weightbearing surface. The blue lines indicate the angle of the hammered-out part of the shoe.

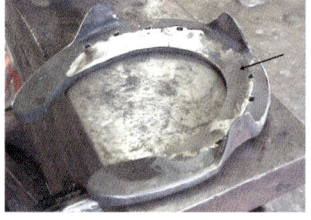

A seated out shoe well hammered out to the nail holes. Three clips prevent pulling off and shifting.

Various horseshoes can be fitted. A good shoe is one that has been hammered-out on the bearing surface (seated out shoe) so that the sole is not borne on the shoe. The shoe is temporarily given three clips until the bearing surface has grown normally. These clips ensure that the shoe will not be pulled off and that the shoe cannot shift. The disadvantage is that the hoof mechanism is temporarily hindered but, in this case, 'necessity rules'! When the hoof has recovered the horse can be fitted with normal shoes.

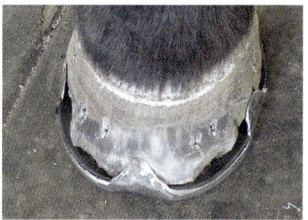

A hoof that has a dropped sole and is shod. It is clear that there is hardly any weightbearing edge on the shoe.

If the sole of a horse has not dropped excessively, then it can be fitted with a hammered out shoe with a low hoof pad fitted in between; this is a special, soft silicone rubber that hardens after 10 seconds. Silicone from a tube usually takes more than 10 hours to harden, so it will get squeezed out as soon as there is hoof pressure. Another advantage of the hoof pad is that there is a constant pressure on the sole so that it no longer changes form.

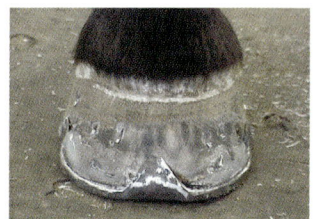

To give extra support to the horny wall, Equi-Thane Hoof Rebuild® is applied.

Puncture Wounds

If a horse treads on a sharp object, such as a nail, and it pierces the hoof, it creates a puncture wound.

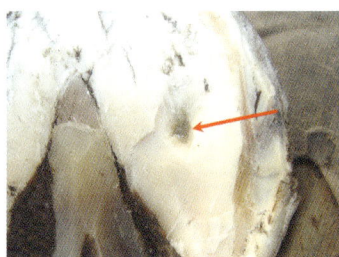

A puncture can occur anywhere in the hoof; it is not necessarily serious but it nonetheless always remains an emergency.

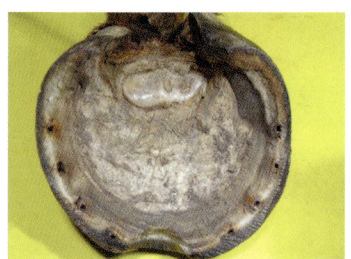

A very serious case: the object went straight into the frog. The pedal bone is removed so that the damage to the navicular bone can be seen.

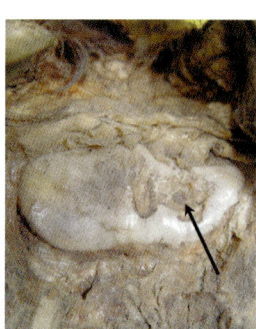

Enormous damage to the navicular bone; the joint capsule is completely damaged.

CAUSE

A puncture wound is caused by the horse treading on a sharp object. The seriousness of the injury depends on the following:

- **Where the sole has been pierced by the object.** The hoof can be divided into three parts: the front – or toe part; the back – or heel part; the digital cushion. A puncture wound from say, a nail, in the font part can cause damage to the sole corium or the pedal bone. If it causes a splintered bone or if a piece of the pedal bone is broken off (chip) then this place can easily be treated. If the puncture wound is in the back part – the heel part – or the digital cushion, the deep flexor tendon can then be pierced through and the synovial sheath or even the navicular bone or the hoof joint can be damaged. This can cause chronic lameness
- **How dirty the object was.** The horse's hoof offers the perfect environment for the development of bacteria. Thus a serious inflammation can develop
- **How deeply the object penetrated.** Usually one can conclude: the deeper the penetration, the greater the damage it causes

A puncture can occur at any time. Frequently, it causes sudden and extreme lameness.

TREATMENT

If a horse has trodden on a sharp object, of course the first thing that must be done is that the object is immediately removed. Observe well at what angle the object entered. Make sure the whole object is removed. Always consult a veterinary surgeon or the farrier; a puncture wound is always an emergency. If anything remains in the hoof, this could cause inflammation. It is also necessary to save the object so that the veterinary surgeon can better judge where the damage might be and how much grime is involved.

Firstly, X-rays must be taken; a probe is put in to judge the depth and the direction of the wound. After this, the area of penetration is deeply cut away. Subsequently, the horse is administered medication for the wound and vaccinated against tetanus.

HORSESHOES

A horse troubled with a puncture wound is usually fitted with a surgical plate horseshoe. This is a normal shoe with four screw holes where a metal plate can be fixed so that no dirt can enter the wound and the ground pressure on the hoof is removed. Also, the wound can be easily examined and treated.

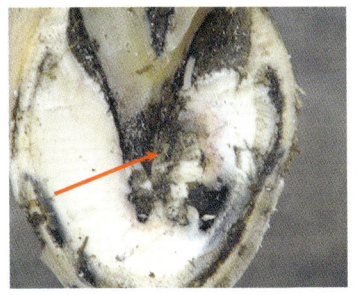

Puncture wound in the sole area next to the digital cushion has caused bruising and inflammation. Penicillin is used for an extensive period.

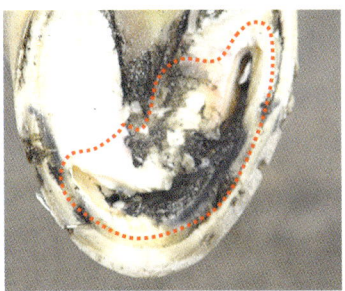

The inflammation has caused a rotting process and the whole marked out area of the sole is undermined and has become loose.

CASE HISTORY 1, PHOTOS THIS PAGE AND OPPOSITE (TOP)

A horse that was presented had trodden on a nail on its lateral cleft and could not stand on its hoof any more. The lower foot was anaesthetised so that the horse would feel no pain while being treated. The spot where the nail had penetrated was cut away and cleaned. Then a flexible probe was inserted in the nail hole for examination; a fine wire thread was passed into the probe so that where the nail had entered could clearly be seen on the front and back views of the X-ray – the nail had indeed penetrated very deeply. It had pierced the frog to the corium, had penetrated through the deep flexor tendon and the synovial sheath (the deep flexor tendon is fixed to the pedal bone in a fan shape) and had finished at a mucus pouch next to the navicular bone. Mucus pouches are bursa filled with lubricant – synovial fluid – that serves to lubricate the joint. On the side view of the X-ray it could be seen that the nail had gone right through the deep flexor tendon and towards the hoof joint; it seemed as if it had penetrated the joint between the navicular and pedal bones but, on the front and back views of the X-ray, it could be seen that the nail had slanted just in front of the navicular bone and exited. Thus the navicular bone had not been damaged, but the nail had touched the joint capsule – which could mean a chance of joint inflammation.

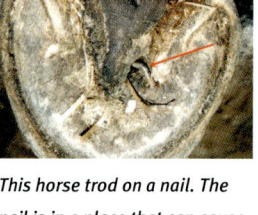

This horse trod on a nail. The nail is in a place that can cause a lot of damage.

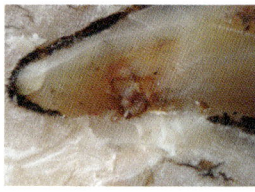

Treading on a dirty, sharp object immediately causes an infected wound.

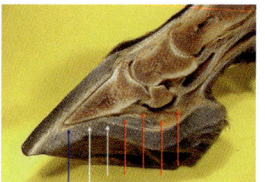

If a puncture wound occurs in the toe (blue arrow), then a piece of the pedal bone can break off. If there is a puncture under the pedal bone (white arrows), then the object can get stuck in the bone. If the object goes in at an angle as well, then a bone splinter can result. This area is easy to reach for treatment. If there is a puncture wound in the back part of the foot (red arrow) the consequences can be much more serious.

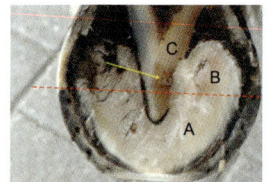

Underside of a hoof which shows the digital cushion, which is extremely flexible. This flexibility is necessary for the expansion and contraction of the hoof – the so-called hoof mechanism. The hoof can be divided into two parts: the front part – or toe part (A), and the back part – or heel part (B). The yellow arrow shows were the nail went in.

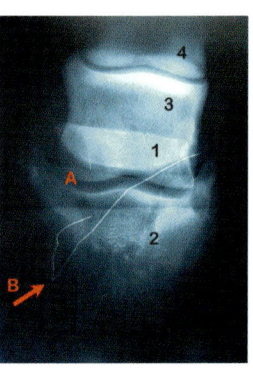
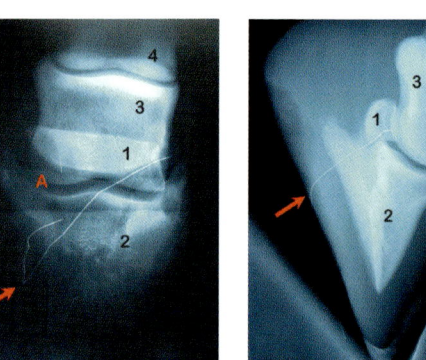

On this front and back view X-ray, taken from the horse's front, can be seen:
1. Navicular bone
2. Pedal bone
3. Short pastern bone
4. Long pastern bone
A. Hoof joint
B. Probe

On this side view X-ray it can be seen that the nail went through the deep flexor tendon and towards the hoof joint.

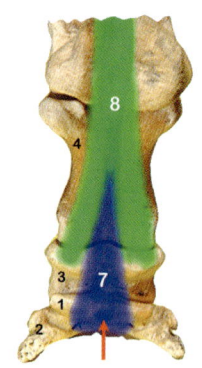

This diagram shows that the superficial flexor tendon (8) is fixed to the underside of the pedal bone (2) and runs over the navicular bone (1). The nail went through the deep flexor tendon (7) (red arrow). It will take some time before the tendon completely heals.

Part 2 – Disorders of the Limbs and Hooves

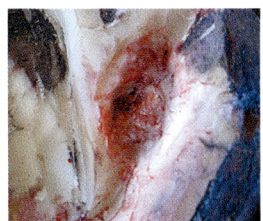

The area where the object penetrated is thoroughly cleaned.

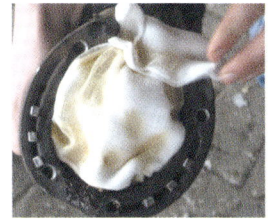

After the operation, the wound is tightly dressed with gauze and Betadine (iodine) to prevent bulging out.

The channel was cleaned as thoroughly as possible and then the hoof was fitted with a surgical plate shoe. This shoe ensures that no dirt can penetrate and the wound stays under pressure so that it cannot bulge out. A puncture wound is a very serious problem that does not always have a happy ending; if the navicular bone had been touched, then the outcome would have been much worse and the horse could have been permanently lame.

CASE HISTORY 2, PHOTOS THIS PAGE

A horse that was presented was seriously lame. It had banged into a wooden bar which caused a splinter to tear open the frog from back to front and had touched the deep flexor tendon. The wound was thoroughly cleaned and the hoof was fitted with a surgical plate horseshoe. This wound could be easily treated and after three weeks it had healed and the horse could return to its owner.

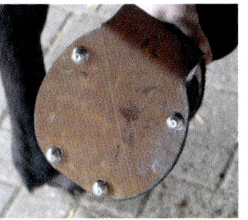

The surgical plate horseshoe is a normal shoe to which a steel plate can be screwed. In this way the wound can be properly checked and treated. As well as this, there is even pressure on the wound, and the horse suffers no additional pain.

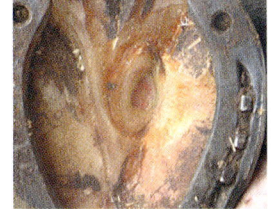

A healthy wound nicely closed up. The hoof must still be protected for a while but the horse may begin slowly with gentle exercise.

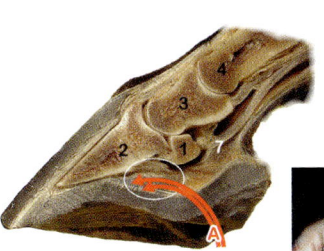

Horses that paw the ground a lot can also do themselves a lot of damage. This horse pawed a wooden pole and received a splinter in the hoof that ripped open the whole frog from the back (A) to the front. The splinter also touched the deep flexor tendon (7).

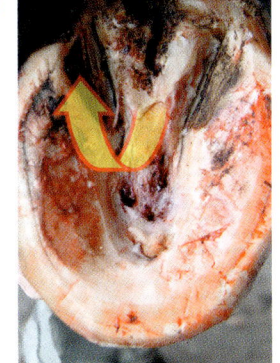

This picture shows how the splinter pulled out the frog.

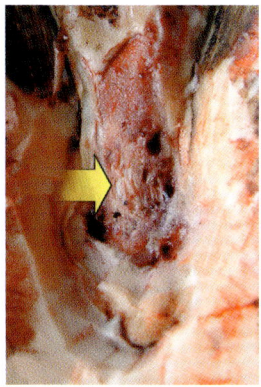

The deep flexor tendon is clearly visible. The area is cleaned and fitted with a surgical plate horseshoe.

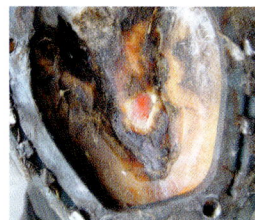

After two weeks of treatment, the wound has healed well and will close in a couple of weeks. The surgical plate horseshoe will remain for a few weeks so that the wound can re-grow horn.

Bruised Sole

A bruised sole is damage of the internal tissue in the hoof caused from an external blow.

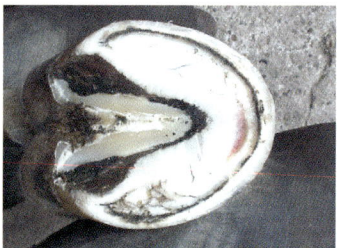

An example of bruising in the toe of the hoof.

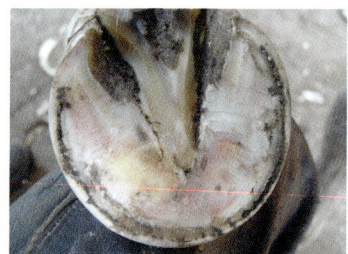

Horses that frequently exercise on uneven terrain or rubble can bruise the whole solar surface. Such horses can best be fitted with a shoe which has been packed with Equi-Thane Hoof Pak® to protect the sole.

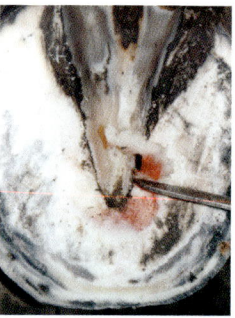

Example of bruising next to the frog. This horse probably stood on a pointed object.

CAUSE

Bruised soles can have several causes:

- Stepping on an object or stone
- Wrong horseshoes, such as shoes that are too short and too small, or where the branches are bent into the heels so that there is faulty pressure on the hoof capsule
- Through diseases such as laminitis or a trauma that causes enormous traction in the coronary band, causing damage in the venous system. Little vessels can rupture, which colours the horny tubules (bruising)

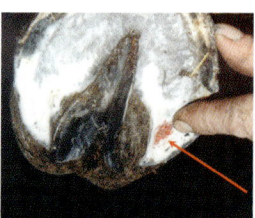

This bruising of the heels has been caused by a stone under the branch of the horseshoe. This can cause serious lameness.

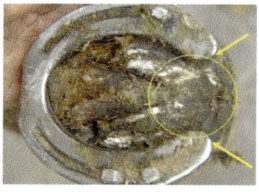

Open-toed horseshoes; both branch-ends push into the sole, and the toe area (yellow circle) is free of weightbearing. This can easily cause painful bruising.

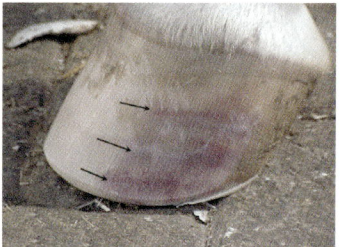

Because this horse constantly kicked its stable wall, the side wall shows bruising coloration from the ruptured blood vessels. This is very common but rarely leads to lameness.

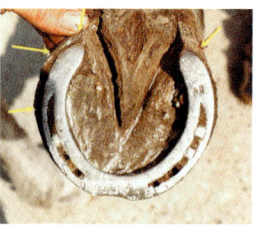

A great cause of bruising in the heel area and sole is shoeing with horseshoes that are too short and too small and with branches that are bent inwards.

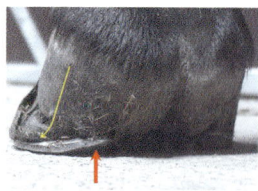

A clear example of a shoe that is badly fitted. The branches of the shoe are too short and the horseshoe is too narrow. Both branches have been bent in under the hoof with disastrous results. This is an extremely badly fitted shoe.

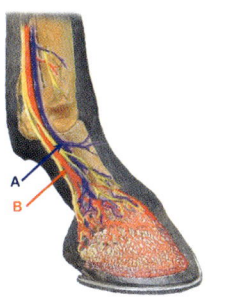

The network of arteries and veins around the pedal bone nourish the hoof.
A. veins; B. arteries

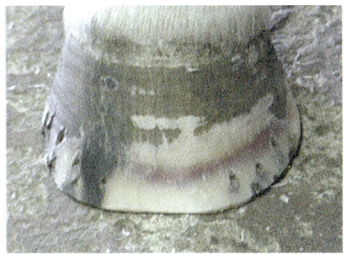

Bruising of the sole shows not only under the solar surface but also in the horny wall. The discolouration caused by lameness or sickness remains visible with hoof growth but does not cause complications.

- A hoof banging against a wall. Thus the capillary system ruptures and the side walls are bruised
- Too much pressure on the digital cushion from the horseshoe. As well as bruising, this can cause sensitive hooves

There is a broad network of arteries in the hoof that nourish the internal parts of the hoof and that make good horn growth possible. When there is tissue damage – for example, by an external blow – the blood vessels in the hoof capsule rupture. Because the vessels bleed, the horny tissue is bruised and dies off. The body reacts by clearing up the tissue; this reaction can be compared to an inflammation reaction.

If the bruised sole is not infected, the consequences are not necessarily serious. However, the horse can have an irregular gait or even display lameness, because some bruises can cause internal pressure. Whether or not bruising is the cause of lameness is often difficult to see immediately because it takes a while before the bleeding – from the blow – causes bruising in the horny cells and tubules. If a bruised sole leads to lameness, it is usually an inflammation of the corium that must be treated.

DIAGNOSIS

People often diagnose a bruised sole before the true cause has been found; actually, bruising is only discovered when the farrier next shoes the horse.

TREATMENT

Although horses should be able to go on every kind of terrain, every now and then a horse steps on a sharp object and hurts itself. Usually, the outcome is not serious and the problem disappears after a couple of days. If the hooves are too short, bruising may more easily occur and a horse should be shod to cope with this problem.

CASE HISTORY 1, PHOTOS BELOW AND PAGE 188

A horse that was presented was lame. After examination of the hoof it appeared that the egg bar shoe that had been fitted was not behind the bulbs but had been placed on the frog. This egg-shaped horseshoe had a

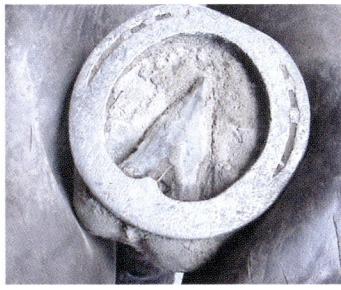

A horseshoe with a curved bar between the branches has more disadvantages than advantages. This farrier had intended to forge an egg bar shoe, but without success.

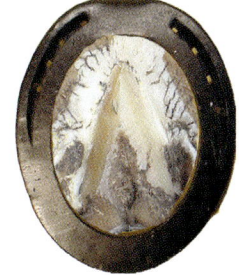

A good egg bar shoe should be egg-shaped. The bar should be behind the frog so that the shoe cannot be brought to bear on the frog.

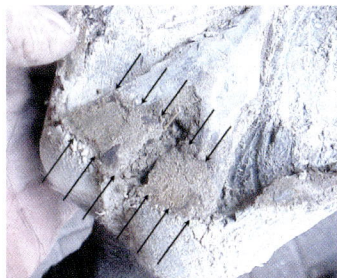

The shoe has bruised the digital cushion and pressed it into the hoof of this horse so deeply that the horse did not dare to put any weight on its foot.

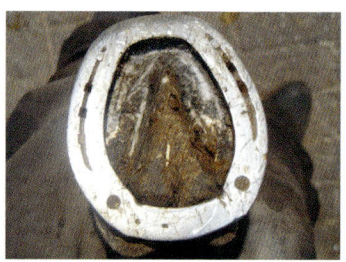
Horseshoes with bars do more harm than good if they are not well fitted.

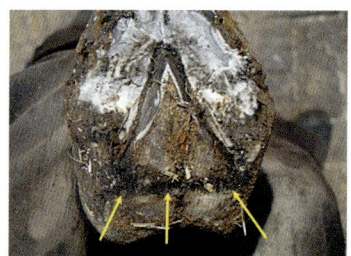
This bar put so much pressure on the bulbs that the horse would move only on its toes. The inside edge of the bar has caused great bruising by pushing deep into the bulbs (yellow arrows).

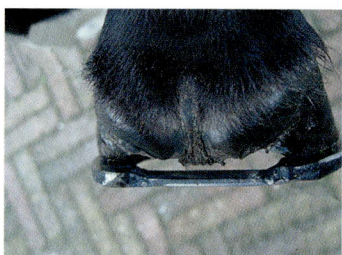
The hoof was shod with a thin bar so that the bar could no longer press on the digital cushion. Only when the hoof is weightbearing will the digital cushion bear on the bar.

round bar welded between the two branches. The back of the shoe lay behind both bulbs. This horse had difficulty in walking because the horseshoe was putting pressure on the frog. The shoe had pressed in the digital cushion just in front of the bulbs so much that the horse did not dare put all its weight on its foot. Treatment consisted of fitting a shoe with a thin bar so that the digital cushion did not rest on the horseshoe.

Cracked Sole

A cracked sole is an interruption in the solar surface going in as deep as the corium.

CAUSE
A cracked sole can be caused by an inflammation in the wall corium. This is usually due to neglect of the hooves. Dirt gets trapped in the crack, cannot escape, and remains there. The build-up of dirt pushes out the horny wall, which gets wider and wider until it cracks open to the corium. In the end, the solar surface – that is connected to the horny wall – also cracks open. This can cause serious lameness in the horse.

TREATMENT
Sole cracks are completely opened up and cleaned until healthy horn attachment in the sole has been reached at all points; afterwards, the hoof can be shod.

CASE HISTORY 1, PHOTOS OPPOSITE
A horse that was presented had a very serious sole crack and was lame. The hoof had to be trimmed to determine the extent of the crack and the manner of treatment. It could then be seen that the crack had caused more damage to the solar surface than was first thought. The crack had to be cleaned and the part of the horny wall that had been affected had to be removed. It then became clear that the cause of the crack was an inflammation of the toe: a black part was visible, which meant that the horny wall and the insensitive and sensitive laminae were inflamed. The

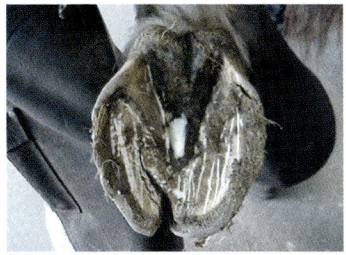
Example of a split which went deep into the sole at the weightbearing edge.

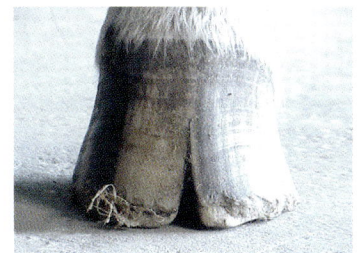
Because the hoof has not been trimmed in good time, the horse collects more and more grime and the wall can split. To determine the seriousness of the split, the hoof must first be trimmed.

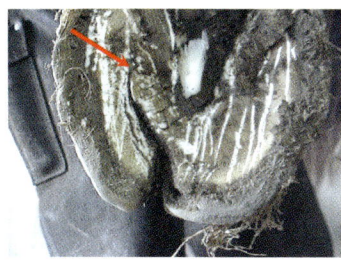
The crack runs half way into the sole.

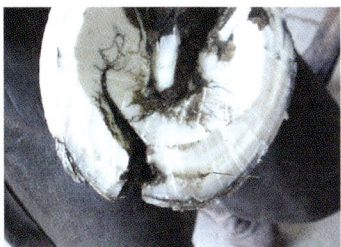
After trimming, it is clear that the crack has caused even more damage than was originally thought.

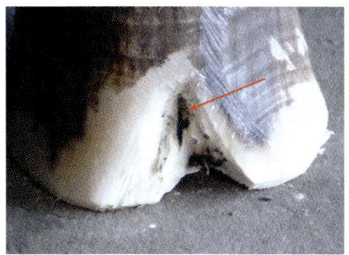
The cause of the crack is an inflammation in the toe. The inflamed insensitive and sensitive laminae are easily visible (black part).

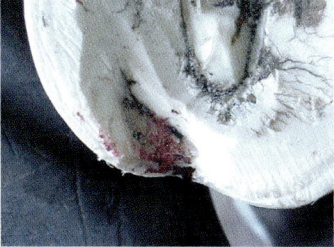
The sole is cleaned for healthy development of the sole and horny wall.

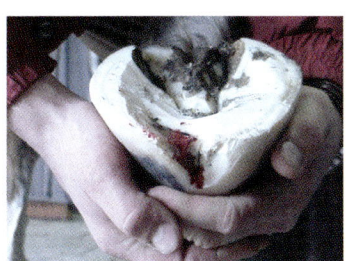
The wound is cleaned to the depth of the corium and dressed with a bandage with a bactericidal; afterwards, the hoof is shod.

solar surface was cleaned until healthy horn was reached so that there could once again be a healthy development of the solar surface and horny wall. The hoof was applied with a Betadine (iodine) solution. As well as this, this horse needed a shoe that would support the horny wall and the sole so that the horny wall would be prevented from cracking further. To protect the wound, a back 'brushing' shoe was fitted which had a broad toe part. To prevent infection, the hoof had to be dressed with a bandage with disinfectant. Afterwards, a piece of gauze was put between the shoe and the wound to prevent dirt getting in. The hoof had to be checked daily. After treatment, the horse was no longer lame.

4 THE HOOF: HOOF CAPSULE

Infected Crack

An infected crack is an interruption in the horny wall due to infection. The causes are, for example, kicking against stable doors, kicking side walls when feeding, or banging against poles when jumping, with a trauma of the wall corium as a result. Getting little stones or dirt caught in the white line can also cause inflammation. Infected cracks vary depending on where they are: they can occur anywhere in the hoof capsule. Every crack has a different effect: a normal, small crack in the toe, for example, could be due to an internal cause which can lead to big problems and to serious lameness.

TREATMENT
An infected crack must be filed down to the corium. This is usually under anaesthetic and with the absence of blood in the lower foot; the hoof is then temporarily tied off with a ligature to block the blood flow.

CASE HISTORY 1, PHOTOS RIGHT AND PAGE 191 TOP
A horse that was presented had trouble with an infected toe crack. The white line had become thick and had been forced back; it had also taken on a defective shape. This clearly indicated a bacterial infection accompanied by a fungus. These characteristics often point to serious problems in the hoof capsule. In treating, the wall was temporarily removed; the wall corium was infected and had to be cut away. Behind the horny wall on the corium a broad, yellow wall corium was uncovered. A horseshoe nail could be inserted into the horny wall in this spot because the wall had become separated by the infection. For the sake of clarity – this horse did not have seedy toe. The infection had, though, loosened 2 to 3 centimetres of sensitive and insensitive laminae. The area was cleaned up as far as the coronary band so that healthy horn could develop again. By stimulating the coronary corium, the growth of the horny wall is also stimulated.

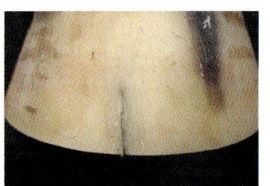

A crack in the horny wall on the front of the hoof; the line of the crack indicates a fungus.

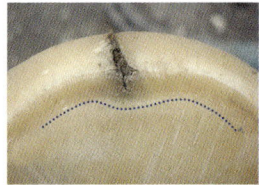

Infected toe crack seen from under the hoof. The white line is slightly thickened and pushed back (blue line).

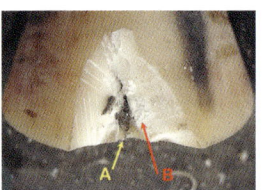

Having removed a piece of wall, it is clear that the wall corium is infected (A, yellow arrow). The red arrow shows that there is indeed a fungus present which will affect the horny wall further.

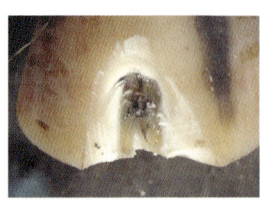

Because the wall corium is infected and a fungus is present, the lower part of the hoof capsule must be cleaned.

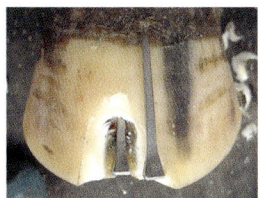 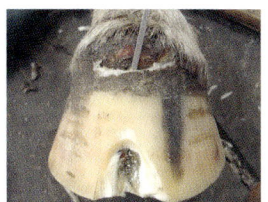 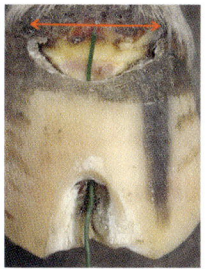 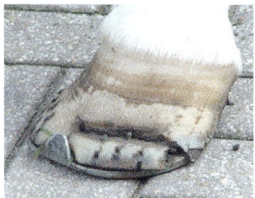

A horseshoe nail can be inserted up into and behind the horny wall, as the wall has been loosened by the infection. This nail can reach as far as the coronary corium.	*The coronary band has to be thoroughly cleaned so that it can make a new and healthy horn structure.*	*Due to the irritation of the inflammation, the coronary corium will grow a thicker horn wall. In further treatment this will be left untouched because it gives extra strength to the hoof capsule. The interruption in the horny wall is called a horn fissure.*	*After seven to nine months, the horn fissure has grown down and a normal broad shoe is fitted. The horn above the fissure is normal and the coronary band has retained its original shape.*

Thicker horn was necessary to strengthen the hoof capsule. In order to keep the connection with the hoof capsule intact the horny wall was not removed any further. Thus the coronary band could not collapse. After several months the coronary band had resumed normal horn growth. The horse was shod with a bar shoe; a shoe with a bar between the branches to prevent movement in the shoe and to keep the hoof capsule as stable as possible.

White Line Disease

White line disease is a sudden deterioration of the white line in the hoof or horny wall. In very serious cases this leads to a whole or part wall cavity. The affected area is characterised by a granular structure.

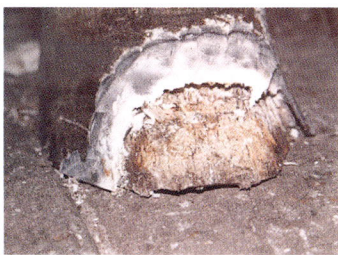 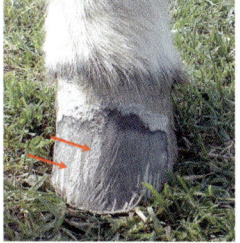 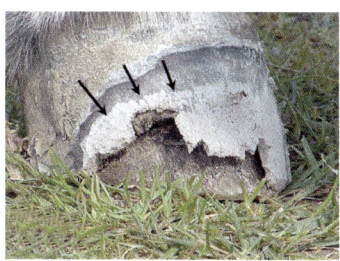

Example of a separating wall caused by a fungus.	*The vertical, lighter parts in the wall are a sign of deterioration as a result of a fungus.*	*As soon as the wall is touched, pieces fall off. The horny wall appears to be completely pulverised.*

The Hoof – Hoof Capsule

CAUSE

White line disease is caused by a fungus accompanied by a bacterium. The fungus and the bacterium are found everywhere in stables and outdoors and are thus called environmental bacterium and fungus. Actually, the name 'white line disease' is misleading because the disease affects not only the white line but other parts of the hoof capsule too. Above all, it is not a disease of the white line but a result of collaboration between the bacterium and the fungus.

White line disease always begins underneath in the hoof capsule and is usually a result of damage or an interruption in the hoof wall or the white line which, unfortunately, is nearly always discovered too late. Because the natural immunity of the horn is interrupted, even non-pathogenic bacteria cause infections. A number of bacteria grow optimally in an aerobic environment. This group is the most troublesome with *Pseudomonas aeruginosa* and *Staphylococcus aurius*. The worst kind are the clostridium kind; the sort that develop in an anaerobic environment – a warm, damp, dark and oxygen-free place such as is found in a hoof – and cause the dying of tissue in the location. The combination of aerobic and anaerobic bacteria ensures that the fungus type geotrichum develops well. Bacteria multiply faster than fungi by their cell division, but fungi produce spores that spread rapidly and are more difficult to combat than bacteria. Deep in the horny wall, fungi form their mycelia – a network of fungal threads on which the spore-forming organs of fungi can build. Fungi develop by preference in a warm, damp, dark and oxygen-free environment – elements found pre-eminently in the hoof interior.

White line disease begins mostly with a crack, an irregularity in the white line or in a nail hole. Because the white line is extremely soft, it offers the perfect place for the start of an infection. The fungus that causes white line disease is immediately present in an infection because it is an environmental fungus.

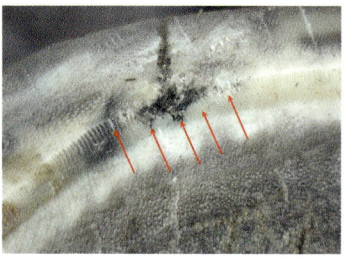

There is an inflammation behind the crack in the wall. Next to it a fungus is present.

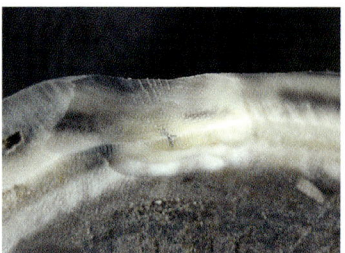

If the farrier is alert, he can prevent things getting worse. The crack and the inflammation with the fungus are removed. The farrier will ask the owner to spread honey over the area.

TREATMENT

It is of the utmost importance that the farrier removes the affected tissue completely. Afterwards, the spot must be sprayed with a Betadine (iodine)/alcohol solution to combat the *Staphylococcus aurius* bacterium. Then a piece of cotton wool soaked in 3 percent hydrogen peroxide or Bocasan powder (natriumperborate with natriumhydrogenartrate) is applied because the bacterium such as the clostridium needs oxygen. This dose must be repeated several times. Finally, a natural product of bees is applied so that fungi such as geotrichum do not have a chance. Bees know how to keep the nursery of the queen's eggs clean: they make honey, which contains the substance propolis. Finally, provide good hoof care to keep the pseudomonas bacterium at bay; that is to say; pick out the hooves, brush dry and maintain good stable hygiene.

In a period of about six years, my twin brother and I, together with various others, set up a programme for curing white line disease. We discovered that the fungus could be killed with honey because of the substance propolis – a fungicidal agent. In recent years, many horses have been treated successfully. Often the veterinary surgeon or the

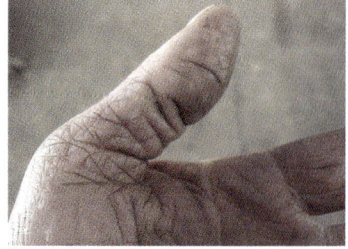

The fungus can aggressively affect the skin of people and dry it out; it causes many fissures and cracks.

farrier will first remove the horny wall to take away the fungus, but this is not necessary in all cases. The horny wall should be preserved as much as possible: the more horn there is, the stronger the hoof. Unfortunately, white line disease often goes unnoticed; this is why we try to issue as much information about it as possible.

HORSESHOES

Well-fitted shoes are of great importance in white line disease. Whether the horse can continue to function is dependent on the farrier. There are many remedies available for white line disease but so far there is no proof that they work. Fungi are very aggressive and can easily return: usually, rigorous treatment is the only way to regain a healthy hoof.

CASE HISTORY 1, PHOTOS BELOW

A horse that was presented was lame when putting weight on a hoof during lungeing on the circle. An inflammation in the side wall had been treated previously by a farrier, but without follow-up treatment. Thus the fungus had affected a great part of the wall. Treatment consisted of removing part of the weightbearing edge and removing the affected

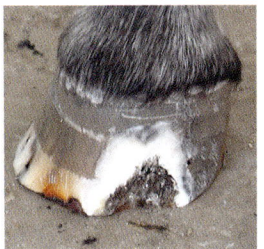
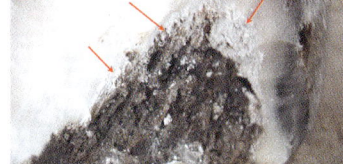
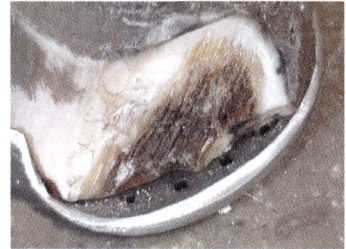

An inflammation has loosened the horny wall. Afterwards, the fungus has affected a great part of the wall; the affected part has a granular texture.

The side of the wall had to be completely removed from this hoof. The horny wall is removed until healthy horn attachment on the corium is reached. The place will be treated with honey.

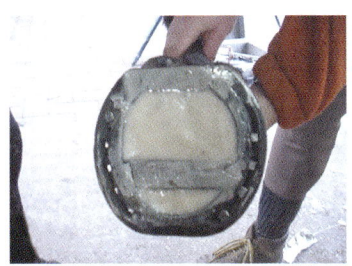

Because a great deal of the wall has been removed, Equi-Thane Hoof Pak® is packed between the bar and the solar surface. This allows the ground pressure to be distributed over the whole hoof so that the remaining weightbearing edge is not stressed unduly.

tissue. The horny wall was removed up to healthy attachment. The hoof was fitted with a bar shoe to prevent movement in the horseshoe. Equi-Thane Hoof Pak® was put in between the bar and the hoof to distribute the weightbearing over the whole hoof. The horny wall can be closed by making an artificial wall but this is strongly advised against because there is a big chance that spores are still present and the problem can thus arise again.

CASE HISTORY 2, PHOTOS PAGE 194 (TOP)

A horse that was presented had a crack in the horny wall caused by an inflammation. The fungus was present with the inflammation. The fungus was not only in the white line but also in the horny wall – thus, on the outside. The affected wall and the white line, where the pulverising, fat-like substance of the fungus was situated, could be scraped away with a horseshoe nail. As a matter of fact, the fungus is also very contagious for humans.

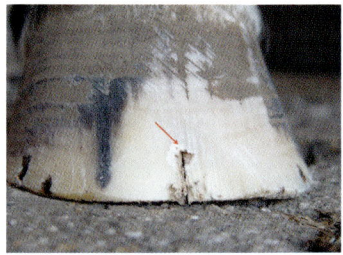 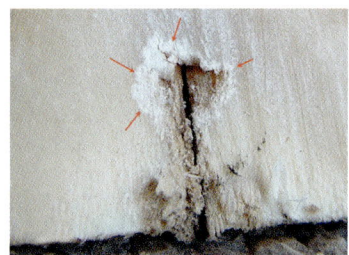 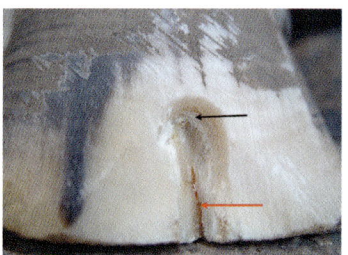

A crack in the front of the hoof always indicates an underlying cause. A fungus is present with this inflammation (white structure); it is the cause of the white line disease.

The affected horny wall (red arrows) is a clear sign that the fungus has left traces of its spore throughout.

The whole area is cleaned carefully. It is now clear where the inflammation was (red arrow). There is an opening in the sensitive laminae where dirt can enter.

CASE HISTORY 3, PHOTOS BELOW AND OPPOSITE

Horn cracks usually run down in the same direction as the horny tubules. A horse that was presented had a crack that was wavy. The wavy line indicated the presence of a fungus with a bacterium. These cracks can also be as a result of insufficient trimming but in this case it was white line disease. The treatment consisted of removing the crack in its entirety as the fungus had to be removed from the whole area. The spot was cleaned carefully; the horny wall was cut away until healthy attachment was found between the horny wall and the wall corium. During treatment, the network of vessels – which are very close to the area being treated –

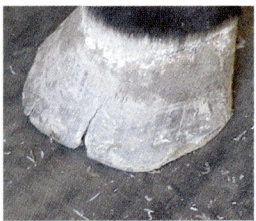 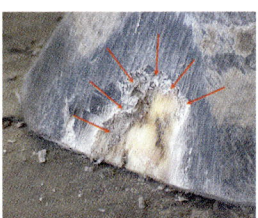 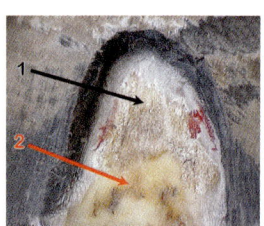

'Just a wavy crack' in the horny wall is always the result of a deeper problem. This is a recognisable sign of white line disease.

As soon as a piece of horn is removed, the pulverised mass caused by the fungus becomes visible.

The inflamed spot (red arrow). The corium is dark yellow and smooth. Above the inflammation, the fungus has done its destructive work (black arrow). The fungus, with its development of spores, completely loosened the horny wall.

should be avoided to prevent heavy bleeding. After cutting away, the hoof capsule was in two parts so the hoof had to be fitted temporarily with a fore shoe with two side clips. This shoe prevented the hoof capsule from expanding further. In this way the hoof could easily be kept clean and treated with honey. It is important that enough oxygen reaches the fungus; the fungus can be quickly eliminated with oxygen so the area should never be closed up. It is pointless to fit a horseshoe with double

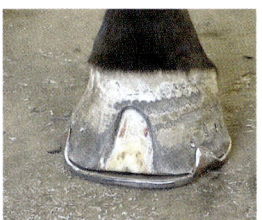 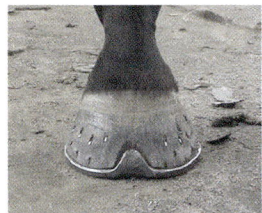 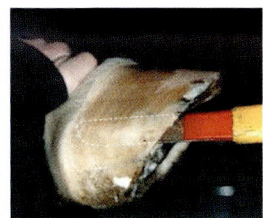 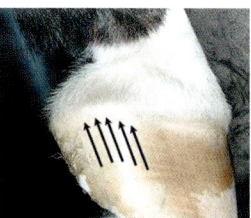

Because part of the horny wall is removed, the hoof becomes weak. To prevent the wall collapsing, the hoof is fitted temporarily with double clips to protect it.

After six months, the hoof capsule has grown again and the hoof can be fitted with a normal shoe.

The whole of the side wall of the hoof is loose. A hoof knife can be inserted between the horny wall and the corium (dotted line).

The wall has been loosened by the fungus. Pressure from the ground has pushed up the wall together with the coronary band and pushed it outwards (black arrows). The wall has changed shape.

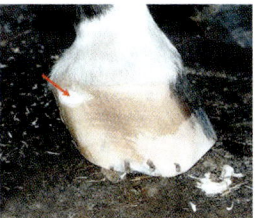 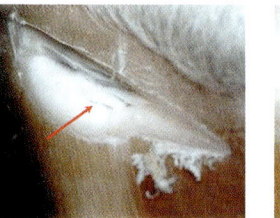

Above in the foot, just under the coronary band, a groove is made in order to reach the corium.

Exactly the right spot is cut away. The fungus has done its destructive work. Above the fungus is a healthy horn attachment to the corium.

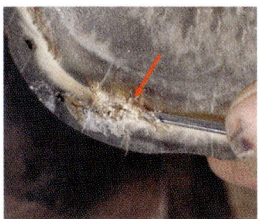 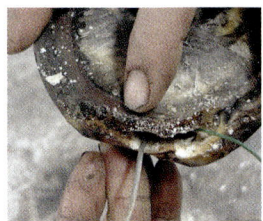 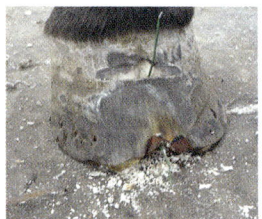 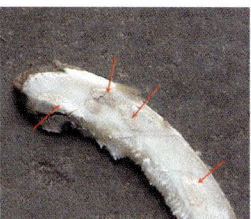

Under the hoof, near the white line and the horny tubules, the fungus can be scraped off with a horseshoe nail.

The place is cleaned and it is now apparent that the spores of the fungus have affected the corium more than was first thought.

The fungus has caused much damage: the horny wall under the groove is not removed, so that the strength of the hoof is preserved. A drain is placed in the horny wall so that the fungus can be treated with the shoe in place.

That the fungus is not only in the white line of the hoof can be seen on the trimmed part of the horny wall; the horny tubules can also be affected.

clips in order to hold the split together, as this does not get to the root of the problem. After six months, the hoof had re-grown and was fitted with a normal horseshoe so that the hoof mechanism could work optimally. The farrier continued checking the horse; this is very important in the prevention of further problems.

CASE HISTORY 4, PHOTOS RIGHT

White line disease can lead to serious lameness. The fungi can completely loosen the wall from the corium. A horse that was presented had fungi that had been present for a long time in the coronary band. The hoof capsule is internally connected to the coffin bone and cannot normally change position. Because this wall had been loosened by the fungi, the ground pressure had pushed up the wall, with the coronary band, to the outside. Thus the wall took on another shape. Action had to be taken to stop the wall remaining loose. The fungi had to be eliminated so that further damage to the hoof capsule was limited. The horny wall was not completely removed otherwise the hoof would have been weakened. Up above in the hoof, where the fungi were situated, a groove was made in order to reach the healthy corium; the affected tissue was removed until a healthy attachment to the horny wall was reached. The wall under the filed out groove could be used as temporary strengthening for the whole hoof capsule and to prevent problems with shoeing. As soon as the wall had grown down again, the farrier could nail above the crack again. In this way, the form of the hoof capsule would not change in the course of the treatment.

DONKEYS

White line disease affects donkeys as well as horses. In Holland, white line disease is common in donkeys because they are usually overweight, a situation which can easily cause laminitis. The horny walls of donkeys are softer than those of horses and thus more susceptible to a fungus. A donkey's hoof is long in shape and it is less mobile than that of a horse. Horny walls of donkeys are more easily handled; the donkey is not disturbed by treatment and above all can function easily on the solar surface.

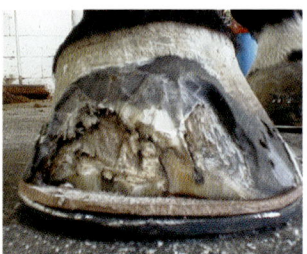

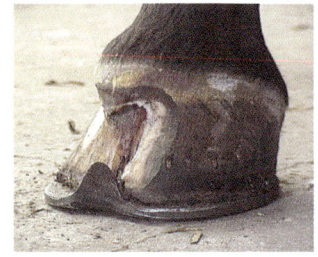

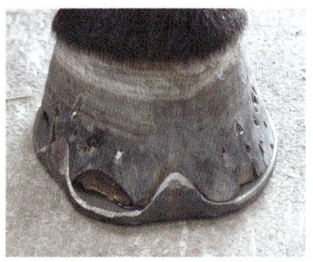

The treatment of white line disease is long but the results are rewarding.

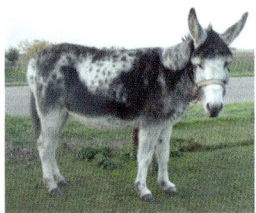

Donkeys frequently have white line disease.

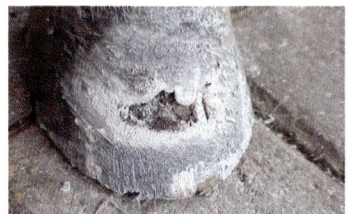

White line disease is worse in donkeys than horses because of the soft quality of their horn; the whole wall can be affected.

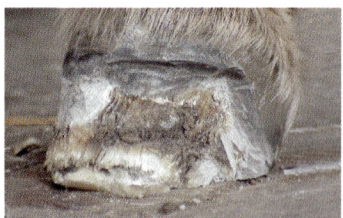

The only solution is the removal of the horny wall. Donkeys can very easily bear weight on their hooves, which is not the case with horses.

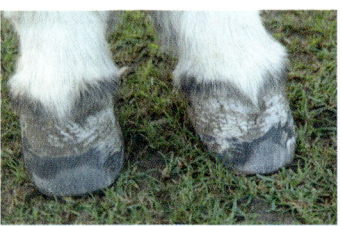

After eleven months, both hooves are completely re-grown.

4 THE HOOF: PEDAL BONE

Chip Fracture of the Pedal Bone

A chip fracture is when a small piece of bone breaks off.

CAUSE
A chip occurs when a horse treads on a sharp object or because the hoof lands on a stone or hard object. When there is pressure on a tiny spot, a piece of the pedal bone can spontaneously chip off. The small piece of

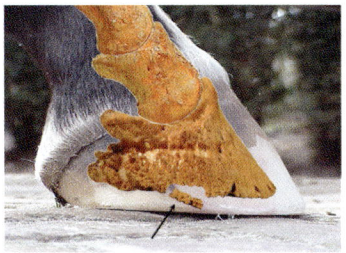

Example of a pedal bone with a chip fracture.

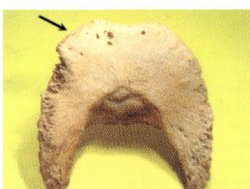

Underneath view of a pedal bone. The edge is clearly dissolved and pieces of bone break off spontaneously.

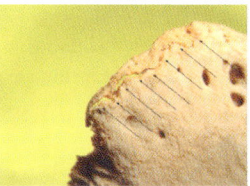

The disintegration and dissolution of the edge of the pedal bone happens extremely slowly.

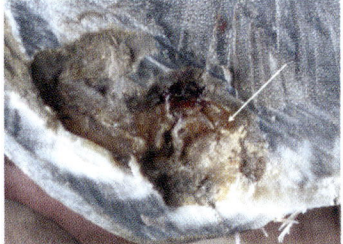

Pedal bone fracture where the piece of bone is wrapped in connective tissue. This piece of bone can no longer cause inflammation in the hoof.

bone can cause very serious inflammation in the hoof with grim consequences for the horse. If an inflammation is developed caused by the piece of bone, the horse becomes lame and this is followed by worse lameness. There is not always inflammation with a chip fracture of the pedal bone; sometimes the body reacts by surrounding the bone with connective tissue. In the most unexpected places, the encapsulated piece of bone can rest against the sole corium and, subsequently, exit the body in a natural way. The farrier may come across these pieces when he is trimming the hoof. As soon as the piece is removed, the sole continues to grow normally and no inflammation is caused in the hoof nor is any lameness caused.

SYMPTOMS
When a horse has a chip fracture of the pedal bone it will not fully bear weight on its hoof and, if possible, it will move on the toe of the hoof.

DIAGNOSIS

A chip fracture can only be determined with the help of an X-ray. On an X-ray it is clear to see that a piece of bone has broken off from the pedal bone (see photos right).

TREATMENT

It is only with the help of an operation that the cause of the inflammation and the lameness – the chip fragment – can be removed. For the operation a rubber band – a ligature – is tied around the hoof so that the operation can take place in the absence of blood. In the operation, the solar surface where the chip is situated is removed. Then the pedal bone is examined for a loose bit of bone; when it has been located, the whole piece is removed. The edge of the pedal bone is examined and cleaned up – the bone is filed clean. After the removal of the chip, the hoof is shod with a shoe that can have a metal plate screwed on to it, a so-called surgical plate horseshoe. Under this plate, a bandage is placed to give counter-pressure and to staunch the flow of blood. As well as this, the use of a surgical plate shoe is economical, as otherwise the hoof has to be dressed daily with expensive bandages.

After a week, the wound should be dry, which indicates that all the fragments were removed in the operation. If a piece of bone had been

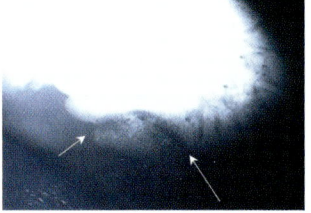

A chip fracture is clearly visible on the X-ray.

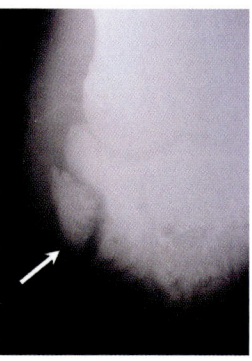

This X-ray shows a chip fracture.

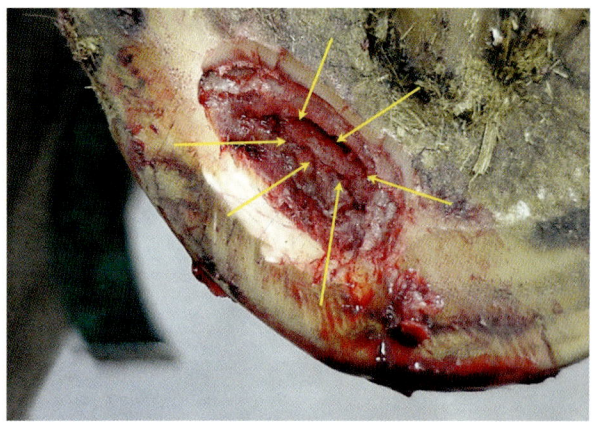

After removing part of the sole, the pedal bone is searched for the chip fracture.

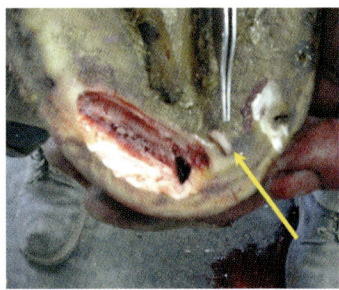

Here, the yellow arrow shows the piece of bone that has broken off from the pedal bone.

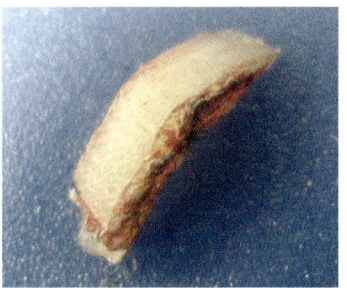

The piece of bone removed from the pedal bone.

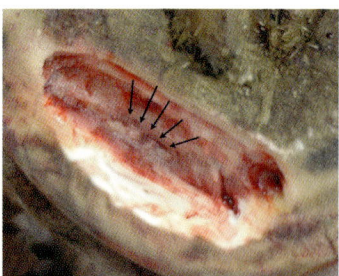

It is clear to see where the piece of bone has been removed from the pedal bone. It is important to examine the area around the chip fracture to check for the possibility of other pieces of bone.

overlooked in the operation, there would be an inflammation reaction; the wound would not be able to close and the healing process would be slow. In the case of a satisfactory healing process, the wound is protected by a thick layer of horny sole after eight or ten weeks.

Sometimes it is not a fragment of bone that is chipped off but a large piece. This is then called a pedal bone fracture. When this concerns a

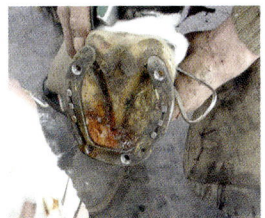
A surgical plate horseshoe has four screw holes for attaching a metal plate.

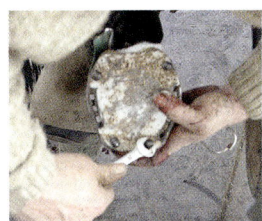
The metal plate is screwed under the hoof.

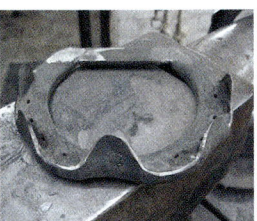
Example of a horseshoe with several clips. This shoe is used when a large piece of bone has broken off the pedal bone.

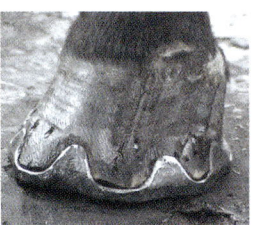
A horseshoe with several clips fitted to the horse's hoof.

young horse and the piece of bone is in the right place, the first thing to do is to try to force the piece back to a correct position and immobilise it with the help of a good horseshoe. The shoe should be fitted as exactly as possible with three, four or five clips (as deemed necessary) so that there is immobility in the lower shoe. The placing of the clips depends on the location of the fracture.

CASE HISTORY 1, PHOTOS LEFT AND BELOW

A horse that was presented was seriously lame. Treatment consisted of filing a hole into the horny wall to locate the inflammation so that the lameness could be cured. This, however, did not work: the horse was still lame and the inflamed corium bulged out of the bored-out hole. Because a pungent-smelling fluid oozed from the hole, the whole wall was removed in order to clean up the corium. During the cutting away of the wall, there appeared to be a loose piece of pedal bone. After its removal, the hoof was dressed with a compress to put pressure on the corium to stop it bulging out. The hoof was shod with a bar shoe to immobilise movement in the shoe. The piece of bone that was removed had encapsulated itself. After two weeks, the wound had healed beautifully. The horse was no longer lame and white edges were visible around the cut away part which indicated that no pieces of bone had been left behind. The complete healing would take a number of weeks.

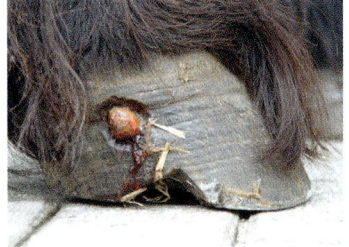
The piece of bone removed from the pedal bone.

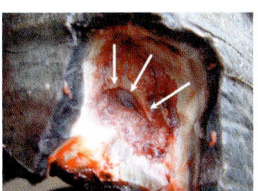
During the filing away of the wall and corium a loose piece of bone is discovered.

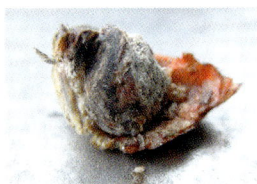
Piece of bone with coagulated pus.

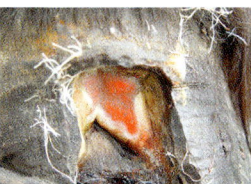
The wound is healing beautifully after the operation. Around the filed away part, white edges can be seen; this is proof that all the pieces of bone have been removed in the operation.

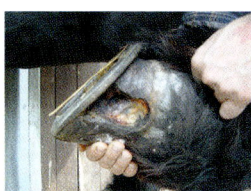
The wound is completely closed and hardened off. The horse can commence light exercise.

Pedal Bone and Navicular Fracture and Fissure

A fracture is another word for a broken bone. Usually, a bone breaks in two, but it can also have multiple breaks. Fissures are cracks – an incomplete break – in the bone tissue.

CAUSE
Fractures and fissures are caused by an awkward step, by blows or stumbling, or by an uncontrolled movement of the horse. Immediately after a fracture or fissure, the horse cannot put weight on its hoof because of pain.

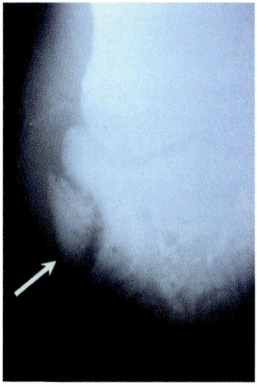

The arrow shows the place where there is a fracture in the pedal bone. This will be treated by fitting a special horseshoe.

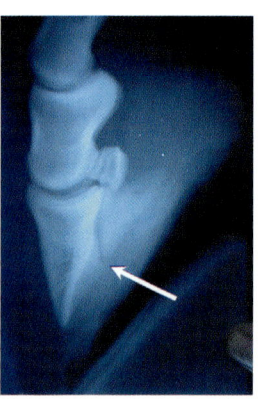

This X-ray clearly shows a fracture of the pedal bone (arrow).

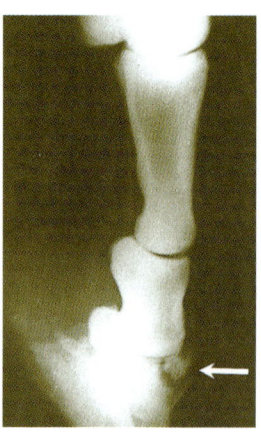

One of the most frequent types of fracture is the fracture of the coronary rim of the pedal bone (arrow). The extensor tendon is attached where the coronary rim is situated; through a sudden force of traction the coronary rim can crack off.

DIAGNOSIS
When a horse has a fracture or fissure in the pedal bone, it is not immediately obvious. Only with the aid of X-rays can fractures and fissures be seen. A clear dividing line between the two (or more) bone parts is visible with fractures. A fissure is more difficult to see because the break is incomplete and the dividing line is less visible.

The diagnosis of a fracture or fissure requires thorough examination: the whole lower foot must be checked for possible inflammation of the hoof, as this displays the same symptoms as those of a fracture or fissure, that is, acute lameness. If inflammation is not found, then an X-ray is taken to determine whether there is a fracture or fissure.

TREATMENT
The treatment depends on where the fracture or fissure occurred. A fracture of a pedal bone lateral cartilage can very well be held in place by a horseshoe which keeps the hoof immobile; a fracture of the coronary prominence of the pedal bone, however, cannot be immobilised by a horseshoe. The problem is that this spot is near the coronary band and this is where the flexor tendon is fixed – the tendon that allows the horse to bring its hoof forward.

The hoof capsule can be immobilised by fitting a horseshoe with three to five clips and a cast – a firm plaster bandage. After treatment, the horse must be rested for a period to allow for healing. After fitting this type of horseshoe, the horse is clearly far less lame but this does not mean that the problem is not very serious. After eight weeks, an X-ray is taken to see if both pieces of bone are in place. The hoof is re-shod with the same type of shoe so that there is no difference in pressure.

OTHER FRACTURES AND FISSURES IN THE HOOF

Breaks are also seen in the pedal bone lateral cartilages. Hoof cartilage is found on the pedal bone lateral cartilages; it has an important function in the hoof mechanism. When the hoof cartilage hardens – or ossifies – it can easily break. This is called a fracture in the outside lateral cartilage or inside lateral cartilage of the pedal bone. If a horse has such a fracture, it can cause lameness.

Navicular bone fractures or fissures heal very badly because the navicular bone is a very small and thin bone that is part of the hoof joint.

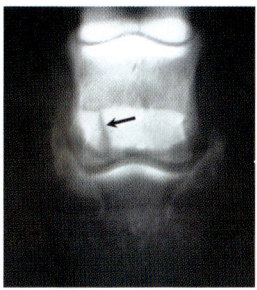

Fracture of a pedal bone lateral cartilage.

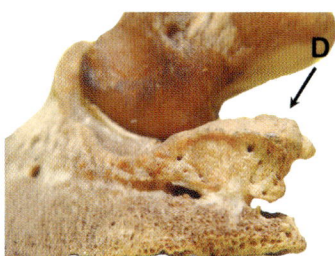

The X-ray view of the back of the pedal bone. The fracture in the navicular bone is clearly visible.

If the cartilage (D) becomes ossified – harder and bigger – and continues to grow as well, it can easily break off.

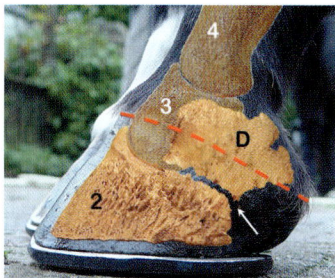

A normal hoof with serious ossification of the cartilage (D). The red dotted line indicates the coronary band. The elastic movement of the short and long pastern bones (3 and 4) will be painfully impeded. The white arrow shows the break.

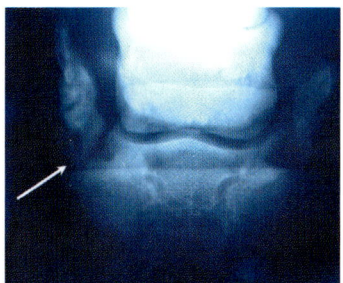

The white line shows an ossified cartilage that has been broken by an external blow. Ossification of the cartilage is frequently seen in horses such as harness horses that are exercised on hard surfaces.

Fractures and fissures in the navicular bone cause damage in the joint capsule. On this spot, too, the deep flexor tendon runs over the navicular bone, bringing great pressure to bear. This explains why the chances of a complete healing of navicular bone fractures and fissures are small and that the condition can have an unfavourable outcome. On its front surface, the navicular bone is closed in between the pedal bone and the short pastern bone and at its rear it is bound in by the deep flexor tendon and ligaments. This spot is extremely difficult to immobilise completely, in contrast with the pedal bone that is enclosed by the hoof capsule and easier to keep in a fixed position by a horseshoe.

To achieve good results in the treatment of fractures or fissures requires a professional team consisting of veterinary surgeons and farriers. Although the treatment for fractures and fissures require long-term treatment of at least six months, they can be successfully treated with current knowledge and medicine. Sometimes an operation is necessary; the results of such are variable.

CASE HISTORY

A foal was frolicking about and suffered a break in the pedal bone and was very seriously lame. An X-ray was taken to determine the place of the fracture. Afterwards, a horseshoe was made with multiple clips and a bar in order to close in the area and immobilise the hoof. In this way, the piece of broken pedal bone could be kept in place and the break could heal. In fitting the shoe, the farrier had to make sure that he did not place a clip where the break line was and he had to ensure that there could be no movement.

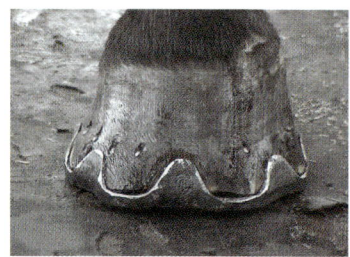

Example of a hoof with five clips to immobilise the hoof.

Laminitis

Laminitis is a metabolic disease which results in the inflammation of the insensitive or sensitive laminae that form the connection between the hoof capsule and the pedal bone. Just as with other inflammations, swelling develops between the hoof capsule and the pedal bone, which causes the horse extreme pain. Laminitis is an extremely serious disease which often starts if there are problems elsewhere in the body other than in the feet. This complaint occurs mostly in the fore limbs but also appears regularly in the hind limbs.

Laminitis has various causes:
- Over-eating of carbohydrates from, for example, oats, horse nuts, young grass or apples; a horse that escapes from its stable and gorges at the feeding bin in the night
- Excessive condition: the horse is too fat. This is mostly seen in ponies that are kept as companions where they are not asked to do a stroke of work and are put out in rich pasture. If this is supplemented by silage, then there is a high possibility of laminitis
- Not – or not completely – getting rid of the afterbirth in foaling
- Various processes of disease of horses with fever and pain. Usually, with these serious illnesses, toxic substances are deposited in the bloodstream
- Some medicines, such as corticosteroids, can have damaging side-effects which develop a heightened sensitivity to laminitis in horses
- Overtaxing: by riding too long, by an untrained horse being suddenly heavily taxed or by long-distance transportation where the horse must stand still for a long time and cannot rest its hooves. Also a horse that has long-term lameness in one limb can overtax the opposite limb
- Stress and emotional factors
- A trauma that affects the hoof. Accidents where the hoof capsule is pulled off. Hoof operations and/or hoof problems
- A puncture wound from treading on a sharp object that penetrates deeply into the horse's hoof. Because the healthy hoof is overtaxed, it can become laminitic
- Toxic substances, such as dry seeds, grasses, plants and shrubs
- Neglect
- Cushing's disease (tumour of the pituitary gland)

This horses places its limbs in front of the vertical and clearly has laminitis. The hind limbs are placed far under the body, and thus carry the greater part of the bodyweight.

ACUTE LAMINITIS AND FOUNDER

Laminitis can be acute; from the very beginning the symptoms appear suddenly and to a serious degree. If acute laminitis is not treated, it develops into a chronic (continuous) form of laminitis. A horse that is troubled by acute laminitis displays intense pain and lameness. If both fore limbs are affected, it tries to unburden its fore hooves. The fore limbs are placed far in front of the vertical, the perpendicular line that runs down from the horse's shoulder. The hind limbs are placed far under the body and carry the greater part of the bodyweight. In movement, the horse endeavours to keep the fore limbs out in front. It endeavours to set the heels down first, in order to unburden the painful toe area. The horse has difficulty remaining standing, and wants to lie down stretched out. The affected hooves and coronary band feel warm to the touch and the pumping of the arteries in the pastern cavity can be clearly felt. The horse displays obvious pain and it begins to sweat. It has an increased heart beat and sometimes a high temperature.

WHAT SHOULD BE DONE WHEN THERE IS AN ACUTE ATTACK?

Laminitis is an emergency, and the cure depends on the cause and on whether or not there has been speedy intervention. In a case of acute laminitis, the veterinary surgeon or farrier may decide to take an X-ray to determine the seriousness of the laminitis and to get a picture of the extent to which the pedal bone has rotated (for which the horse can be immediately shod). It is usually recommended that the hooves are cooled down straight away with running water. As the horse is standing still, the area becomes warm and this is disadvantageous. Also, pressure from the ground on the sensitive sole is a problem for the horse, so ensure that the horse has space enough with plenty of straw so that it can lie down. A good farrier can help a horse to get back on its feet quickly. He can ensure that the pain is reduced by removing the front part of the hoof capsule in whole or in part. Thereby the fluid is drained off, which takes the pressure off and thus reduces the pain. Subsequently, the sole can be protected with a special horseshoe.

WHAT HAPPENS TO THE FOOT?

Before going further, the reader ought to know something about the hoof itself. A hoof has several different types of corium and, depending on their position in the hoof, they are known as the periople, coronary, wall or frog corium. Together they form one whole that encloses the internal part of the hoof. The pedal bone is situated in the interior of the hoof: it lies firmly encapsulated against the hoof capsule. Two tendons are attached to the pedal bone: at the back, the deep flexor tendon, and at the front the extensor tendon. These tendons bring a contracting tension – or traction – to bear. The tendon that is attached at the front of the pedal bone is called the extensor tendon or pedal bone extensor. The tendon that is attached to the back of the pedal bone is called the deep flexor tendon or the pedal bone deep flexor. The traction of the pedal bone extensor is less strong than that of the pedal bone flexor. Working together, the pedal bone extensor and the pedal bone flexor keep the

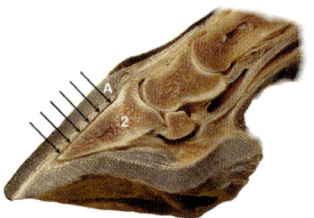

Whenever the connection (black arrows) between the horny wall (A) and the pedal bone (2) is broken due to aseptic inflammation, the pressure from the flexor tendons and the weight of the horse cause the pedal bone to come loose from the wall and rotate.

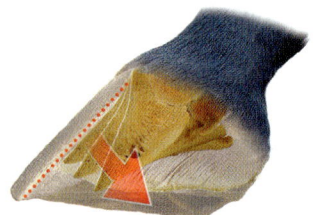

The aseptic inflammation that is caused by laminitis occurs in the corium (red dotted line). The corium contains many blood vessels and nerves. The pressure of the pus loosens the laminae so that the pedal bone, which is connected to the horny wall internally, comes loose. When this happens, the pedal bone rotates (red arrow).

pedal bone in the correct position in the hoof.

In laminitis, an aseptic inflammation of the corium causes the connection between the horny wall and the hoof corium of the pedal bone to be broken down. The traction of the deep flexor tendon and the weight of the horse then cause the pedal bone to be torn away from the horny wall and begin to rotate. The extent to which the pedal bone rotates determines the seriousness of the laminitis.

FOUNDER

When acute laminitis is not treated, it develops into a chronic form of laminitis called founder. In founder, the symptoms of acute laminitis continue to progress. Among these, there is also another clearly visible symptom – the flipping up of the toe at walk, to the extent that, standing in the front of the horse, the soles are become visible. As well as this, the shape and the growth of the hoof change drastically.

In chronic laminitis, the pedal bone is rotated, which can have the following serious effects:

1. The horse suffers extreme pain. The rotating of the pedal bone causes more pressure on the solar surface, and the arteries in the lower foot close off.
2. In an advanced stage, the pedal bone can punch through the sole – the so-called break in the sole. In a break in the sole, the point of the pedal bone breaks through the sole, which can cause extensive inflammation. Between the pedal bone and the horny wall a 'false' horn develops that still gives some grip to the pedal bone. In such serious breaks in the sole, the horse can usually no longer be cured.
3. As well as rotating, the pedal bone can also drop down vertically in the hoof capsule – so-called sinker. In a normal situation the epiphysis – the highest part of the pedal bone – is at the same level as the coronary band. In sinker, the epiphysis is clearly dropped down even so much that it comes below the coronary band. This causes the germinating layer – the root of the hoof capsule – to be pulled down as well. This seriously hinders the healing process.

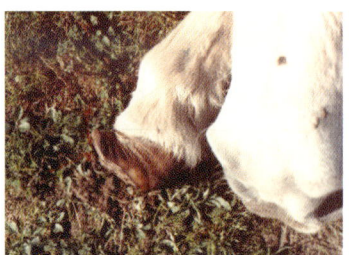

A pony that is repeatedly laminitic can be regarded as a victim of animal abuse.

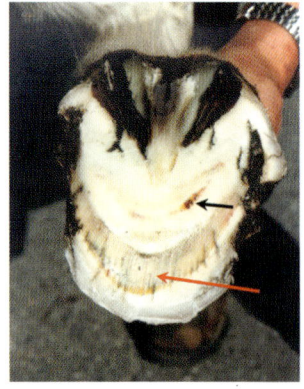

This horse's hoof shows an extremely widened white line (red arrow) due to the rotating of the pedal bone. The white line is inflamed. The rotating of the point of the pedal bone puts pressure on the sole. This has caused bruising (black arrow).

Part 2 – Disorders of the Limbs and Hooves

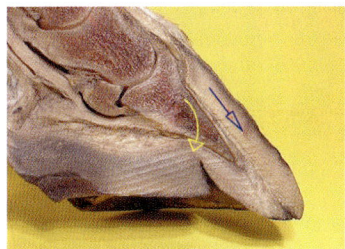

First stage: when the corium is inflamed, the interplay of forces is disturbed and the pedal bone can rotate (yellow arrow) because the pedal bone flexor pulls strongly on the pedal bone, tearing the pedal bone from the horny wall.

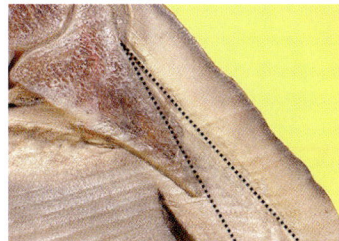

Second stage: the point (front side) of the pedal bone begins to point in the direction of the sole. The hoof feels warm to the touch and the horse clearly demonstrates pain when the wall is tapped or when pressure is put on the sole in front of the point of the frog.

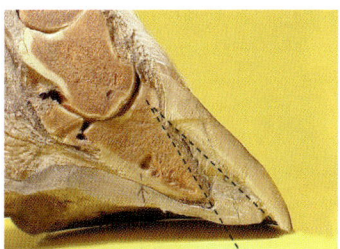

Third stage: the pedal bone is no longer attached to the horny wall. The point of the pedal bone puts pressure on the sole, causing the whole weight of the horse to be on the sole. This causes intense pain. The horse lies down stretched out and has a high temperature.

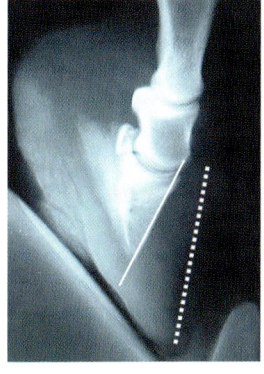

The X-ray shows that the pedal bone is rotated in relation to the horny wall. The front side of the pedal bone should be parallel with the horny wall.

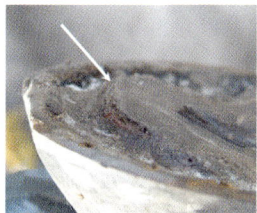

This is an example of a pedal bone that, because of rotation, has come through the sole.

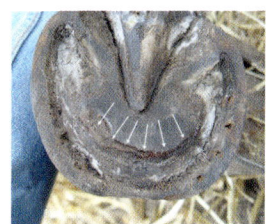

The shape of the pedal bone (white arrows) is clearly visible and forms a centre for bacteria.

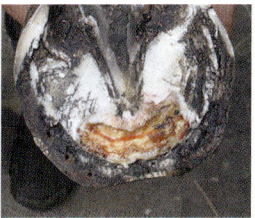

A piece of the solar surface has been removed; a completely inflamed sole corium is revealed.

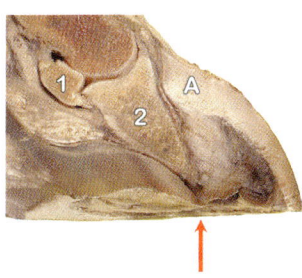

The pedal bone (2) breaks through the sole (red arrow) and an inflammation centre has developed and the horny wall develops a 'false' horn or necrosis (A). This still allows a little grip on the horny wall. Very little can be done for a horse in this situation.

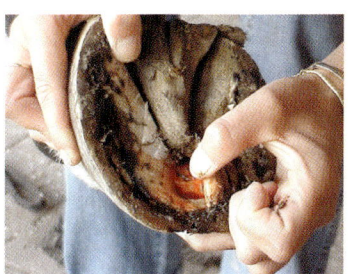
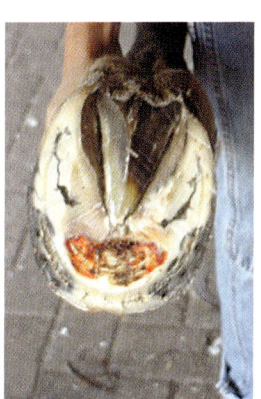

Pressure of the pedal bone on the sole causes enormous bruising. These patients can be treated as long as the pedal bone has not pushed through the sole.

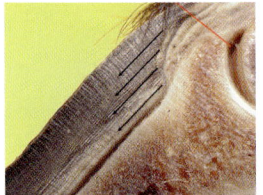 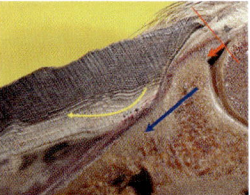 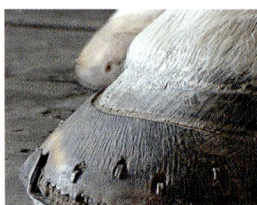 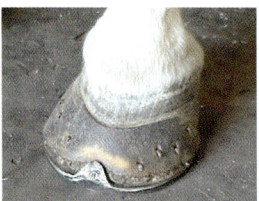

The picture on the left displays normal horn growth. The hoof capsule is developed from a healthy germinating layer of the coronary corium and grows down along the pedal bone to the ground surface. The coronary rim is at the level of the coronary band (red line). The picture on the right displays sinker. Horses that get past this stage have defective horn growth; because of the enormous force of traction of the pedal bone, the coronary corium (which develops the horn growth) can no longer grow down with the pedal bone but instead grows in a horizontal line to the outside (yellow arrow). It can also be seen that the coronary rim of the pedal bone has dropped below the coronary band.

This hoof displayed sinker. There is 43 centimetres of good horn growth from the coronary band. An extremely pronounced ring of horn is visible.

A hoof which had sinker eight weeks after being shod. The horn under the ring of horn has a tendency to grow outwards. This picture shows clearly that the coronary band has dropped down.

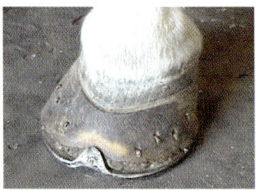 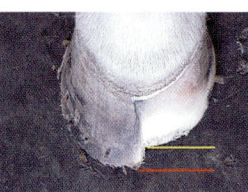

At each trimming session, the horny wall is rigorously removed (yellow and red arrows, right picture). The foot axis must be respected in a laminitic hoof, and so the hoof capsule cannot be taken as the guide. At every shoeing session the horny wall is trimmed until it is straight. By reducing the thickness of the wall, the ground pressure is reduced and the horse can move the hoof forward more easily.

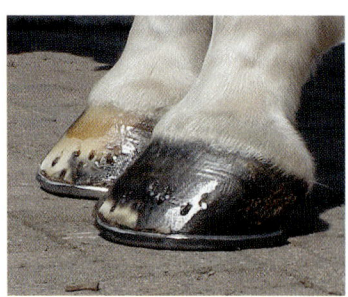

Result of good treatment. This is thanks not only to the farrier but also to the good care of the owner.

4. The hoof changes shape. In laminitic horses or ponies, where the growth of the horny wall is not properly looked after, a distorted hoof develops. The horn development of the germinating layer no longer grows down next to the pedal bone but, from the germinating layer onwards, grows forwards. A distorted hoof hinders forward movement and leads to a faulty traction at the coronary band. A farrier can correct this fault. In distorted hoof development, the hoof has to be resolutely pared down to a normal shape. Sometimes this means that the toe area of the hoof capsule must be removed.
5. Because of the enormous pressure that the pedal bone exercises on the sole of the foot, the point of the pedal bone can become deformed. The rounding that develops can be seen on an X-ray after the laminitis is cured. This rounding of the point of the pedal bone is called the 'hat brim effect'.

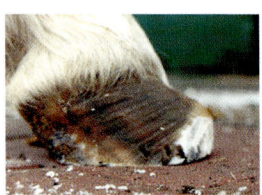 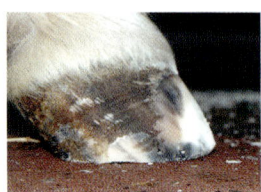

Example of a horse with a distorted hoof.

The distorted hoof after treatment. With this kind of deformation the hoof must be brought back to its normal shape.

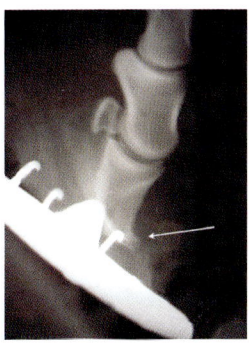

This X-ray shows that the shape of the point of the pedal bone has changed because of the extreme pressure.

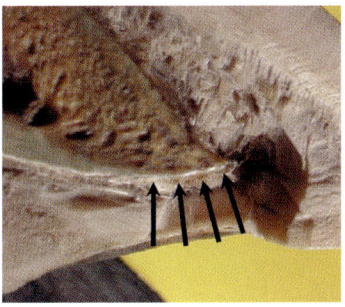

Because the pedal bone rotates, the pressure on the point is greater, and it becomes distorted.

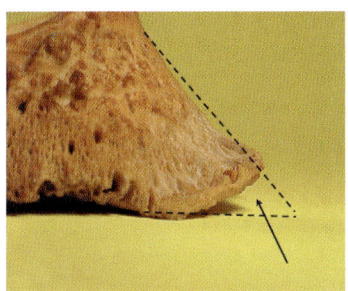

The pedal bone distortion is called a 'hat brim'. The dotted line shows where a normal shape would be.

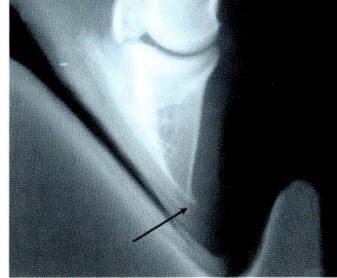

This X-ray clearly shows a 'hat brim'.

RESECTION OF THE HORNY WALL

After the laminitis has been treated by a veterinary surgeon, the farrier can still make a valuable contribution to the treatment. In most cases, resection (cutting away) of the whole of the front of the hoof capsule seems to work well.

CASE HISTORY 1, PHOTOS PAGE 208 (TOP)

A horse that had laminitis had been given a resection where the bulging white line had become visible. A bulging white line indicates that the pressure from pus – from the inflamed laminae in the hoof capsule – is excessive. Resection – or cutting away – of the horny wall removes the pressure because the pus can escape. As after resection the pus no longer put pressure on the pedal bone, the horse felt less pain. In some cases, it is necessary to remove the whole of the horn. When the toe area was removed, the pus escaped, as well as the blood of the sensitive laminae which had caused the pressure in the hoof capsule. Using the correct horseshoe is extremely important in these cases. The remaining horny wall had to be well supported and the painful area protected. The whole hoof was dressed with a Betadine bandage to repress the bacterial growth, to dry out the sensitive laminae and to create an artificial wall.

The Hoof – Pedal Bone

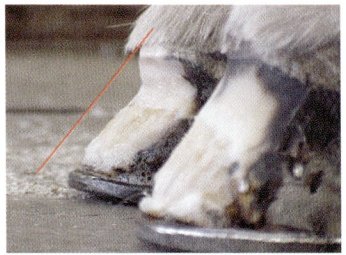
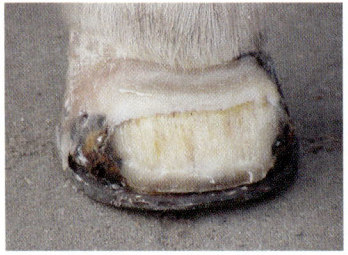
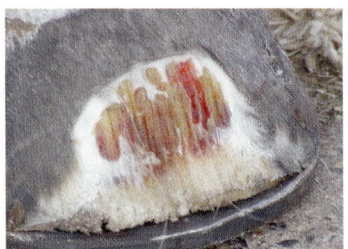

The trimming of the horny wall (red line) reduces the pressure on the hoof nerves because the pus is released.

When the horny wall is removed, the inflamed laminae and the release of blood can be seen clearly. Healthy insensitive laminae should be white.

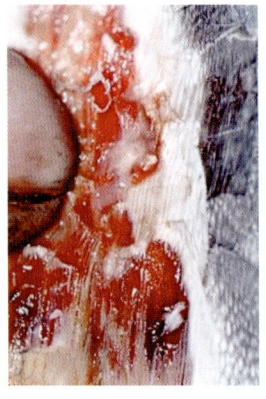

A macro shot of the wall corium clearly shows both the blood of the sensitive laminae and the pus that is caused by the pressure in the hoof capsule.

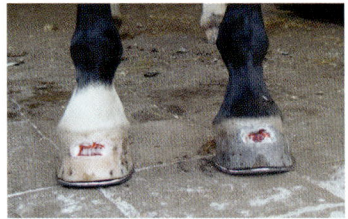

In cases of acute laminitis, making a large opening in the horny wall can somewhat reduce the horse's pain.

OPEN-TOED HORSESHOES

A horse with laminitis had been put in open-toed horseshoes. These shoes, however, have more disadvantages than advantages:

- Open-toed horseshoes are shoes placed back to front, and thus the heels do not fit properly on the shoe
- Neither the toe nor the sole is protected

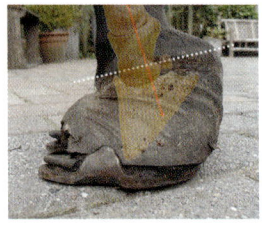
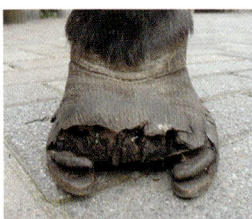
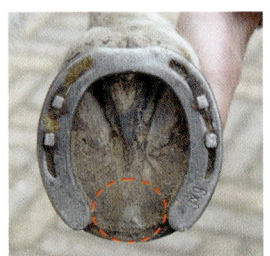

The unprofessional treatment of laminitis in combination with the fitting of open-toed horseshoes gives this horse very little chance of getting better. The coronary band is lower than the bulbs (dotted line) and at the front of the coronary band horn growth is, due to the great pressure, impossible.

Front of the hoof with an open-toed shoe where even a leather pad has been added – a typical example of incompetence.

An open-toed shoe. It was thought that putting a horseshoe on back to front would unburden the painful area, but because of loading on the hoof, the ground pressure is unimpeded. The horse can no longer move on these horseshoes. This is outright animal cruelty.

- The branches of the horseshoe are pressed into the hoof at the toe
- The ease of the hoof rolling over is hindered
- The horseshoe causes serious deformation of the hoof
- The front of the hoof capsule, where it is the most painful, is not protected against ground pressure in soft going

Open-toed horseshoes can have disastrous consequences for horse's hooves because the place where the pedal bone puts pressure on the sole – the most painful spot of a laminitic hoof – cannot cope with pressure from the ground.

THE CORRECT HORSESHOE

The Hoofcare® Breakover horseshoe offers protection to the painful areas. The shoe is wide in the toe area and is forged out in a wedge shape to protect the painful parts from ground pressure. The rocker toe is in the horseshoe and is not trimmed into the hoof, so the effect is doubled. The horseshoe supports the horny wall only and can roll over as easily sideways as forwards, as the horse or pony wants. The horseshoe

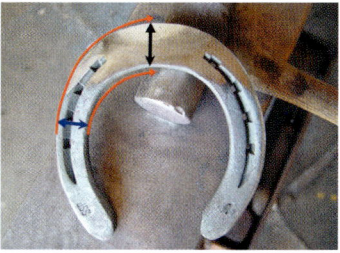 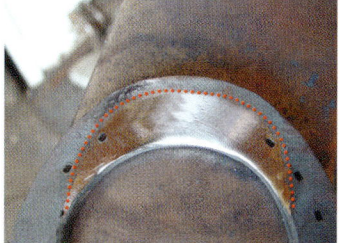

The Hoofcare® Breakover horseshoe has been developed by my twin brother and me. It can be of great support to the laminitic horse or pony in both acute and chronic cases. It is a requisite that the hoof is trimmed according to the foot axis. The front of the shoe must be broad and thinly forged towards the front, so that a wedge-shape is formed. The surface that the hoof stands on is made concave in the toe area, so that the painful part of the sole is not pressed on by the shoe.

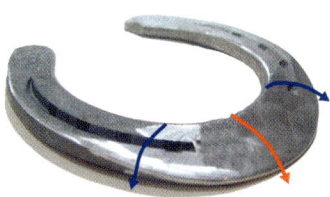

The advantage of the Hoofcare® Breakover horseshoe is that the laminitic horse or pony can roll its hoof over in the way it wants to. Even a sideways breakover point is possible.

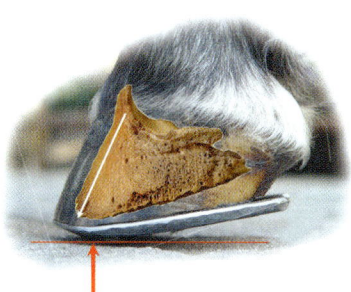

This shoe allows the hoof to roll over further back, and will reduce the pressure on the point of the pedal bone and the sole. Because the shoe is forged out to be broad and concave, the painful areas are protected from ground pressure. If there has been a total resection of the horny wall, this horseshoe provides relief.

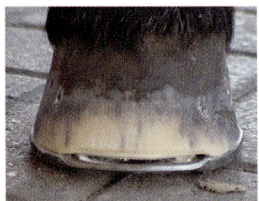 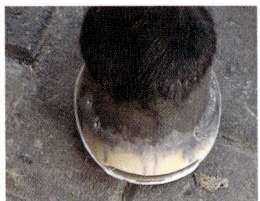 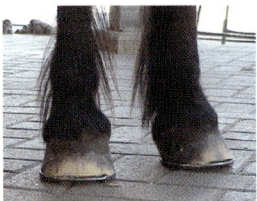

The painful front of the horny wall and the solar surface are completely free; there is space between the hoof and the horseshoe. Seen from above, the round form of the coronary band is mirrored in that of the horseshoe. Both hooves have been fitted with a long shoe with a sufficient rocker toe.

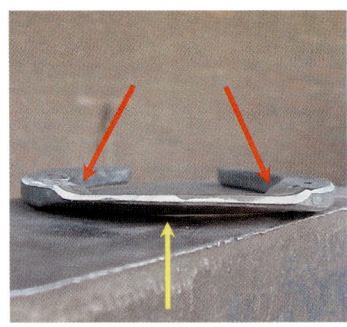

There are many variations in horseshoes but the crucial point is that the painful point must always be protected from ground pressure because every stage of laminitis is treated differently. In acute laminitis, a horseshoe can be fitted that completely relieves the painful area. The hoof capsule is supported from the point of the red arrows. A rocker toe will be brought into the shoe so that the hoof can easily roll forward (yellow arrow).

can be fitted wide and long, so that the whole hoof can be thoroughly supported. The illustrations clearly demonstrate the advantages of this horseshoe.

RECURRING LAMINITIS

Above, we have indicated what the various causes of laminitis can be. Laminitis is a serious condition but it can be treated. If nothing is done about the cause of laminitis, the condition will recur.

CONCLUSION

Every case of a horse with laminitis is different. Take care that the toe area under the sole is burdened as little as possible, because it is there that the pain is greatest. Through lack of knowledge, a lot of mistakes are made in the treatment of horses and ponies with laminitis. Owners are often told that nothing more can be done for their horse or pony. However, nothing is less true. If the owner is alert and calls in the help of both the veterinary surgeon and the farrier, laminitis can be treated and the horse can be spared much suffering.

For years, a solution has been sought for this painful and serious disease; over the years there have also been many horseshoes invented, such as the heart bar shoe, shoes that put pressure on the frog, shoes with hoof pads and shoes with soles. All these horseshoes prevent the pedal bone from rotating but do not give, or hardly give, relief and they can, if they are not correctly fitted, even lead to outright animal abuse.

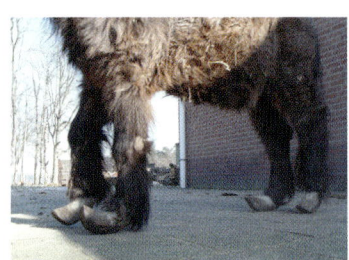

After laminitis, horses and ponies have accelerated horn growth and must be trimmed more frequently by the farrier. If this is not complied with, there can be serious consequences.

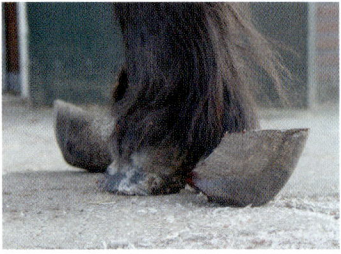

The result! The hoof was trimmed radically so that the pony could regain a normal conformation.

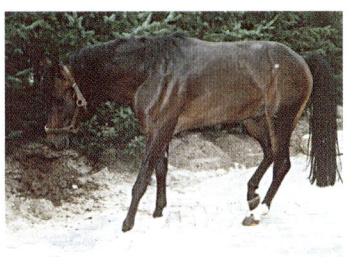

A horse that has laminitis puts its weight on its hind limbs and holds its fore limbs as far forward as possible.

Sinker

Sinker is a serious form of laminitis. In sinker, the pedal bone does not rotate from the wall, as in normal laminitis, but instead the whole pedal bone drops down vertically. Laminitis is itself a big problem but sinker is an even greater one. The farrier can, when the pedal bone rotates (laminitis), reduce the pain by shoeing and by cutting away the horny wall. Sinker, on the other hand, causes pressure on the horny wall and the solar surface. The chance is great that the solar surface will burst open from this bulging out.

There are various causes of sinker:

1. Every year the laminitis recurs, or the horse is always too fat from too much feed or too rich a pasture. This must be brought to the owner's attention in both cases. A horse absolutely need not get laminitis every year, or become too fat. When this situation is constantly repeated, this is animal abuse.
2. If a mare has foaled and the afterbirth has not come away in good time this causes a poisoning in the womb. This is a frequent cause of acute sinker. As soon as the mare has difficulty in moving, then the farrier is called in, but it is by then mostly too late: sinker can start on the first day. It would be good practice, for mares in this situation, to take preventive measures and shoe from the first day on; however, it cannot be said with certainty that this would save the horse.
3. Acute poisoning, for example by eating poisonous plants.
4. Too rich feed, that horses cannot digest.
5. Treatment by corticosteroids.

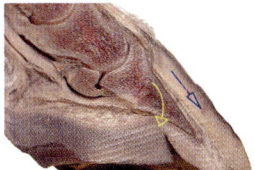

Hoof of a laminitic horse. The pedal bone has begun to rotate (yellow arrow) because of the inflammation in the wall corium, and is being pulled from the corium. The blue arrow shows the horny wall.

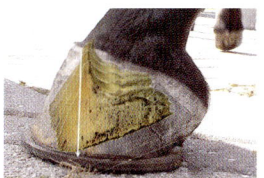

In sinker, the pedal bone will not only rotate but will also drop down in the hoof capsule.

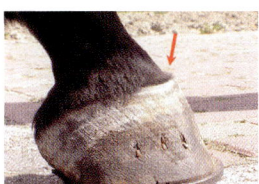

With sinker, the pedal bone drops down and pulls the coronary corium with it. An indentation will appear on top of the coronary band.

When a horse has sinker the complete corium is inflamed. This causes the suspension of the pedal bone on the horny wall to come away completely – usually the pedal bone and the sensitive laminae are attached to the insensitive laminae of the horny wall. The pedal bone drops vertically down in its totality and completely puts its weight on the solar surface. This causes the blood circulation to be partly closed off. The horse has a dreadful amount of pain with sinker because the pedal bone puts the whole solar surface under pressure. The horse does not want to stand on its hooves and does not – as is usual with ordinary laminitis – lean on its hind hooves but stays standing straight up on all

The Hoof – Pedal Bone

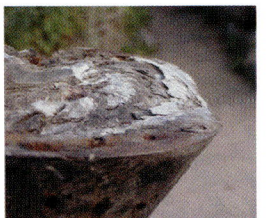
The solar surface bulges out from the weightbearing edge because of the enormous pressure from the pedal bone.

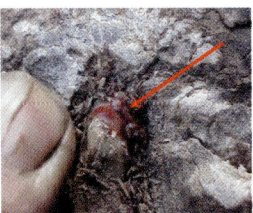
In the end, the sole can no longer support the pressure and will spontaneously burst open at the point of the frog.

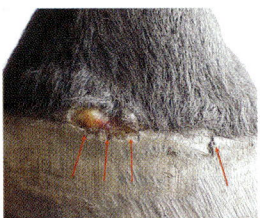
The coronary corium is pulled down with the dropping of the pedal bone. This causes inflammation at the coronary band.

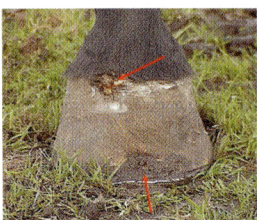
The inflammation can affect the whole hoof and it may then 'de-hoof'.

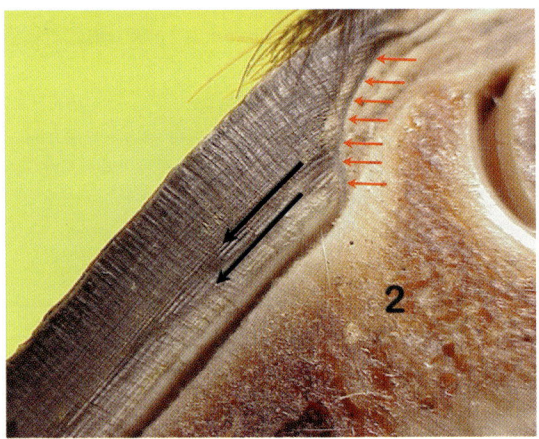
In a normal situation, the horny wall grows down along the pedal bone to the ground surface (black arrows). The coronary corium (red arrows) is responsible for the making of new horn.

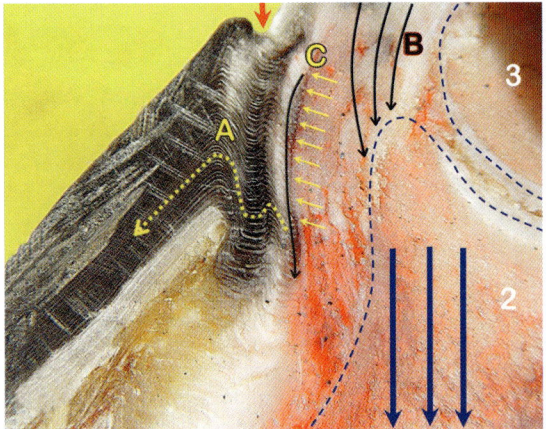
When there is sinker, the pedal bone (2) will pull the coronary corium (C) down so that the direction of the horny tubules is disturbed (A). The beginnings of sinker (black arrows at B and C). The pedal bone has dropped vertically and the coronary corium (yellow arrows, C) is pulled down with it. Thus the horny wall no longer grows down along the pedal bone. Due to the enormous force of traction from the pedal bone, the direction of the horny wall growth changes (dotted yellow arrow, A). This causes an indentation above the coronary band (red arrow). This horse will not survive.

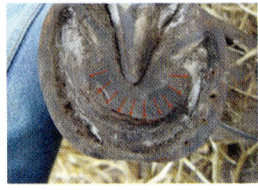
The pedal bone will break through the sole with an acute case of sinker.

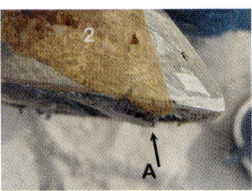
The point (A) of the pedal bone (2) will emerge from the weightbearing edge and cause unbearable pain.

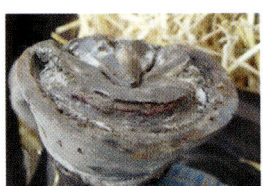
The shape of the pedal bone is visible from the front. The whole area is inflamed.

four hooves. The solar surface rapidly bulges out under the pressure of the pedal bone. In the worst cases there is a break in the sole. The only solution is a horseshoe that enables the ground pressure on the solar surface to be reduced. When the pedal bone drops down, the coronary corium is pulled down with it. This causes inflammation in the coronary band. The whole coronary band becomes thicker and swells up. The pain gets worse, and by degrees the whole coronary band begins to open up. The dropping down of the pedal bone means that no more normal horn growth takes place from the coronary corium. The horse has extreme difficulty in moving forward on soft going, and on hard going it has to be forced to go forward with difficulty.

This is a very frustrating condition for the veterinary surgeon and the farrier as they cannot give a verdict nor predict a cure. In the case of sinker, one can only work hard at it, wait and hope that the treatment brings results.

HORSESHOES

The horseshoes for a horse with sinker must be completely forged out or smoothed off on the bearing surface so that the dropped down sole is not carried by the shoe – even if there is not yet any bulging out of the solar surface. Two broad bars are welded on the underside of the horseshoe so that there is a lot of space between the bars and the hoof: this reduces the ground pressure on the sole.

CONCLUSION

When a horse has very serious sinker, it is important to ask oneself if it is ethically responsible to continue treatment. If the healing process does not begin, or lasts too long, it is better to put the horse out of its misery.

Encapsulated Bone Fragment

An encapsulated bone fragment is a loose bit of bone that, after chipping or a fragment loosening, is encapsulated by connective tissue. An encapsulated bone fragment can be recognised by a sudden break in the sole, containing a round, shiny hard piece of tissue: the encapsulated bone fragment.

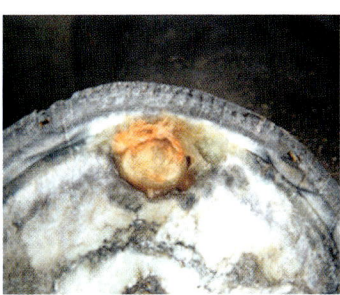

Example of an encapsulated bone fragment.

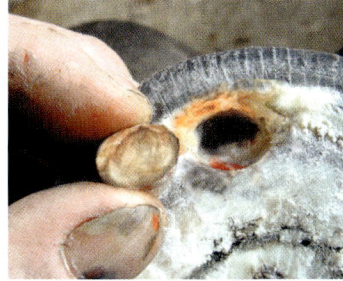

After the removal of the encapsulated bone fragment, a cavity remains.

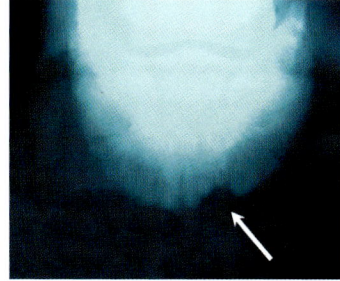

It is clear to see on the X-ray where the bone fragment was situated. In the course of time, the body will fill the cavity with tissues of another structure.

CAUSE

If a horse treads on a sharp object, a piece can spontaneously break off from the pedal bone (see Chip Fracture of the Pedal Bone). Usually this is followed by an inflammation of the hoof and the horse becomes lame. However, sometimes the horse's body reacts by wrapping (encapsulating) the piece of bone so no inflammation takes place. The encapsulated bone fragment consists of extremely strong, smooth tissue. The horse is not bothered by it and does not become lame, because the bone fragment with its wrapping of tissue is separate from other horn tissue and can move together with the hoof. The encapsulated bone fragment remains in the connective tissue and at the same time grows downwards with the horn of the hoof until it is discovered just under the solar surface by the farrier at the time of trimming.

DIAGNOSIS

An encapsulated bone fragment is visible and must be taken note of. Whenever there is an encapsulated 'ball' just under the surface of the sole of the foot, it can be presumed that it is an encapsulated bone fragment.

TREATMENT

The encapsulated bone fragment can be removed easily by a veterinary surgeon or a farrier. A cavity remains at the place where it has been removed. In time, the cavity gets filled with tissue of another structure; until then, the cavity must be kept clean. A piece of gauze soaked in a Betadine solution is packed into the cavity to prevent dirt getting in.

HORSESHOES

The whole area is protected from ground pressure with the help of the horseshoe. A shoe has to be fitted that still allows checking and cleaning of the cavity. For this, a normal horseshoe can be used that, at the area where the encapsulated bone fragment was, has been forged thinly (flat) and wide so that one can continue to check. After a while, the horse can have normal horseshoes.

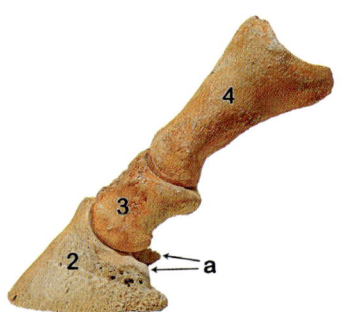

2. Pedal bone
3. Short pastern bone
4. Long pastern bone
a. Lateral cartilages of the pedal bone

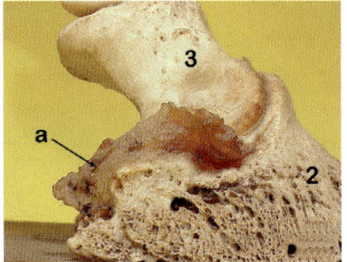

On top of both lateral cartilages of the pedal bone (2) there is a very strong, resilient and mobile cartilage between which the short pastern bone (3) lies. When the horse is moving, the short pastern bone moves down and both cartilages are pushed to the outside.

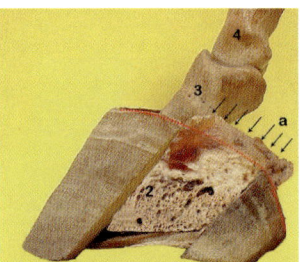

Both cartilages (a) are positioned half in the hoof capsule. The top half rises above the coronary band and lies under the skin in the area of the bulbs. This half gives shape to the heels.

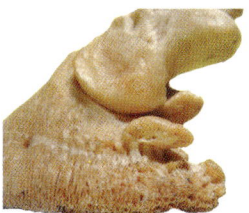
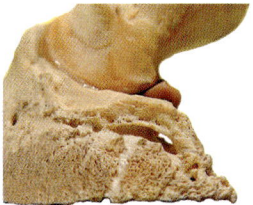
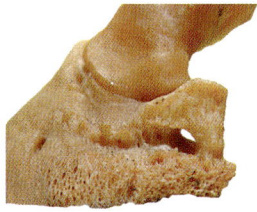
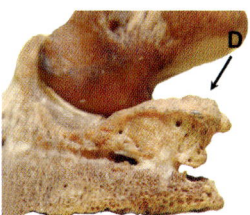

The cartilage ossifies through calcification. First phase: the start of enlargement of the pedal bone lateral cartilages.

Second phase: the growth of the calcification on the pedal bone cartilage extends steadily upwards.

Third phase: a quite serious calcification. This obstructs the movement of the short pastern bone downwards between the lateral cartilages of the pedal bone.

Fourth phase: this extremely advanced calcification of the lateral cartilages of the pedal bone (D) causes lameness.

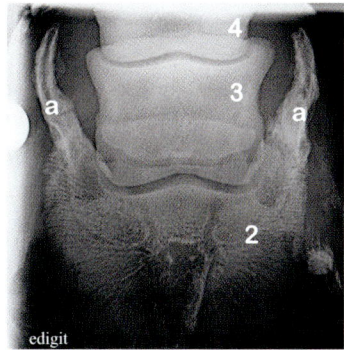

This X-ray clearly shows that the calcified lateral cartilages have curved inwards, which will obstruct the movement of the under part of the hoof.

Side-bone

When both lateral cartilages of the pedal bone become hard due to calcification, this is called side-bone. (See photos this page and opposite)

CAUSE

The pedal bone is a single bone. On both sides of the pedal bone there is cartilage. This lateral cartilage is exceedingly strong, elastic and mobile. Good mobility of this cartilage is of great importance for the hoof mechanism and for good venous circulation of the hoof. Healthy cartilages have no calcification.

The calcification of the lateral cartilage is a gradual process. First, the lateral cartilage calcifies, followed by the calcification of the connecting tissue between the lateral cartilage and the pedal bone. It is above all in these last stages that the mobility and functioning of the hoof mechanism are reduced and consequently the venous circulation of the hoof depleted. If the lateral cartilage is completely ossified, the short pastern bone and the long pastern bone can no longer descend between the lateral cartilages of the pedal bone. This causes the horse to move more carefully: it tries to relieve pressure on the heels as much as

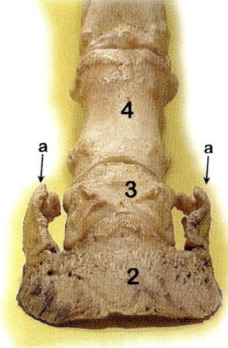
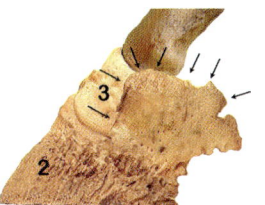
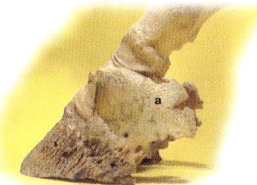
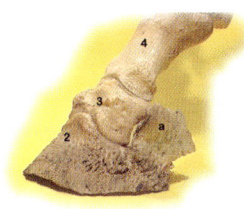

Both calcified cartilages stand straight up, curve in toward the area of the heels, and will not be able to move any more.
2. Pedal bone; 3. Short pastern bone; 4. Long pastern bone; a. The two calcified cartilages of the pedal bone

Calcification can become extremely large.
2. Pedal bone; 3. Short pastern bone; Black arrows: calcified or ossified cartilage

In some cases, calcification can be extremely large. The downward movement of the short pastern bone – and sometimes even that of the long pastern bone – is impeded and results in serious lameness.

possible and no longer steps through well. The horse's paces become shorter and stiffer, and the hoof narrows and develops a narrow frog and long heels.

Cases have been known where completely ossified pedal bone lateral cartilages have broken due to the intense pressure caused by the descending of the short and long pastern bones. This can happen at exercise or when the horse is required to make an extreme weightbearing step such as landing after a jump. As a result of this, such horses have fewer problems with moving. The process of ossification of the lateral cartilage cannot be prevented. In the end it results in a horse that moves with shorter and stiffer paces; it can no longer be used as a sport horse and it can only do light work.

Side-bone is more common in some breeds than others. Side-bone is seen regularly in Friesian horses, the Dutch warmblood and the Dutch draught horse and, to a lesser degree, in ponies and pedigree horses. Age also plays a role.

In some breeds, side-bone begins above a certain age – mostly over the age of twelve. Certain breeds are more affected. Side-bone is also seen more often in horses that work on a hard surface. In the past, side-bone was far more prevalent than today: in the past, horses had to work a great deal on hard surfaces. Nowadays, horses are usually worked on a soft ground surface.

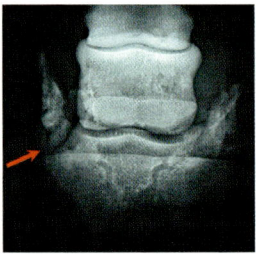

An X-ray showing that both cartilages are seriously ossified. It is clear that there is a fracture of the inside lateral cartilage (red arrow).

DIAGNOSIS

Side-bone can be identified with the help of X-rays. The farrier can apply various techniques when shoeing, which can offer some improvement:

1. The side walls can be made thinner so that they become more mobile. The big disadvantage of this is that, in time, the hoof collapses. This sets up an even greater problem because it weakens the hoof wall.
2. In the buttresses of the heel, long vertical grooves are made from the ground up to the coronary band. They ensure that the horn wall is weakened so that it can be more mobile, and thus the pastern bone can more easily descend between the two lateral cartilages of the pedal bone. Such treatment of the side walls can seriously weaken the coronary band, which can lead to cracks in the hoof wall.

Unfortunately both these treatments cause more problems than solutions.

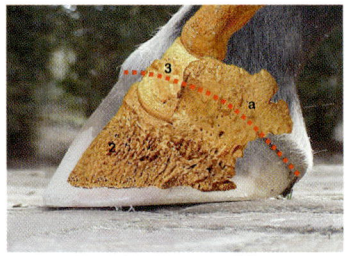

The calcified cartilages (a) are partly enclosed in the hoof capsule. The red line (3) indicates the coronary band. The growths can best be felt on both sides of the bulbs of the heels. The horn capsule is very rigid and cannot expand to create space for these growths.

HORSESHOES

In nearly all cases, good shoeing can bring solace. It can reduce lameness but not, however, make it disappear. A farrier can apply a shoe with broadened branches to give as much support as possible to the buttress of the heels. Lameness can also be reduced by welding a bar between the shoe branches, making the shoe more stable and rigid. A shoe with a leather pad or a leather band between the horseshoe and the hoof can reduce concussion to the under side of the foot.

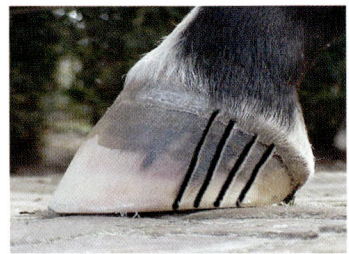

'Rainures' or deep grooves in the horn wall on both sides of the horn wall sometimes provide somewhat more movement in the horn capsule. The disadvantage of this is that the horn wall is weakened in the area of the heel buttresses; this can cause other problems.

4 THE HOOF: NAVICULAR

Navicular Disease

Navicular disease (podotrochlitis) is an inflammation process in the area of the navicular bone. A horse with navicular disease shows no outward signs on its limb. The inflammation is visible only on an X-ray. An X-ray shows if the channels that nourish the navicular bone have been enlarged or if there are defects present such as prominences ('spur formations') at the sides or if the profile of the bone is correct.

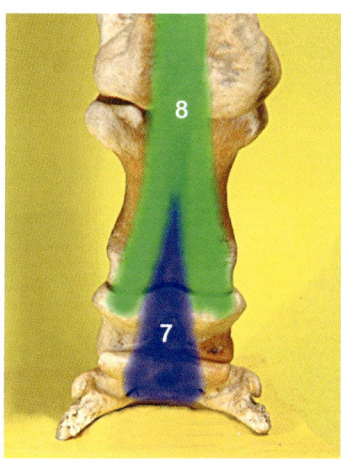

Example of a fore limb, as seen from the rear. The deep flexor tendon emerges here (blue, 7); it runs visibly over the navicular bone and then attaches to the underneath of the pedal bone. The superficial flexor tendon (green, 8) is in the shape of a tube. It divides and is attached to the rear of the small pastern bone. The deep flexor tendon has a fan-shaped attachment on the under side of the pedal bone and runs up through the tube of the superficial flexor tendon.

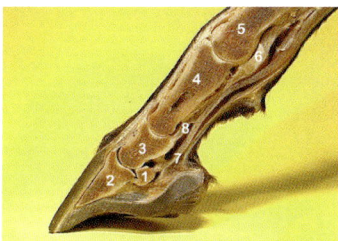

Anatomy of the lower foot of the horse.
1. Navicular bone; 2. Pedal bone; 3. Short pastern bone; 4. Long pastern bone; 5. Cannon bone; 6. Proximal sesamoid; 7. Deep digital flexor tendon; 8. Superficial flexor tendon

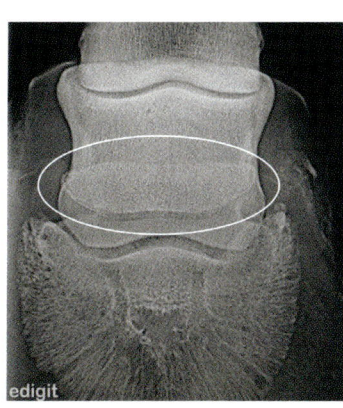

A healthy navicular bone (circled). The X-ray is taken from behind, towards the front.

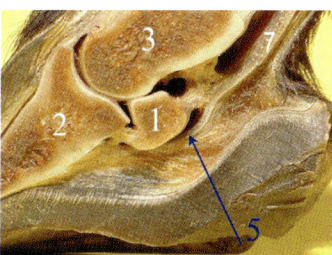

The deep digital flexor tendon (7) glides over the back surface of the navicular bone (1). This gliding surface of the navicular bone is covered with smooth cartilage, which allows the flexor tendon to glide over easily when flexing and stretching. The gliding over is made easier by a lubricant (synovial fluid) that is released by a mucus pouch situated between the rear area of the navicular bone and the deep flexor tendon. The mucus pouch looks like a flat pocket (5).

THE DEVELOPMENT OF NAVICULAR DISEASE
Various factors can play a role in the development of navicular disease:

- Heredity
- Diet
- Time of commencement of training
- The build of the hoof
- Overtaxing
- The condition of the horse
- The horseshoes
- Too much time in the stable; too little exercise
- Bad hoof care
- Irresponsible administration of medicine for influencing performance

Horses that are lame are often too quickly presumed to have navicular disease. What is meant by the navicular area is the area in the hoof which includes the navicular bone, the mucus pouch and the deep flexor tendon. An inflammation in this area is called navicular disease.

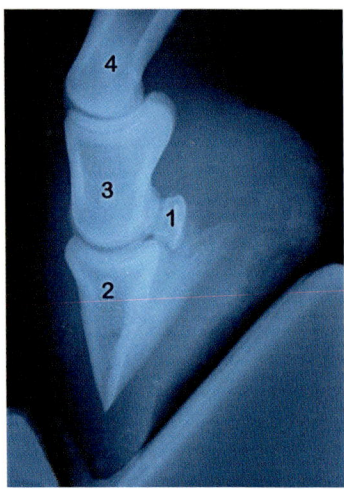

X-ray of the anatomy of the lower foot of a horse.
1. Navicular bone; 2. Pedal bone; 3. Short pastern bone; 4. Long pastern bone. Between 1 and 3 is the hoof joint and between 3 and 4 is the coronary joint.

CAUSE
There has been much research into the causes of navicular disease. It has been concluded that a disturbed blood supply to and from the hoof plays an important role. The flow of blood ensures the supply of building materials for good development of tissue, and oxygen (fuel) so that the tissue process can function well. During exercise the blood circulation of the horse is optimal, but if the horse is merely returned to the stable afterwards, the blood circulation is considerably diminished. The disturbances in circulation that result can lead to degenerative processes, that is to say, irreversible changes in cells and tissues which affect their normal functioning.

SYMPTOMS
Navicular disease reveals itself in an indistinct, sporadic lameness that, with time, gets gradually worse. The lameness often changes from the left limb to the right limb. The horse stumbles, bumps itself more, and its gaits become shorter. As well as this, the horse points – putting its toes forward – in order to relieve its hoof. As the condition worsens, the smaller the frog becomes, the narrower the hoof, and the more concave the sole. The growth of the hoof stagnates.

Some horses with navicular disease are very stiff when they come out of their stable but gradually improve while exercising because they work through their lameness. The opposite also frequently occurs. It is of paramount importance that the owner properly evaluates the qualities and capacity of the horse and then uses these in a responsible manner. It is

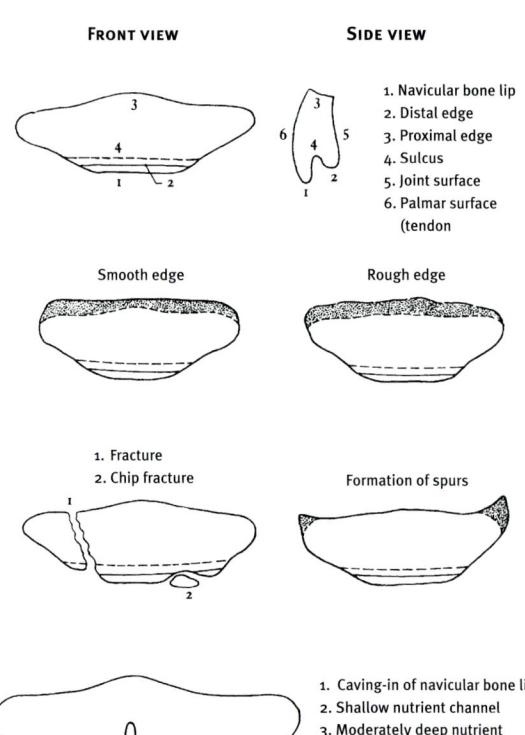

These are examples employed for the diagnosis of the seriousness of navicular disease.

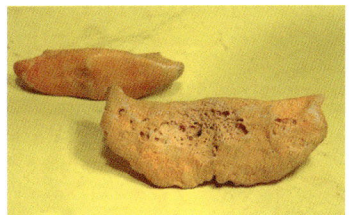

A cyst is a serious form of deterioration of bone tissue in the area of the gliding surface of the navicular bone. The horse suddenly displays an extremely serious lameness but the next day moves normally. This form of lameness will reappear frequently and will finally become permanent as the cyst gains in size.

particularly show jumping horses that are driven beyond capacity; this is usually for financial reasons, at the expense of the horse.

DIAGNOSIS

An examination often used to determine navicular disease is the performance of flexion tests. These consist of firmly flexing and relaxing the lower foot and, after a few minutes, requiring the horse to trot away without showing lameness or irregularities. It is a dangerous and crude method of examination. Above all, this test must be taken with a big pinch of salt because many other parts of the lower foot are flexed that have nothing to do with the navicular area. The performance of flexion tests by inexperienced people is an extremely unreliable way of determining navicular disease. What is more, an unprofessional flexion test can be extremely dangerous because it can cause a horse to become lame.

If one suspects that a lame horse has navicular disease then it is best if one switches to a thorough examination of the lower foot under local anaesthetic. By anaesthetising the lower foot from underneath to above, it can be determined exactly where the lameness is. As soon as this is established, X-rays are taken; with these, a veterinary surgeon can ascertain if it is navicular disease. Some horses are found to have a bad navicular bone according to the X-rays made at a veterinary examination, yet have never been lame. In many cases, such horses have been declared unfit, because it is difficult to forecast if it will cause lameness in the future.

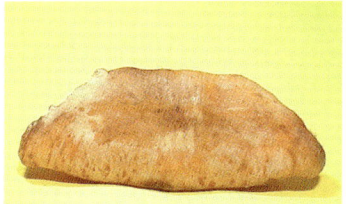 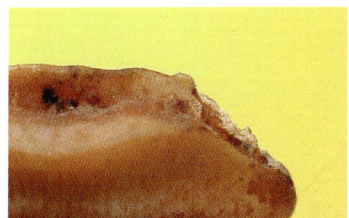 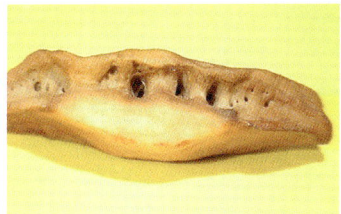

Navicular disease can come in various degrees of seriousness. To get a better picture of a bad or a good navicular bone, see these examples. Left: the deep digital flexor tendon moves over the whole width of the healthy navicular bone. Centre: on the gliding surface of the navicular bone, a small amount of extra bone growth is visible and the side surface is rough. The deep digital flexor tendon is irritated by this. Right: a navicular bone with extremely large nutrient channels, which have an adverse influence on the blood circulation; the pressure and the propulsion of the blood are lost, causing a reduction in the flow of nutrients.

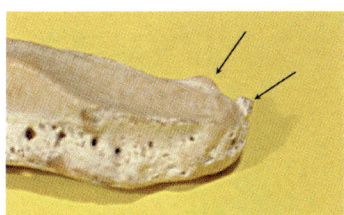 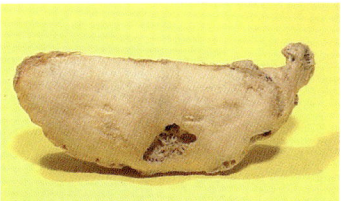 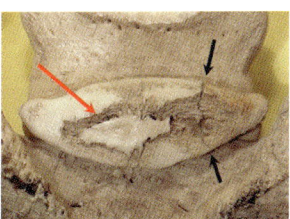

Left: Proliferation of bone growth on the edge of the joint surface of the navicular bone causes discomfort to the horse when turning. As well as this, the bone tissue has degenerated. Centre: A big spur on the side and a cyst on the gliding surface of the navicular bone. Right: A disastrous case; total dissolution of bone tissue (red arrow) and a fracture in the bone (black arrow).

The Hoof – Navicular

TREATMENT

Through the years there have been various treatments to 'cure' navicular disease. There are even those who swear that they can completely cure horses of navicular disease with special exercises or alternative medicine. Nevertheless, navicular disease remains a condition that cannot be cured.

With thoroughly good shoeing, correct weightbearing which does not force the horse into an unnatural conformation, and with sufficient time spent out at grass, the development of navicular disease can be prevented. Horses with this condition do not have to be written off but can, with suitable horseshoes and the correct exercise, still be used. Horses with navicular disease can be shod in various ways. Below, several are mentioned.

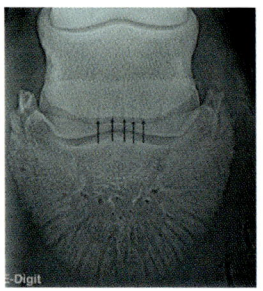

Example of a bad navicular bone. At the side are spurs (B), many of the nutrient channels are widened (C) and on the top surface there is the commencement of a seam (A).

WEDGES

In the past, horses with navicular disease were usually shod with shoes that had wedges between the shoe and the hoof. However, a horse with navicular disease wants to weight its hoof normally according to a straight foot axis. Horseshoes with wedges cause the axis to be broken forward. As horses always want to stand with a straight foot axis, most of the weight falls on the wedges, which causes the heels to press into the wedges and to become fixed. This obstructs the hoof mechanism and thus the flow of blood back and forth. Formerly, it was thought that the back part of the hoof should be raised with a wedge or a calkin so that the flexor tendons can be relaxed more and so curb the inflammation. In

On the X-ray of the navicular bone the far too widened nutrient channels can be seen.

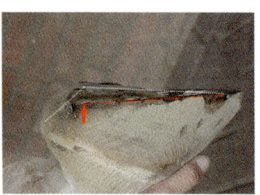

The heels have been pushed away by the wedges. This has caused the frog of the hoof to be higher than the heels.

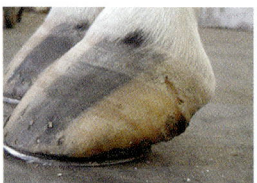

This horse clearly has a problem. The farrier has tried to raise the heels by putting a wedge under the hoof. This causes so much pressure on the rear of the hoof (heels) that the wedge is pushed into the hoof. This only makes navicular disease worse.

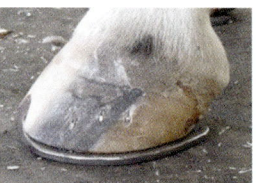

After corrective treatment, the hoof is positioned according to the foot axis and the hoof has returned to its former shape; the horse has a healthy hoof again.

practice, this has long been considered outdated. The farrier who shod the horse in the photos tried to raise the heels by fitting a wedge. By trying to raise the hoof in this manner, the pressure on the heels becomes greater and the heels will be completely pushed in or away, so that they can no longer perform their function well. Allowing a horse to move in this way only makes navicular disease worse.

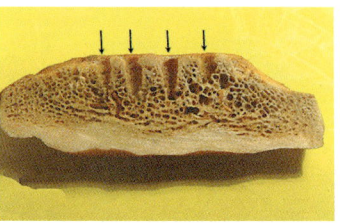

This navicular bone has been sawn in two and clearly shows the enlarged nutrient channels which cause reduction in blood pressure.

Part 2 – Disorders of the Limbs and Hooves

FIXED CALKINS

A horseshoe with fixed calkins is another example of faulty shoeing for a horse with navicular disease. Horseshoes with fixed calkins have a heightened piece of iron welded on the end of each branch. The shoe gives too much weight to the back of the hoof, which means kinetic energy is released when the hoof is in forward flight. This has a counter effect on the deep flexor tendon, because the weighted branches have more kinetic energy than the toe part. When the hoof is set down, the branches of the shoe are preceded by the rest of the hoof. This gives a shock to the inflamed area, which makes it even more difficult for the horse. As well as this, a horseshoe with calkins makes the foot axis break forward, which taxes the hoof capsule even more.

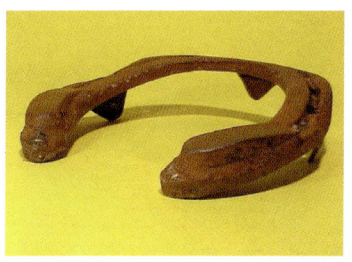

A horseshoe with fixed calkins. This is a disaster for every horse's hoof because the weight on the end of the branches gives rise to kinetic energy which results in problems for the tendons.

HOOF PADS

A third example is a shoe with a hoof pad. In this horseshoe a hoof pad (elastic rubber) is placed between the hoof and the shoe. The idea of the hoof pad is to distribute the ground pressure evenly over the whole hoof including the solar surface and the frog. The disadvantage of a horseshoe with a hoof pad is the weight of the shoe, and also some horses cannot stand the pressure on the solar surface and the frog, which are directly connected to the navicular bone.

In place of a hoof pad, many farriers put silicone between the shoe and the sole. The silicone, however, does not have the required effect. Silicone takes 24 hours to harden; in that time the horse has trodden with its hoof hundreds of times and the silicone is pressed out of the horseshoe. The hoof pad hardens much faster and the pressure is constant without becoming weaker. The hoof pad is spread in the hoof

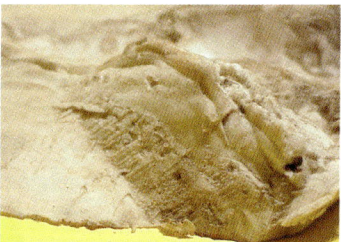

A hoof pad (a kind of rubber which hardens rapidly) is placed between the horseshoe and the hoof so that the pressure on the hoof is evenly distributed.

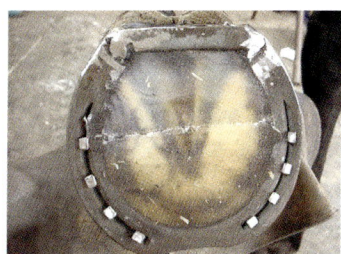

A much better padding is Equi-Thane Hoof Pak®. It can be applied without an artificial sole between the horseshoe and the hoof, and it will produce extremely satisfactory results.

before the horseshoe is nailed in place and is already hardened before the horse puts its hoof on the ground.

EGG BARS

A fourth example of horseshoes for horses with navicular disease is an egg bar shoe. An egg bar shoe is an egg-shaped shoe. The bar must lie in a vertical line from the bulbs without touching the frog. A disadvantage of egg bars is the addition of kinetic energy to the hoof. When the hoof is placed on the ground, the kinetic energy makes the back of the bar touch

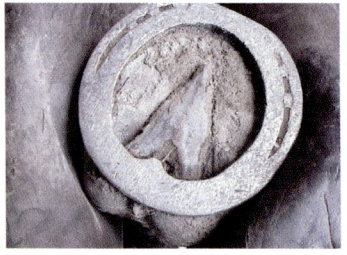 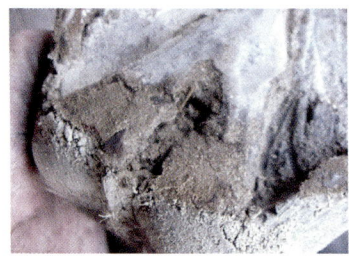

An extremely bad example of an egg bar horseshoe. The bar has been made round on a normal horseshoe (left). The bar was so forged that it pressed onto the frog (right). The result of this was lameness.

An egg bar horseshoe is often used for horses with navicular disease, but there are no indications or proof that this horseshoe can solve the problem or improve the condition.

the ground first and the hoof follows. It can be compared to walking in ski boots.

BAR SHOES

A final, and up until now the best, horseshoe for horses with navicular disease is a broad and long shoe with a straight, thin bar that immobilises the shoe. By preventing movement in the shoe the hooves will be loaded equally when turning. What is more, by placing a leather edge between the shoe and the hoof, concussion will be absorbed. The Hoofcare® Breakover horseshoe can be of help because the hoof can be brought forward more quickly.

CONCLUSION

Navicular disease comes in serious and less serious forms but each form needs particular treatment and particular horseshoes. One horse does well on bar shoes and another on shoes with a hoof pad. No general rules apply; each horse must be considered separately. In this, close cooperation between the veterinary surgeon and the farrier is of the greatest importance.

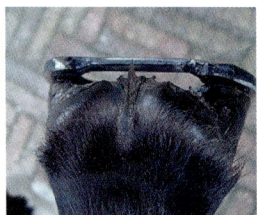 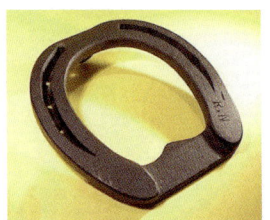 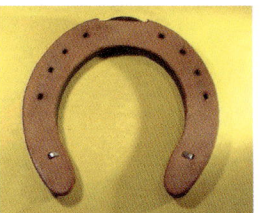

Correct Belgian horseshoe that puts pressure on the frog only when the horse puts weight on its hoof in movement.

A horseshoe that respects the foot axis and a straight, thin bar that immobilises the horseshoe. This is a wide and long horseshoe on which the hoof can function properly.

Sometimes a leather sole is put on the horseshoe to reduce concussion.

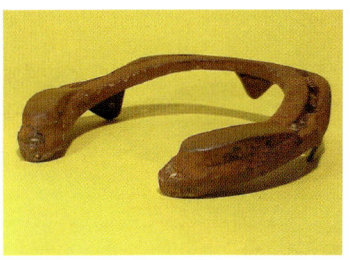

A horseshoe with fixed calkins. This is a disaster for every horse's hoof because the weight on the end of the branches gives rise to kinetic energy which results in problems for the tendons.

FIXED CALKINS

A horseshoe with fixed calkins is another example of faulty shoeing for a horse with navicular disease. Horseshoes with fixed calkins have a heightened piece of iron welded on the end of each branch. The shoe gives too much weight to the back of the hoof, which means kinetic energy is released when the hoof is in forward flight. This has a counter effect on the deep flexor tendon, because the weighted branches have more kinetic energy than the toe part. When the hoof is set down, the branches of the shoe are preceded by the rest of the hoof. This gives a shock to the inflamed area, which makes it even more difficult for the horse. As well as this, a horseshoe with calkins makes the foot axis break forward, which taxes the hoof capsule even more.

HOOF PADS

A third example is a shoe with a hoof pad. In this horseshoe a hoof pad (elastic rubber) is placed between the hoof and the shoe. The idea of the hoof pad is to distribute the ground pressure evenly over the whole hoof including the solar surface and the frog. The disadvantage of a horseshoe with a hoof pad is the weight of the shoe, and also some horses cannot stand the pressure on the solar surface and the frog, which are directly connected to the navicular bone.

In place of a hoof pad, many farriers put silicone between the shoe and the sole. The silicone, however, does not have the required effect. Silicone takes 24 hours to harden; in that time the horse has trodden with its hoof hundreds of times and the silicone is pressed out of the horseshoe. The hoof pad hardens much faster and the pressure is constant without becoming weaker. The hoof pad is spread in the hoof

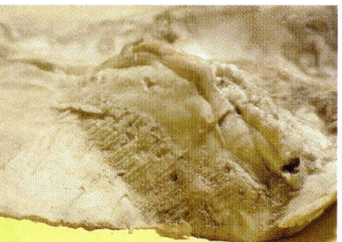

A hoof pad (a kind of rubber which hardens rapidly) is placed between the horseshoe and the hoof so that the pressure on the hoof is evenly distributed.

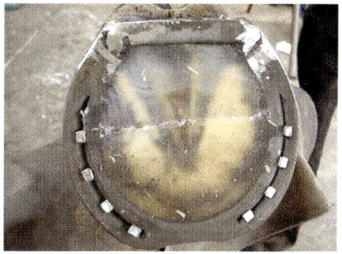

A much better padding is Equi-Thane Hoof Pak®. It can be applied without an artificial sole between the horseshoe and the hoof, and it will produce extremely satisfactory results.

before the horseshoe is nailed in place and is already hardened before the horse puts its hoof on the ground.

EGG BARS

A fourth example of horseshoes for horses with navicular disease is an egg bar shoe. An egg bar shoe is an egg-shaped shoe. The bar must lie in a vertical line from the bulbs without touching the frog. A disadvantage of egg bars is the addition of kinetic energy to the hoof. When the hoof is placed on the ground, the kinetic energy makes the back of the bar touch

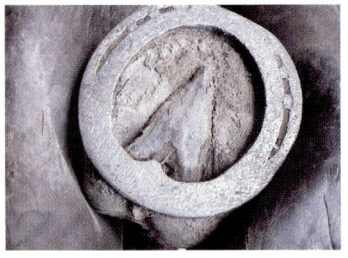
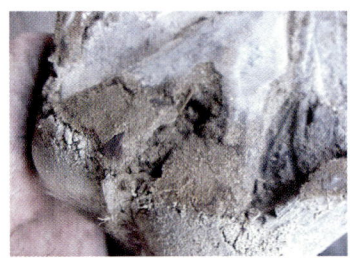

An extremely bad example of an egg bar horseshoe. The bar has been made round on a normal horseshoe (left). The bar was so forged that it pressed onto the frog (right). The result of this was lameness.

An egg bar horseshoe is often used for horses with navicular disease, but there are no indications or proof that this horseshoe can solve the problem or improve the condition.

the ground first and the hoof follows. It can be compared to walking in ski boots.

BAR SHOES

A final, and up until now the best, horseshoe for horses with navicular disease is a broad and long shoe with a straight, thin bar that immobilises the shoe. By preventing movement in the shoe the hooves will be loaded equally when turning. What is more, by placing a leather edge between the shoe and the hoof, concussion will be absorbed. The Hoofcare® Breakover horseshoe can be of help because the hoof can be brought forward more quickly.

CONCLUSION

Navicular disease comes in serious and less serious forms but each form needs particular treatment and particular horseshoes. One horse does well on bar shoes and another on shoes with a hoof pad. No general rules apply; each horse must be considered separately. In this, close cooperation between the veterinary surgeon and the farrier is of the greatest importance.

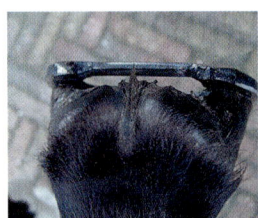

Correct Belgian horseshoe that puts pressure on the frog only when the horse puts weight on its hoof in movement.

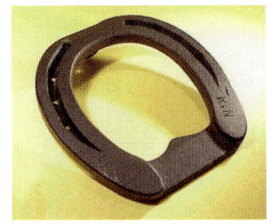

A horseshoe that respects the foot axis and a straight, thin bar that immobilises the horseshoe. This is a wide and long horseshoe on which the hoof can function properly.

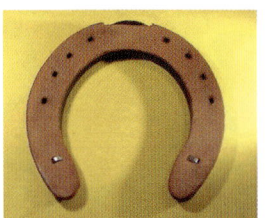

Sometimes a leather sole is put on the horseshoe to reduce concussion.

INDEX

afterbirth, retention 211
annular ligaments 27
arthrosis 12, 71–3
    see also ring-bone, bone spavin

bacterial infections 138, 157–61, 166–73, 192
bar corium 26
bars 169
base-narrow conformation 38, 43
base-wide conformation 38, 43, 165
bear-paw conformation 39
bedding 46, 124
Betadine (iodine) 75, 86, 119, 136, 146, 149, 180, 189, 192
    bandages 207
    compress 135, 160–1
blood supply, hoof 22, 27–8, 187
Bocasan powder 192
bone(s) 11–12, 14
    cyst 97–8
    encapsulated fragment 213–14
    see also named bones
bow-legged conformation 38–9, 44
breakover moment 51, 66–7
bulb corium 25

calkins, fixed 221
canker, frog 173–9
cast, synthetic 95, 96
clasps, for treating cracks 119, 122, 130, 144, 146, 147
clench 57
clips 51, 55
    double/multiple 63, 103, 112, 124, 129, 156, 182, 194–5, 199
club foot 32–3, 93–6
collateral ligaments 17
conformation, see limb conformation
corium 23
coronal suture 22
coronary band
    damage/injury 74–5, 115–17, 126
    irritation 113–15
    septic breakout 161
coronary corium 23–4
    displaced 88
    indentation 211, 212
    irritation 114–15
cow hocks 43
cracks 26, 27, 46
    full thickness 144–9
    full thickness complete 127
    grass cracks 128–9
    infected 190–1
    remedies for 46
    sandcrack 118–22
    sole 188–9
    superficial 142–3
    superficial complete 126–7
    treated with plates/clasps 119, 122, 130, 144, 146, 147
    treated with scoring/burning 129

cyst, bone 97–8

digital cushion 179
donkeys 141–2, 196
dumping 59

Equi-Thane Hoof Pak ® 95, 104, 138, 154, 155, 164, 182, 186, 193, 221
exercise 45

false quarter 135–6
fissure
    horn 191
    navicular bone 200–1
    pedal bone 198–9
flat foot 31
flexion tests 106, 107, 219
foal
    hoof development 22–3, 33–4
    limb defects 12, 92–6, 153
    pedal bone fracture 202
foot axis 34–6, 59, 60, 62–3, 150–1, 162–3
    and stride length 44
fore limb
    anatomy 11–18, 217
    conformation defects 36–41
fractures
    lateral cartilages 201
    navicular bone 200–1
    pedal bone 197–9
frog
    canker 173–9
    corium 25
    inflammation 179–80
    paring 53
    role of 25
    thrush 47, 133, 171–3
fuller 49
fungal infections 138–9, 190–6
fungicidal agents 139, 192, 194, 139

grass cracks 128–9
greasy heel 89–90
growth plates 12

hammer
    nailing 48
    turning 48
heels 162–70
    greasy 89–90
    inflammation 166–8
    low 128, 150–7
    over-reach injury 86–7
    rolled-under 162–4
    sheared 31
    support of horseshoe 57, 156–7, 165
    under-run 31, 164–6
hock joint
    bone spavin 79–84
    conformation 42, 43
honey 139, 192, 194

hoof
    blood supply 22, 27–8, 187
    chipped 125
    cracks, see cracks
hoof capsule 19–21
    development 22–3, 33
    pigmentation 26–7
hoof care 45–7
hoof corium 23
hoof mechanism 27, 28, 45, 129
hoof pads 98, 182, 216, 221
hoof shape 29–34
    deformed 87–8
    laminitis 33, 206–7, 210
Hoofcare ® Breakover horseshoe 63–8, 164
    advantages 66–7
    use in laminitis 209–10
    use in ring-bone 109–10
horn
    characteristics of 20
    fissure 191
    glass-like 105, 126
    poor quality 46, 123–5
    rings 132–3
horny tubules 23, 26, 87, 123
    fungal infection 195
horny wall
    bruising coloration 186, 187
    cracks, see cracks
    fungal infection 193–6
    resection 207–8
    separating 137–42
    uneven thickness 152–3
horseshoes 50–3
    back to front fitting 103–4
    bar 104, 134, 165, 180, 181, 187–8, 193, 199, 216, 222
    Belgian bar 155, 165, 222
    with bridge 140–1
    'brushing' 84, 86, 189
    characteristics 50–1
    clips 51, 55
    double or multiple clips 63, 103, 112, 124, 129, 156, 182, 194–5, 199
    Dutch bar 154–5
    egg-bar 187–8, 221–2
    fitting 56
    forged/seated out 170, 182, 213
    forging 55
    for full thickness cracks 145–7
    history of 47
    Hoofcare ® Breakover 63–8, 109–10, 164, 209–10
    leather pads 98, 216
    length of branches 57–8
    loss of 58, 62, 125
    measuring 54
    nailing on 56, 128
    nails 52, 57
    open-toed 186, 208
    poor fitting 186
    purposes 47

horseshoes *cont*
    rocker toe 51, 55, 65–6, 67, 209, 210
    side bar 170
    size of 28, 50, 54, 55, 59–61, 137, 156–7, 164–5, 186
    spavin 84
    surgical plate 167–8, 183, 185, 198, 199
    'therapeutic' 61
    three-quarter 127
    toe extension 92, 94, 95–6
    wedges 82–3, 151, 153–5, 163, 165, 220
    weight 62
hydrogen peroxide 192

injuries
    coronary band 74–5, 115–17, 126
    foot punctures 182–5
    over-reach 85–7
    wire wounds 74–5
    see also fractures

joints 11–13
    arthrosis 12, 71–3
    inflammation 12
    ligaments 18
    nomenclature 13
    see also named joints

keratoma 99–100
    fan-shaped 100–1
    side wall 104–6
    toe 101–4
kicking, stable wall/door 142, 186, 190
knee joint
    arthrosis 72–3
    conformation 39
knife
    drawing 48
    hoof 48

laminae
    inflammation 121, 122, 160
    insensitive 21, 23–4
    sensitive 24–5, 26
laminitis 137
    acute attacks 203
    causes 202
    changes to pedal bone 203, 204, 205
    donkeys 141
    founder 204–7
    hoof distortion 33, 206–7, 210
    recurring 210
    rings of horn 132, 133
    separating wall 140–2
    sinker 181–2, 204, 211–13
    treatment 207–8
lateral cartilages 201
    calcification (side-bone) 201, 214, 215–16
    fracture 201
leather pads/sole 98, 216, 222
ligaments 17, 18, 27
ligature 198
limb anatomy 11–18, 217
limb conformation 91–3

evaluation 34
foals 12, 92–6
fore limb 36–41
hind limb 41–4
and hoof shape 44
ideal 37

mange 92
mare, laminitis 211
metal plates, for treatment of cracks/defects 119, 122, 144, 147
muscles 15–16

nail holes 49
nails
    horseshoe 52, 57
    puncture wounds from 184
navicular bone 14, 22, 217
    changes in navicular disease 218, 219, 220
    cyst 97–8
    fracture/fissure 200–1
navicular bursa 22
navicular disease 217–22
nerves, hoof 22

oiling of hooves 46
older horse, hoof cracks 26, 27, 126
ostitis 110–12
over-reaching 85–7, 151

pastern
    bone cyst 98
    conformation 39–40
    over at 91–3
pastern joint 12
pawing the ground 185
pedal bone 14, 21, 203
    chip fracture 197–8
    encapsulated fragment 213–14
    fracture/fissure 198–9
    'hat brim' effect 206, 207
    ostitis 110–12
    puncture wound 182, 183
    rotation in laminitis 204
    sinking in laminitis 181–2, 204, 211–13
    see also lateral cartilages
penicillin 146, 147, 167
periople corium 23
perioplic ring, irritation 113–15
pes equinus 93–6
pincers, farrier's 48
pododermatitis 135
Pododermatitis purulenta 157–61, 166–8
pritchel 49
propolis 139, 192
Pseudomonas aeruginosa 192
pulse, hoof artery 158, 159, 160
punch 49
puncture wounds 182–5
pus formation
    frog 179–80
    heels 166–9
    toe 157–61

'rainures' 216
rasp, hoof 49

ring-bone 72, 106–10
rocker toe 51, 55, 65–6, 67, 209, 210

sandcrack 118–22
seedy toe 133–4
semi-horny substance 27, 126
separating walls 137–42
shoeing
    advantages/disadvantages 53
    poor practices 60–1, 186
shoes, *see* horseshoes
sickle hocks 42
side-bone 214, 215–16
silicone 182, 221
sole
    bruised 186–8
    cracked 188–9
    dropped 33, 181–2
    puncture 182–5
spasms 76–7
splint 78–9
stabled horse
    bedding 46, 124
    exercise 45
stamp 49
staphylococcus bacteria 161, 192
stones, causing cracks/inflammation 131
stride length 44
stringhalt 76–7

tarring of hooves 47
tendons 16–17
    deep digital flexor 16, 17, 22, 184, 201, 203, 217
    extensor 17, 92–3, 200, 203
    shortened in pes equinus 94–5
    superficial flexor 17, 184, 217
thrush 47, 133, 171
Tildren ® 82
toe 150–61
    horny wall cracks 128–32
    inflammation 157–61
    keratoma 101–4
    length of 62–3, 128, 150–7, 162–3
    seedy 133–4
toe extension shoe 92, 94, 95–6
toe-in conformation 32, 36
toe-out conformation 36–7
tools, farrier's 48–9
trimming 53–4, 59
    inadequate 152–3

ultraviolet light 26, 27

veterinary surgeon 144, 145, 147, 158

walls, separation 137–42
water, hoof 20, 45, 46
wedges (horseshoe) 82–3, 151, 153–5, 163, 220
white line
    change of form 160, 190, 207
    inflammation 135
white line disease 137, 191–6
wire wounds 74–5

zinc ointment 90